Andrew Stanway, MB MRCP, and his wife Penny, MB BS, LRCP MRCS, both qualified in medicine over ten years ago. After three years' practice in the Medical Professorial Unit at King's College Hospital, London, Andrew Stanway decided to devote his career to medical communications and health education, working for major medical publishers and writing for both the scientific and popular press. In 1974 he started his own publishing and film-making concerns, dealing solely with medical subjects. His documentary films are shown worldwide, and in 1975 he produced one of the programmes in BBC's *Horizon* series.

Penny Stanway's career, initially in general practice and then as a Senior Medical Officer to an Area Health Authority, led to her special interest in and commitment to child health problems in the community. She studied developmental paediatrics and the assessment of handicapped children at the Institute of Child Health, London University. She gave up full time practice after the birth of her first daughter and now contributes regularly to *Parents* magazine as well as to the popular press and professional journals. She also runs a mother and toddler group.

Andrew Stanway has written several books including *Taking the Rough with the Smooth* (1976) about dietary fibre and *Breast is Best* (1978) jointly with his wife.

D0228127

Pears Encyclopaedia of Child Health

Andrew Stanway, MB MRCP

Penny Stanway, MB BS, LRCP MRCS

Advisory Editor Aidan Macfarlane MB, B Chir, MA Cantab, MRCP

SPHERE BOOKS LIMITED
30–32 GRAY'S INN ROAD, LONDON
WC1X 8JL

First published in Great Britain by
Pelham Books Ltd 1979

Copyright original series © *Parents*
Magazine 1977
Copyright this edition © Andrew and Penny
Stanway 1979

Published by Sphere Books Ltd 1981

TRADEMARK

Printed and bound in Great Britain by
Fakenham Press Limited, Fakenham, Norfolk

Introduction

'Not another baby book!' we can hear you say. 'Surely there are enough of those already?' There are, and we're not going to add to the pile.

Over the years we have heard from many mothers how difficult it is to find out what they want to know from books, partly because there are usually so many entries in the index on any one subject. In the *Pears Encyclopaedia of Child Health* we have overcome this problem by condensing everything about each subject under one heading. Some subjects are necessarily widely cross-referenced so that matters of interest can be easily followed up. We have tried to write a book which parents can refer to quickly in an emergency; learn from after returning from the doctor; or simply use to check up facts.

To avoid perpetuating mistaken old wives' tales and myths, we have relied heavily on recent medical literature and have enlisted specialist advice when necessary. The proofs were carefully checked by two very different paediatricians: one a father of young children who is responsible for the organization of child health care in a large area of the country, and the other a grandfather who was until recently the head of the Department of Child Health of a major London teaching hospital. We hope that between the four of us we have covered all the topics in as full and as varied a way as our readers will need.

This encyclopaedia is not intended to be a substitute for the family doctor or paediatrician. Parents should always ask their doctor for help with a child if there is any cause for concern. Children often do not have classical signs and symptoms of the disease they are suffering from and can become seriously ill much more quickly than adults.

We hope that by being armed with more information, the reader will worry less when his child has a minor ailment; will understand a little more about the investigations, tests and treatments available; and will be able to help the doctor help the sick child by giving a more informed account of what's happening. Once you've read the entry in the encyclopaedia we hope you'll be in a better position to help your child, the doctor, and yourself.

enlarge. The best example of this is the stretching of pregnancy but even a really big meal fills the stomach and so causes some distension of the abdominal wall. The abdomen also bears the belly button (navel or UMBILICUS), the place at which the umbilical cord dropped off after birth.

See ABDOMINAL PAIN, HERNIA, PERITONITIS, RECURRENT ABDOMINAL PAIN

Abdomen The part of the body between the diaphragm and the pelvis. In everyday speech the back of the abdomen is usually called the loins and the front the belly or tummy.

Inside the abdomen are the organs comprising the digestive system (the STOMACH and intestines), the KIDNEYS, LIVER and SPLEEN. The inside of the abdomen is lined with a thin, moist membrane, the peritoneum, which also envelops almost all the abdominal organs between its layers. This enables them to slip easily over each other as they move and as the body moves. (The bowel, for example, is on the move almost non-stop, passing food along.)

The abdominal walls are formed of muscles which stretch when any of the organs inside

Abdominal pain Almost every child suffers from abdominal PAIN from time to time and the cause may be difficult to establish, especially in young children who cannot explain exactly where the pain is or anything else about it. Because some causes are potentially serious if not treated (such as APPENDICITIS and pyelonephritis), no pain should be ignored, even if the child has previously been subject to pains which disappeared spontaneously. Pain in the ABDOMEN may be caused by infection, inflammation, a change in the activity of the bowel, or obstruction or

The contents of the abdomen, shown from the front and back. a. liver, b. stomach, c. spleen, d. gall bladder, e. pancreas, f. large intestine, g. small intestine, h. kidney, i. ureter, j. bladder, k. rectum.

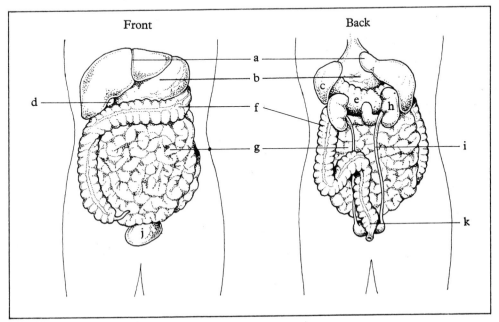

1

distension of the bowel. These conditions, alone or in combination, can accompany many diseases, which is why the doctor examining a child has to consider a wide range of possible underlying causes of the pain.

Although the possible causes are numerous, unless the pain is severe or combined with other symptoms such as vomiting, loss of weight, or pain on passing water, no specific cause will necessarily be found and the trouble is likely to pass.

If you are at all worried about your child's abdominal pain, ask for your doctor's advice. Besides examining the child carefully, he will ask exactly where the pain is felt, how it started, what it feels like, how bad it is, how often it comes, how long it lasts, whether there have been any previous episodes and whether there are any other symptoms, such as DIARRHOEA, CONSTIPATION, VOMITING, or frequency of passing URINE. Sometimes it is necessary to perform an exploratory operation (a laparotomy) to make sure of the reason for the pain, especially if an acute condition such as appendicitis, a twisted HERNIA, a VOLVULUS or INTUSSUSCEPTION is suspected, though as many other tests as necessary will be done beforehand to try to establish the diagnosis.

To give some idea of the many causes of abdominal pain, here are some of the conditions that a doctor may consider when seeing your child: constipation, FOOD POISONING, GASTROENTERITIS, mesenteric adenitis, a urinary tract infection (see CYSTITIS; NEPHRITIS), appendicitis, food allergy, PNEUMONIA, a twisted hernia, a sickle cell ANAEMIA crisis, a twisted ovarian cyst, a twisted TESTIS, ULCERATIVE COLITIS, CROHN'S DISEASE, LEAD POISONING, CYSTIC FIBROSIS, emotional problems, threadworms (see WORMS) and, in babies, a volvulus, an intussusception and three month COLIC.

Abrasion Superficial damage of the skin by hard rubbing against a rough surface.

Most small abrasions aren't serious and don't bleed, but a deeper abrasion may ooze fluid (serum) and blood from broken capillaries.

The best treatment is gentle washing with plain water to remove any foreign matter. An antiseptic cream or solution may aid healing by reducing the likelihood of infection, but abrasions usually heal quickly anyway.

Deeper abrasions may need a non-adhesive dressing or even the attention of a doctor, but most heal best if left open to the air. The exception to this is the abrasion that is likely to get dirty and thus infected. After a serious abrasion, immunization or, if necessary, re-immunization against TETANUS is advisable, especially if the abrasion is contaminated by road dust, soil or animal manure, all of which may contain tetanus bacteria.

Abscess A localized collection of pus in any part of the body. An abscess may be accompanied by local symptoms of inflammation, swelling, constitutional symptoms (especially if it is large), pain and tenderness. It may, however, be dormant.

As with any swelling, the degree of pain produced by an abscess depends on the tightness of the surrounding tissues. A small abscess in a confined area such as the root of a tooth causes considerable pain early on, whereas a lung abscess, for example, can be very large yet produce few symptoms.

An abscess in the skin is called a boil. (*See* BOILS.) Many abscesses are treated by releasing the pus by surgical incision, with or without the use of antibiotics. Any underlying condition which might have caused the abscess will also need treatment at the same time.

See QUINSY

Achondroplasia *See* SMALL CHILDREN

Acne A condition of the SKIN that is so common in young people between the ages of 12 and 20 as to be almost universal.

The pimples, blackheads and pustules of acne are most often seen on the face, neck, back and chest. Acne on the face obviously causes most embarrassment.

Blackheads are collections of pigmented sebum and not, as was previously thought, dirt or oxidized plugs of sebum. Adolescents in particular are affected because of their increased hormonal activity which stimulates the sebaceous glands of the skin to produce

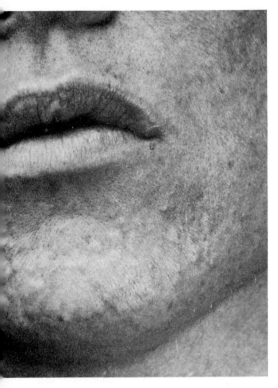

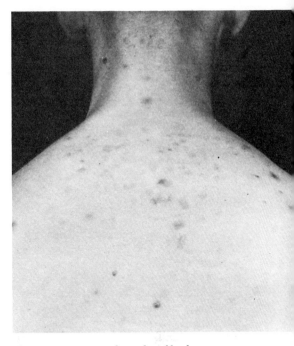

Acne may appear on the neck and back, as here, as well as on the face, where it is most often seen.
Acne may sometimes result in permanent scarring (left).

more sebum.

Pustules (little boils) develop from pimples, probably because of the leakage of sebum into the skin. In mild cases of acne, the pus produced as a reaction to the sebum in the skin is usually not infected with harmful bacteria and only becomes infected if the spots are picked with dirty fingernails.

Acne is often worse in girls at their period time. Many people agree that chocolate, cocoa and coffee aggravate the condition, and that sunlight or ultra-violet light from a lamp alleviate it to some extent. It is now known that sulphur preparations, so long used to treat acne, can themselves cause it, as can some cosmetics and certain soaps and detergents.

Excessive attention to skin cleanliness is now no longer thought to be important but if the spots are squeezed (and whatever doctors say, people will always pick their spots), it is essential that the fingers are clean and that the surrounding skin is damaged as little as possible.

Acne can be very embarrassing for the sufferer, especially as it occurs at a time when children and young adults are most sensitive about their looks. The majority of sufferers seem to get better spontaneously in their twenties or early thirties, though some may need treatment with tetracyclines or hormones. Many girls find that their acne goes when they are on the Pill.

Addiction An overwhelming need for an outside agent (tobacco, alcohol or one of many drugs) which alters a person's life, eventually to its detriment.

Addiction in children is an unusual phenomenon, but there is growing concern about children smoking and drinking alcohol and about adolescents taking certain drugs.

Three main factors influence the development of addiction. First, the child is pressurized or simply influenced by his peer group to take up the addictive habit. Second, the potential addict finds pleasure in SMOKING,

3

DRINKING or taking drugs. This is partly because of the sensations involved (such as a feeling of relaxation when smoking, a loosening of inhibition when drinking and a heightening of sensations when taking certain drugs), and partly because of the pleasant social set-up initially surrounding these pastimes.

Third, alcohol and some drugs are addictive because they affect the body's metabolism so as to make it physically dependent upon them. Gradually the addict finds he needs increasing amounts of the drug to produce the same effect, and this tolerance is a prime feature of addiction.

The most distressing thing is that if the drug is withheld, the addict suffers from unpleasant withdrawal symptoms because the cells of the body need the substance in order to function normally. The body can return to its normal state after a while but the danger of readdiction is always present.

Most parents worry about the possibility of their children becoming addicted to something. This is understandable because smoking and drinking to excess are widespread today in the adult world and both take their toll of health. Because forbidden fruit is always sweeter, many parents allow older children to drink small amounts of alcohol at home. They also take care to explain in a matter-of-fact way the serious threats to health involved in any addiction.

Adenoids Collections of lymphoid tissue lying in the upper part of the space at the back of the mouth and nose (the nasopharynx).

Together with the tonsils and some patches of similar tissue on the back of the tongue, the adenoids form a ring of lymphoid tissue. The function of this ring is thought to be to trap samples of bacteria breathed in through the mouth and nose. Once the sample is taken, antibodies are made by the lymphoid tissue which then fight these bacteria both locally and in the body generally. The enlargement of the adenoids (and tonsils) at this time is a normal and necessary part of the body's fight against infection.

During childhood, the adenoids enlarge

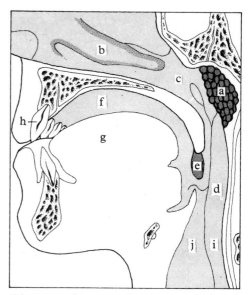

Diagrammatic cross section of part of the head and neck. a. enlarged adenoids, b. nasal cavity, c. nasopharynx, d. pharynx, e. tonsils, f. mouth cavity, g. tongue, h. teeth, i. gullet, j. windpipe.

disproportionately to the nasopharynx and this is considered to be a normal stage in development. At puberty this growth ceases and the adenoids actually shrink.

In some children the growth of the adenoids is so great that the nasopharynx is completely filled by them. When this happens it becomes difficult for the child to breathe through the nose, to eat and even to sleep properly because of snoring. Enlarged adenoids may be chronically infected, giving rise to a snuffly nose and smelly breath. The most serious consequence of this adenoidal enlargement, however, is that the EARS may be affected, either by the infection passing up the eustachian tubes to the middle ears, or by the enlarged adenoids blocking the openings of the eustachian tubes and thus causing deafness and earache.

The decision on whether or not to remove the adenoids is often postponed for a few months (or even years if the symptoms are not too worrying) because they are expected to shrink in the normal course of development. Should the symptoms persist, especially deafness caused by adenoidal enlargement, then the adenoids are removed in an operation known as adenoidectomy. The tonsils may be removed at the same time.

Thousands of people have their tonsils and adenoids removed each year, and of these about 90 per cent are children, mostly between five and seven years old. On the whole, doctors would rather avoid the risks of an operation so adenoids are now only removed if absolutely necessary. A child who has had his adenoids removed may need help in learning to breathe through his nose after many years of breathing by mouth.

See LYMPHATIC SYSTEM; TONSILLITIS

Adrenals There are two adrenal glands, each sitting on top of a kidney. Each gland has two parts: the cortex (outside) and the medulla (inside).

The cortex is stimulated by the hormone ACTH (adreno-cortico-trophic hormone) from the PITUITARY gland to produce its own hormones, the cortico-steroids, aldosterone, and the sex hormones – androgens, oestrogens and progesterone. These regulate the metabolism of carbohydrates, proteins and fats (especially in conditions of mental and physical stress), the salts in the body, and to some extent the sex organs.

The medulla is under the control of the sympathetic nervous system and produces adrenalin and noradrenalin, hormones acting on the blood pressure, glucose release from the liver and the movements of the gastro-intestinal tract, among other things.

The adrenal glands are essential for life. Under- or overactivity can be harmful and calls for specialized treatment. Replacement therapy is helpful for children with under-active glands.

Aggression Attacking or forceful behaviour normal and essential to a child, which is present from birth onwards and enables him to avoid or cope with problems. Each one of us has to learn to control and harness aggression.

Aggressive or demanding behaviour is seen in young babies when their natural desires are thwarted, such as when they are hungry or thirsty and they have to wait to be fed. A hungry baby will scream and wave his arms and legs about because this is the only way he knows of coping with and signalling his needs to his mother. Making a baby wait for food to teach him that he can't always have everything when he wants it is something mothers often do, but is quite unreasonable. A baby whose needs are usually met straight away is far less likely to respond to every frustrating situation as he grows older with screaming and other signs of rage, because he knows that he doesn't have to go to these lengths to get help from his mother. A baby made to wait to have his needs satisfied every time eventually quietens, but his anger and aggression are then either directed elsewhere or contained and expressed internally, according to modern psychiatric beliefs, and may show themselves as a variety of physical and emotional signs, including FAILURE TO THRIVE and DEPRESSION.

An older baby's aggression may take the form of biting or hitting his mother. This is best handled with loving firmness rather than by returned aggression.

A young child frequently reacts aggressively when he is prevented by his mother or anyone else from having or doing something, and he may have TEMPER TANTRUMS. The JEALOUSY of an older child towards a younger brother or sister may show up as aggressive behaviour towards the younger child or to his mother, because too much of her time has to be spent with the young one. This form of 'sibling rivalry' is quite normal, provided it isn't carried to extremes. However, aggressive behaviour needs controlling and channelling into more constructive outlets.

Later in childhood, the aggressive urge is usually exercised to meet the challenge of competition from other children. The adolescent may rebel against the limits imposed upon him by society and by his parents, but he may also use his aggression to gain his independence in a constructive way.

Whatever age a child is, aggressive behaviour needs to be countered not only with control and direction but, more important, with love. There is usually an underlying reason for over-aggressive behaviour – sometimes it can be a response to emotional deprivation. If this can't be sorted out at home, skilled advice and help is available via the family doctor.

See HOSPITAL; LEAD POISONING; MALADJUSTMENT

Albino A child with very blonde, silky hair, fair skin and red pupils in the eyes. The condition is caused by an absence of pigment in the hair, skin and retinae. The irises of the eyes contain some pigment and are usually pale grey. Some people have a localized form of albinism which shows itself as a single white forelock of hair.

Albinism is inherited recessively, which means that the parents appear normal but each carries the genetic code for albinism. This gene is carried by about one person in seventy but only one child in twenty thousand is born an albino because an albino can only be produced if both parents carry the gene.

Albino children may also suffer from severe short-sightedness (*see* VISUAL PROBLEMS), SQUINTS, NYSTAGMUS and hypersensitivity to light.

The only treatment available is avoidance of exposure to sunlight, the use of sunglasses and of an ultra-violet screening skin cream.

See INHERITED DISEASES

Alcohol *See* DRINKING

Allergic rhinitis *See* HAY FEVER

Allergy A person is said to be allergic if his IMMUNITY system over-reacts to a foreign substance entering his body through his breathing passages or mouth, or coming into contact with his skin or mucous membranes.

The basis of an allergic reaction is the interaction of a foreign protein (allergen or antigen) with the body's antibodies and lymphoid cells. Certain pollens, foods, the house dust mite and animal fur can all act as allergens.

About one in five children develop allergies very readily. This is because they produce an excessive amount of one particular antibody (IgE). These children are termed 'atopic' and develop very quick reactions when they come into contact with the antigens to which they are sensitive. More than half the children of atopic parents are atopic them-

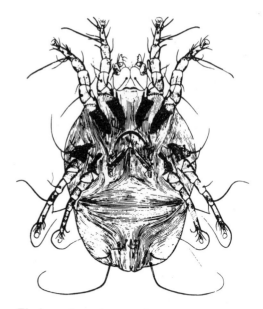

The house dust mite, one of many common allergens.

selves. They are more likely to suffer from repeated infections and may have a family history of HAY FEVER, ASTHMA or ECZEMA and a characteristic biochemical and cellular reaction to foreign proteins to which they are allergic.

Allergic conditions include eczema; asthma; hay fever; allergic conjunctivitis; allergic contact DERMATITIS; allergic reactions to food, insect bites and drugs; and CROUP. Several other conditions including COELIAC DISEASE and MIGRAINE may also have an allergic basis.

Food allergy is a condition which is not well understood yet because the underlying immunological mechanisms haven't been clearly identified. However, certain people produce specific antibodies to certain foods and are adversely affected by them. It seems likely that food allergy is a common but as yet widely unrecognized condition. Food allergies are said by some experts to be responsible for up to 25 per cent of cases of asthma, for example.

Allergic reactions to food include vomiting, diarrhoea, pain and a bloated feeling in the abdomen, eczema, URTICARIA, and asthma. Specific reactions include swelling and urticaria (nettlerash) after eating strawberries, shellfish or eggs, for example; a runny nose (allergic rhinitis), eczema, asthma, behaviour disturbances and COLIC after cows' MILK, and asthma after taking tartrazine, the yellow colouring in orange squash and other foods.

Although a baby's immunity system is working from about 20 weeks before he is born, during the first four to six months of life, babies do not make enough of their own antibodies to protect the gut wall against the entry of foreign proteins, but rely on antibodies in their mother's breast milk to do this. This explains why the incidence of allergy in children who were bottle-fed as babies is so much higher than in those who were solely breast fed. After the first six months, a baby makes enough of his own protective antibodies, but if he has already been sensitized by a particular foreign protein, it is thought that his immunity system is then primed to develop allergy to other foreign proteins later. (*See* BREAST FEEDING.)

If you and your doctor have good reason for believing that your child is allergic to a particular food, try cutting this food out of his diet completely for about four weeks to see if there is any improvement in his symptoms. It may be necessary to cut out and reintroduce it several times to be quite sure whether or not the food is allergenic. Skin testing has limited value in the diagnosis of food allergy, and should not be done if the child has eczema. Blood tests can be of some value.

See ANTIHISTAMINES; HENOCH-SCHÖNLEIN PURPURA

Alopecia *See* BALDNESS

Amniocentesis The removal of a small amount of amniotic fluid from around a baby while it's still in the womb.

A baby is contained in a bag (the amnion) of fluid (liquor) inside the mother's uterus. The fluid comes from the placenta and the membranes around the baby and circulates through the baby's lungs and kidneys. The baby also swallows the liquid and then passes it out as urine. A foetus under 14 weeks of age has too little amniotic fluid for the doctor to be able to get to it but after this time the volume increases considerably until there is so much that the baby can literally swim around in it.

Having an amniocentesis is much like having an injection. The doctor takes an ordinary syringe with an ordinary blood-taking sized needle and inserts it in the mid-line between the navel and the pubic hair line. The skin is sterilized first to ensure that no bacteria are introduced into the baby's world. A local anaesthetic may be used. Although it is not essential, many doctors prefer to scan the abdomen with an ultrasound machine so as to localize exactly the greatest area of amniotic fluid and so be able to insert the needle into that and not into the baby. This is especially important in early pregnancy, when there is little fluid, and in mothers with rhesus negative blood in whom any bleeding in the baby (caused by the needle) could provoke rhesus disease (*see* BLOOD GROUPS).

Amniocentesis does not hurt much and there is no leakage of amniotic fluid as the needle hole is so small. There is a tiny (one per cent) risk of the baby being born prematurely if the procedure is carried out early in pregnancy but the later it is done, the less the risk. The main danger is that the placenta may be punctured. This is unlikely to occur if the doctor has ascertained by ultrasound the position of the placenta before inserting the needle.

There are many ways in which a sample of amniotic fluid can help doctors help mothers. Perhaps one of the best publicized is that of foetal abnormality detection. Many pointers may make the mother or the doctor suspect that the foetus may be abnormal. If it is likely to be, the parents may wish to have the pregnancy terminated. Ideally an abnormal foetus should be aborted as early as possible, so the earlier the amniotic fluid sample can be obtained, the better. This is difficult before 14 weeks but the sample needs to be taken as soon as possible after this.

Amniocentesis can help doctors diagnose an abnormality in several ways. The fluid extracted contains cells that have been shed from the body of the foetus. As each body cell contains a replica of all the genetic material of the body, doctors can tell from one cell if the foetus has a major chromosomal abnormality such as mongolism (DOWN'S SYNDROME). This can be useful if the mother has already produced such a baby, or in older mothers because it is known that women over the age of 35 are more likely to produce Down's babies than are younger women.

It is possible to tell the sex of the foetus from the cell studies, and this is a pleasant bonus to most mothers, but there are certain conditions such as HAEMOPHILIA in which this information is really helpful. Haemophilia is known as a 'sex-linked' disease because it is seen only in males. Females act as carriers but don't suffer from the disease. If there is a family history of a sex-linked genetic disease, it helps to know the sex of the foetus. Cells from the amniotic fluid can be obtained and examined for the presence of sex chromatin (the Barr body). Absence of the Barr body indicates a boy and thus a child with a 50–50 chance of having the disease. The parents are asked to decide before the amniocentesis whether they want the foetus aborted if it is a male, on the understanding that it would have a 50–50 chance of suffering from the disease if they do not.

Disorders such as SPINA BIFIDA and ANENCEPHALY can also be detected early by measuring the level of a substance called alpha-fetoprotein in the amniotic fluid.

The maturity of the foetus can be very important when the mother is uncertain of her dates or when a planned premature delivery is being considered. Newborn babies weighing less than 2500g are at risk because immature lung function may lead to the RESPIRATORY DISTRESS SYNDROME, and it's therefore vital to ensure that babies aren't delivered too early unless absolutely necessary. Both the cells and the amino acids in the amniotic fluid can help in this respect. The larger the number of greasy skin cells (shed by the foetus in increasing numbers as pregnancy progresses), the more mature the foetus. Sophisticated measurements of naturally occurring substances (lecithin and sphingomyelin) reflect the maturity of the foetal lung.

The rhesus positive foetus of a rhesus negative mother who has rising levels of rhesus antibodies during her pregnancy is in danger of becoming severely ill even before birth. Amniocentesis enables the amount of bilirubin in the amniotic fluid to be measured, giving doctors a guide as to whether to induce the labour early.

Amniocentesis is one of several techniques enabling doctors to predict the birth of damaged or severely ill babies. Parents may wish to avoid such births. It is, however, relatively expensive in that highly trained staff are needed to carry out the test and to analyse and interpret the changes in the fluid. This explains why amniocentesis is not available at all hospitals. At present amniocentesis is only justifiable when there are medical reasons for suspicion about the outcome of the pregnancy.

See BLOOD GROUPS; CHROMOSOMES; CONGENITAL ABNORMALITIES; INHERITED DISEASES.

Anaemia A condition in which there is either a reduction in the number of red BLOOD cells or in the amount of haemoglobin (the iron-containing pigment that makes red blood cells red and carries oxygen), or both.

Mild degrees of anaemia cause no physical signs or symptoms – the child looks and feels quite well. The most obvious sign of a very anaemic child is tiredness, though loss of appetite and irritability may develop. Anaemic children are also more likely to get infections and have pale lips, conjunctivae and fingertips. It's important to remember, however, that not all children with pale cheeks are anaemic. Severe anaemia from a heavy loss of blood or in the later stages of a blood disorder can cause a fast pulse, breathlessness and even heart failure.

The causes of anaemia fall into three main groups:

1) *Blood loss,* which may be acute, after an injury, severe NOSE BLEED, or bleeding from the placenta, for example; or long term, due to heavy periods, ULCERATIVE COLITIS or chronic dysentery, for example.

2) *Excessive breakdown (haemolysis) of red blood cells,* due, for example, to severe rhesus haemolytic disease of the newborn (*see* BLOOD GROUPS), certain drugs (in sensitive individuals), infection, poisons, or abnormality of the haemoglobin (such as sickle cell disease and thalassaemia).

3) *Lowered production of red blood cells,* due to a lack of the necessary blood-forming materials (such as iron, protein, vitamin B_{12}, thyroxine,

vitamin C and folic acid), a bone marrow deficiency, LEUKAEMIA, poisons (such as lead), radiation, or chronic infection or illness, for example.

Iron deficiency anaemia is the commonest blood disorder affecting children. Anaemia due to insufficient iron in the diet is unusual in the first four to six months of life, but is seen more often from nine months to two years. Breast milk contains enough iron for the first six months at least, but modified cows' milk formulae have to be fortified with iron to provide for the baby's needs. The iron in breast milk is absorbed better than that in cows' milk. Once a baby is started on solids, there is a chance that he may become short of iron if he doesn't eat enough iron-containing foods (meat, eggs, wholemeal bread, apricots, flour, cereals, potatoes and other vegetables). A premature baby may have lower iron stores and your doctor may check his haemoglobin level from time to time, whether he is breast- or bottle-fed.

Interestingly, about a third of children with iron deficiency anaemia have had a long-standing blood loss from their gut which has caused their anaemia. This blood loss is now recognized as being caused by a certain protein present in unmodified, 'doorstep' cows' milk. The anaemia is not cured by giving the child extra iron but has to be prevented either by heating the milk or by reducing the milk intake to a pint or less a day. This condition is known as milk intolerance or 'allergy'.

Iron deficiency anaemia is treated by altering the child's diet to contain enough iron-containing foods and by giving iron medicines. Large amounts of cows' milk should be avoided because milk may not only decrease the amount of iron absorbed by a baby's gut but can also reduce a child's appetite for iron-containing foods.

Sickle cell anaemia is seen in some black Africans, Indian and Mediterranean peoples. About half of the red blood cells are sickle-shaped and live for only 15 to 60 days as opposed to the normal 120 days: their premature destruction causes anaemia. The abnormal blood is also more likely to clot and can cause many different and painful conditions depending on where the clotting has occurred.

Children with sickle cell anaemia are more prone to infection than other children and are usually underweight in later childhood, although adequate treatment enables them to grow normally. Unfortunately, many die before they are 20 years old because there is no specific treatment.

If a person has only one recessive gene for sickle cell disease he is said to be a carrier, and a small proportion of his red blood cells are potentially abnormal. If two carriers produce children, one in four will suffer from sickle cell anaemia. (*See* CHROMOSOMES.)

Thalassaemia is an inherited type of anaemia in areas around the Mediterranean. Severely affected children develop severe anaemia in the first year of life and need regular blood transfusions. Growth is impaired, puberty rarely occurs, and diabetes and heart disorders are common.

See BLEEDING; LOW BIRTH WEIGHT; WEANING

Anal fissure If a child cries when passing motions or if he is reluctant to open his bowels at all, the cause may be a small but painful fissure (crack) in the skin lining the anal canal (back passage). A fissure arises during the passage of a large, hard motion. Because of the pain caused by stretching the fissure the child is reluctant to open his bowels, so he becomes more constipated, thus setting up a vicious circle. This vicious circle is further compounded because the fissure may bleed and the bright red blood may alarm both parents and child. The bleeding is never serious.

Local treatment consists of lubricating the anal canal with petroleum jelly or a similar substance, preferably just before the bowels are opened. The doctor may also prescribe a mild LAXATIVE to keep the motions as soft as possible until the fissure heals. However, the most important thing is to pay attention to the diet so that CONSTIPATION is prevented. A recurrence of the anal fissure is then most unlikely.

Analgesic Any drug or substance that relieves pain without causing a loss of consciousness. The best known analgesics are aspirin and paracetamol. Analgesics are most often taken to relieve common aches and pains such as headaches and period pains.

Stronger painkillers such as pethidine and morphine suffer from the disadvantage of being addictive. This is why they are not used for everyday minor pains, even though they are more powerful than the medicines available over the chemist's counter.

Young children rarely complain of pain unless they have severe disease, so when they do it is wise to seek medical help. Try to prevent your older children from taking analgesics for the slightest ache or pain. Whilst the commonly used painkillers will do them no harm in the correct dose, it is probably best to let the body heal itself without painkillers if possible. Never give analgesics to babies under three months without consulting a doctor.

Analgesics, like any other drugs, should be kept out of the reach of children and only given as directed on the container. Ideally, all analgesics should be kept in child-resistant packs or containers.

Aspirin is the common name for acetylsalicylic acid, the most widely used drug in the world. This painkiller was first manufactured in a laboratory in Germany at the end of the last century and today the average person in the United Kingdom consumes one hundred tablets in a year.

Although aspirin is most widely used for reducing pain, it also has other clinical properties. Its action in reducing raised body temperature makes it useful in treating FEVER, and its anti-inflammatory actions make it a useful drug for the treatment of arthritis and similar conditions.

Until 1971 it was not known how aspirin worked but British research has now provided the answer. Aspirin acts by preventing the body from making a group of naturally-occurring substances called prostaglandins.

Because aspirin is so commonly found in the home medicine cabinet, it's often taken by children without their parents' knowledge. This is very dangerous as children can appear relatively well immediately after taking the aspirins, yet fall ill very suddenly without any warning. If your child takes three or more aspirins, you must take him to a doctor or casualty department as soon as possible.

With the introduction of unit packaging in foil, which makes it almost impossible for children to take handfuls of tablets, accidental poisoning should no longer be such a hazard to children. Even so, aspirin should be kept out of reach of children and stored in child-resistant containers.

Some doctors are concerned that aspirin causes bleeding into the stomach. Certainly, aspirin does cause the stomach and small bowel to bleed very slightly but this blood loss is only twice that lost every day by the bowel as a natural process.

In spite of critics' warnings against it, aspirin is still the best drug treatment for most of the minor aches and pains of childhood. A soluble form is probably best because it acts faster. Aspirin, like any other drug, should only be given in doses recommended by your doctor or on the packaging itself.

A final word of warning: don't give your children aspirin at bedtime to help them to sleep. There's nothing in it that causes sleep, so this unnecessary drug intake is hard to justify. It's also worth remembering that you shouldn't get your child to place an aspirin against his gum for a toothache as this can ulcerate the gum and cause more pain.

Paracetamol is a pain-relieving and fever-reducing drug similar to aspirin but with fewer gastric side-effects. Paracetamol does not cause blood loss from the stomach, as does aspirin.

However, paracetamol is more dangerous than aspirin if taken in excess, and recent research has shown that surprisingly few tablets can cause serious and irreversible damage. Paracetamol becomes bound to tissues very quickly and in overdose can damage the liver so much that it is not treatable even by the best modern methods. It's therefore imperative to keep paracetamol tablets out of the reach of children.

Anatomy of children From the anatomical point of view, children are not just scaled down versions of adults. Their arms and legs are comparatively shorter and their heads comparatively larger than those of adults, the differences becoming less as they grow older.
See GROWTH; HEIGHT; WEIGHT

Anencephaly In this congenital abnormality, the skull is incompletely formed, part of the brain is exposed and the cerebral hemispheres are absent. The defect occurs towards the end of the first month after conception.

Affected babies die at, or soon after, birth. This malformation causes about one in eight of all stillbirths and affects more girls than boys. The numbers of children stillborn with anencephaly vary widely throughout the world and throughout Great Britain, being especially high in Ireland.

Anencephaly shows similarities to SPINA BIFIDA in its embryological development and geographical distribution. The cause of both conditions is as yet unknown but it seems likely that both genetic and environmental factors are important.

A mother who has had a child with anencephaly or spina bifida has an increased chance of having subsequent affected babies. An ultrasound scan can detect anencephaly early in pregnancy, as can tests for raised levels of alpha-fetoprotein in serum and amniotic fluid. Parents of an affected foetus may wish to have the pregnancy terminated.

Anorexia The medical term for the loss of APPETITE for food. This is a common condition in children, as any parent knows, and although most children lose their appetites for perfectly simple reasons, others may be suffering from an underlying disease.

Perhaps the commonest cause in children is infection. It's important to encourage children with infectious illnesses to drink as much as possible, because this not only maintains their fluid level (which can get very low if they are sweating with a fever) but also provides a means of giving the child some nourishment. Some childhood infections such as thrush and tonsillitis actually make eating painful, so don't force food down.

Never force a child to eat at any time. Children eat when they are hungry and don't eat when they are not. If your child seems well and has no fever, don't fuss about food. Mealtimes can all too easily become battlegrounds and this produces short and long term problems for you and the child. Unless your child is ill, there is almost no chance of him starving himself.

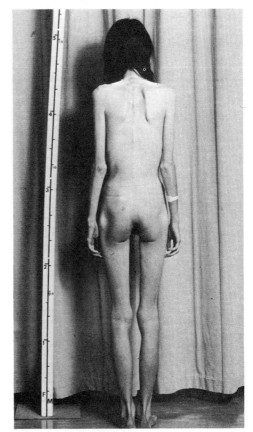

A teenage girl suffering from anorexia nervosa, most commonly seen in this age group.

Some children, like some adults, go off their food when under stress. Disharmony at home, examinations at school, or problems with friends can all cause anorexia.

More serious causes include diseases of the liver, intestine, kidney and thyroid gland, but these are all very rare.

See ANOREXIA NERVOSA

Anorexia nervosa A potentially very serious condition usually seen in teenage girls or young women. It consists of a severe loss of appetite with no obvious physical cause, drastic weight loss, constipation and cessation of periods. It often starts as an attempt to slim but may also be triggered off by an emotional shock.

Many treatments have been tried and most of the girls get better. Success is usually based on the treatment of underlying psychological problems causing the condition.

Anoxia   *See* ASPHYXIA

Antenatal care   Caring for a baby should start even before he is born, while he is still inside the womb. This will give him the best possible chance of optimal development and alert medical and nursing teams to anything which might prejudice a normal and safe delivery.

The pregnant mother provides her growing baby with all his nourishment, supplies him with oxygen, removes waste products, keeps him at the right temperature and protects him from physical damage. If she doesn't eat a well balanced diet, her own body will suffer, making her less able to cope physically with the strains of pregnancy. Advice on sensible eating patterns is available from many sources. It's worth pointing out that if her diet contains sufficient iron-containing foods, there is no need for her to take iron tablets and, if she doesn't like cows' milk, there are other calcium-containing foods which can take its place. Babies of mothers who smoke are likely to weigh less than babies of non-smokers, so the incidence of LOW BIRTH WEIGHT with all its possible complications is increased.

Whoever undertakes a woman's antenatal care, and wherever it is done, the same questions

Measuring the blood pressure is one of the routine checks carried out during the antenatal period, so that any potential problems can be detected early.

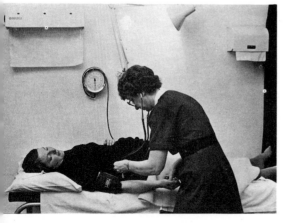

are asked and the same tests carried out. Routine measurements include those of the weight and the blood pressure; the urine is examined regularly for the presence of protein; and examinations of the abdomen are made to check the baby's position and rate of growth. At the initial visit a full medical examination is carried out and the mother's blood is tested for its haemoglobin content and group (including the rhesus factor). A routine blood test for syphilis is also done because, although this disease is rare, treatment of an infected mother before the twentieth week of pregnancy will prevent harm to the foetus. At intervals during pregnancy, further haemoglobin tests are done and, if the woman is known to be rhesus negative, tests for rhesus antibodies are carried out. (*See* BLOOD GROUPS.)

Several other sophisticated tests are available to find out more about the state of the baby in certain circumstances, and these include AMNIOCENTESIS, ultrasonic scanning, X-rays, electronic foetal heart monitoring and foetoscopy.

Traditionally, the breasts are always examined antenatally to assess a woman's chances of breast feeding successfully. Inverted nipples may be helped by wearing breast shells, but no other preparation of the breasts has been shown to be useful.

For various reasons, such as worsening or severe rhesus haemolytic disease in a baby, or diabetes or pre-eclamptic toxaemia in the mother, the labour may be induced before term with hormones or by breaking the waters. The main drawback with induction is that it is not always possible to be sure of the maturity of the baby, and the more immature the baby, the greater the chances of the RESPIRATORY DIS-TRESS SYNDROME. The obstetrician's task is to balance all the pros and cons of the situation, taking into account both the baby's and the mother's condition, with the help perhaps of an ultrasonic scan and various tests on the amniotic fluid to ascertain the maturity of the baby and the likelihood of the respiratory distress syndrome.

Although in many ways it is more pleasant to be delivered at home, many places do not have adequate flying squad facilities should an emergency occur during or after labour.

It seems sensible for most mothers to have their babies in hospital, where expert obstetric, surgical and paediatric facilities are immediately available, and to go home as soon as their condition and that of their baby permits, which might be within a few hours. Before the baby is born it's sensible to make sure that domestic arrangements are made to ensure that the mother's absence and return are as trouble-free as possible.

Improved health and social circumstances of mothers, together with advances in obstetric care, have contributed to the lowering of both maternal and foetal mortality over recent years.
See CHILDBIRTH; PERINATAL MORTALITY

Antibiotics When Alexander Fleming discovered penicillin in 1928, a new era in medicine began. Penicillin was soon followed by other antibiotics and today it is difficult to imagine modern medical treatment without them. Penicillin, tetracycline, streptomycin and others have prevented much suffering and saved many lives.

Antibiotics are used to fight infectious diseases. They work either by stopping the growth and reproduction of the infecting organisms (the bacteriostatic antibiotics), or by actually killing them (the bactericidal antibiotics).

Each antibiotic is effective against a certain range of BACTERIA only and even then certain bacteria may become resistant to the antibiotic's action. To avoid this, antibiotics should not be used indiscriminately for minor infections. Also, it is important to take them exactly as prescribed and to finish the prescribed course even if the infection is apparently already cured, otherwise partially resistant germs may survive and result in re-infection.

Penicillin is an antibiotic produced naturally by a fungus, Penicillium. Today, penicillin is made in large quantities by drug companies and is often made semi-synthetically. Because so many people have taken penicillin over the years (it was first widely used clinically during the second world war), some bacteria have become accustomed to it and instead of being killed as they used to be, they actually *need* penicillin in order to live.

This alarming state of affairs means that the pharmaceutical industry is constantly searching for new types of penicillin that will kill these resistant bacteria.

Some penicillins are inactivated by the stomach's acid and so have to be given by injection, but most are available in tablet or capsule form.

Unfortunately, most of the penicillins in use today can cause side effects, including diarrhoea, skin trouble and allergies. Allergic reactions to penicillin are not uncommon in children who have a history of asthma, eczema or hay fever. Application of penicillin to the skin (now rare) is especially likely to cause a reaction. Allergic reactions to penicillin can be severe and deaths have occurred, though rarely. If your child ever gets a rash or itching after taking penicillin, tell your doctor. If this is an allergic reaction, you must ensure that he never has penicillin again in any form. There are perfectly good alternatives available.

Tetracycline is an antibiotic drug that kills many bacteria and a few viruses. It is active when given by mouth and is a very safe drug. Tetracycline shouldn't be given to young children because milk teeth can become permanently stained yellow-brown and made more susceptible to dental decay. For the same reason, tetracycline is not a good drug to take during pregnancy. Ideally, no child under the age of 12 should receive tetracyclines.

Penicillin and tetracycline are two of many antibiotics available for doctors to choose from.

Anti-convulsants *See* EPILEPSY

Antihistamines Histamine is a substance made in specialized cells (mast cells) found all over the body and is released during the body's response to allergic stimuli. In the skin, released histamine causes a local reddening (because of enlargement of small blood vessels); a blister or weal (because of the release of tissue fluid); and itching (because of the stimulation of nerve endings). Histamine is also released in other parts of the body in response to allergic stimuli.

Antihistamines are drugs which antagonize the effects of histamine. They are used in creams and can be taken as tablets or syrups. Repeated use on the skin can give rise to an allergy to the cream itself in some people.

Drowsiness is the major side effect, which is why people taking antihistamines shouldn't drive or operate machinery. Fortunately, there are many different types of antihistamine and as people's reactions to each vary so much, there's a good chance that a doctor will be able to find one to suit each patient.

Because they cause drowsiness, antihistamines are often used as mild sleeping medicines for children, though sometimes they produce the opposite effect and cause excitation instead of sleep.

Perhaps the most common everyday use for antihistamines is in the prevention of MOTION SICKNESS but some cold medicines and hay fever preparations also contain them. They are useful in some other allergic conditions.

See ALLERGY; BITES AND STINGS; URTICARIA

Anxiety An emotion which we all feel from time to time, and there is evidence that the anxiety we feel before we take an examination or compete in a race, for instance, is associated with other changes in our bodies which help prepare us for the challenge. These are all due to the release of certain hormones. It is only when the responses of the mind and body to this hormone outflow are so great that they interfere with our ability to carry out a task that anxiety actually becomes a problem.

There is no reason to believe that children do not get acutely anxious just like adults and some children may reach an acute anxiety state with feelings of nausea, palpitation, dizziness and weakness. If this occurs in response to something which one would normally expect to produce anxiety, simple reassurance may be all that is needed. But if an acute anxiety state arises in a child in a situation which should not normally provoke fear, for instance going to school, travelling on a train, or going to stay with a friend, then a more detailed enquiry has to be made to try to find out the cause. In severe cases referral to a psychologist or psychiatrist may help.

Anxiety can show itself in the form of physical symptoms such as RECURRENT ABDOMINAL PAIN or recurrent vomiting, recurrent limb pains, headaches or even recurrent episodes of raised temperature. Such a child needs reassurance and someone to sort out his problems, which may be at home, at school, or with his friends. He is not necessarily emotionally disturbed but is simply reacting to stress in his own way. He probably doesn't even connect his anxiety with his physical symptoms.

Apgar score A New York anaesthetist, Dr Virginia Apgar, developed this marking system – see below – for newborn babies (indicating their state of health) which is now used all over the world. The obstetrician gives marks from 0 to 2 for each of five signs of life.

	0	1	2
Heart rate	Absent	Below 100	Over 100
Respiratory effort	Absent	Slow, irregular	Good, crying
Muscle tone	Limp	Some flexion of extremities	Active motion
Response to stimulation by catheter in nostril	No response	Grimace	Cough or sneeze
Colour	Blue, pale	Body pink, extremities blue	Completely pink

A total of 10 marks indicates that the baby is in the best possible state. These marks are given one minute after birth but the score may be re-estimated at intervals.

An Apgar score of under 7 indicates that something may be wrong, while a score between 4 and 0 indicates that the baby's life is in danger. Individual parts of the score are more important than the total.

Appendicitis An inflammation of the appendix. The appendix lies in the right side of the abdomen and is a blind, narrow, worm-like tube opening into the bowel near the junction of the small and large intestines.

For a long time it was thought that the appendix was a useless part of the body, but recent research suggests that this may not be so. The wall of the appendix contains a lot of lymphoid tissue and this may play an important role in the production of antibodies.

Why inflammation so often occurs in the appendix is not known for certain but it is known that small, hard pellets of food (faecaliths) can obstruct the narrow opening of the appendix into the bowel and thus cause inflammation. Appendicitis is very much less common in people who eat a large amount of roughage and so have softer intestinal contents with no faecaliths. Indeed, it is almost unknown in parts of the world where the diet is rich in high-fibre foods.

ABDOMINAL PAIN in children can be due to a variety of causes but if your child complains of pain in the tummy for more than two hours, if his temperature is slightly raised and if he vomits, then you should call a doctor as quickly as possible. While waiting, no medicines, food or drink should be given.

The pain in appendicitis frequently starts around the umbilicus and then settles in the lower right side of the abdomen. The younger the child, the less likely the signs are to be typical but appendicitis is in any case rare in children under a year old. There may be diarrhoea, constipation or no bowel upset.

Acute appendicitis is always dangerous because the appendix can burst. Should this happen, pus will pour into the abdominal cavity and lead to PERITONITIS, which can be fatal. Many conditions mimic acute appendicitis and the diagnosis is often difficult to make.

Children and adolescents are the most frequent victims of appendicitis. Indeed the most common emergency operation in these age groups is appendicectomy. This operation may be performed as soon as the diagnosis has been made or may be postponed at the discretion of the doctor.

The so-called 'grumbling appendix' is not in fact caused by disease in the appendix but is usually found to be due to constipation, wind, anxiety or mesenteric adenitis.

Appetite Just why we feel hungry is not completely understood but there seem to be two main reasons. First, a sensation of emptiness of the stomach itself probably tells the brain that it's time for food and, second, the brain centre that monitors hunger is adversely affected by the low blood sugar level that occurs when we're hungry.

Right from their earliest days, babies have very different appetites. Not only do different babies eat very different amounts but any individual baby eats varying amounts under different conditions, just like an adult. A common mistake with breast feeding is to assume that four-hourly feeds are somehow suitable for every baby and that any demand the baby's appetite makes outside these times should be ignored. Contented breast-fed babies often feed at very much shorter intervals than four hours because their appetites tell them to eat often. This is what nature intended because frequent feeds encourage the breasts to produce more milk and because human milk passes out of the stomach more quickly than cows' milk.

Besides letting a baby breast feed as often as he wants to, let him feed for as long as he wants to. Having a breast feed is like having a meal and it should be the baby who decides how long the meal should last.

Babies have relatively large appetites compared with their size. The appetite often increases suddenly at about six to eight weeks along with the growth spurt that is so common at this time. By about six months a baby's rate of growth slows down and his appetite stops increasing so fast.

Because your baby is growing, it doesn't mean that his appetite necessarily goes on doing so. If you become unduly concerned about his appetite your anxiety can easily lead to a feeding problem. Most children are heavier and taller today than they have ever been, and many children are overweight, so worrying about underfeeding is usually unnecessary. One of the most common times for a child to lose his appetite is in his second year. His rate of growth, which was so fast in the first year, slows down and as a result one-year-olds actually seem to need less food than before.

If your toddler goes off his food for a short time yet seems otherwise well, don't worry – he won't starve to death. Don't make mealtimes a battle of wills simply because your idea of his appetite differs from his. Of course, if your toddler goes off his food completely for more than a few days you should talk to your doctor.

Very many children only want to eat a limited range of foods and some are so choosy that they only seem to eat one or two types of food for a while. This sort of child often changes the foods he fancies, so one month he may ask for ice cream all the time, while in another he may only be interested in bread and butter. For the mother trying to give her child a balanced diet, this can be very worrying, but few children come to any harm by eating such a limited range of food for a short time. If the child's diet is looked at carefully, it's usually found that he is in fact having a wider range of nutrients than was thought. He may, for example, be drinking a lot of milk, or having frequent small snacks between meals that are just as nutritionally sound as 'proper' meals.

There is no real reason, except that it is convenient for the mother, for making children eat only at mealtimes, so it seems sensible to let your young child eat when he is hungry, even if this will spoil his appetite for his next meal. Meals then become less important both to mother and child and battles are less likely. There's nothing worse than preparing a beautifully cooked meal for a child who just turns up his nose at it!

Children are highly influenced by the appearance of their food and some refuse food if it looks unattractive. Small portions are more appealing to the child with a small appetite, as are foods which are not too hot. Children don't have to eat meat or cabbage, for example, in order to be healthy, provided the nutrients are replaced by other foods. Often the sight of a plate of brown meat and gravy puts a child off his meal altogether, and the more a mother insists on the child eating it up, the more she will put him off meat in the future.

Some children are more likely to eat if they are not made to sit at the table. Many more are more likely to have a good appetite if other people are eating with them. Playing with food is a normal pastime for babies and one-year-olds and is more likely if the child is not hungry.

There is no need to make a child finish the food on his plate, though it can be annoying if he has actually asked for more and then doesn't eat it. The child who follows his appetite and eats only as much as he wants is more likely to keep his weight within normal limits later on than the child who gets used to eating everything put in front of him even if he doesn't need it.

Yet other children are actually made ill to some degree by certain foods such as cows' milk. If a child seems to dislike a particular food, it's far better to stop giving it to him. If his dislike is purely the result of a food fad, he will probably eat the food again one day of his own accord, but if it really makes him feel ill, then he'll probably avoid it thereafter. A problem arises here if a child is made unwell by a certain food but neither he nor his parents recognize the relationship between the food and the symptoms it produces. This happens quite often and detailed dietary counselling may be necessary.

See ALLERGY; ANOREXIA; ANOREXIA NERVOSA; DEHYDRATION; OBESITY

Arthritis Pain in one or more joints, often accompanied by swelling of the joint.

Joint pains in children, unlike those in adults, usually get better. Some children have aches and pains in their joints when they have infectious fevers but these soon disappear and are of little importance.

The most important cause of painful joints in children is RHEUMATIC FEVER. Some parents worry that their child has rheumatic fever when he has simple 'GROWING PAINS', but two things may put their minds at rest. First, rheumatic fever is now very uncommon and second, growing pains are felt in the muscles between the joints (particularly in the calf or thigh) and not in the joints themselves.

GONORRHOEA is the commonest cause of arthritis in adolescents and occurs most frequently in girls. It is rare in children under the age of ten years.

Children may develop RHEUMATOID ARTHRITIS and it has been estimated that in one in twenty adults with this condition, the symptoms began in childhood.

Arthritis may also be caused by an injury to a joint.

See HENOCH-SCHÖNLEIN PURPURA

Artificial respiration *See* KISS OF LIFE

Asphyxia The medical name for the condition resulting from a lack of oxygen (anoxia) when a child suffocates or chokes. When a baby is born, he may suffer from a lack of oxygen during labour or immediately afterwards if the onset of breathing is delayed. The brain cells are the most sensitive to oxygen lack of all the body's tissues, and can withstand only a short time without oxygen before being permanently damaged. (*See* CEREBRAL PALSY; FOETAL DISTRESS.)

It's impossible to tell how much BRAIN DAMAGE is actually done by a few minutes' lack of oxygen at this stage as it is known from experience that most children who don't breathe for even as long as two minutes still grow up to be perfectly normal. Some children develop normally after even longer periods of oxygen lack.

If your baby chokes on a piece of food that goes down the wrong way, lift him up by the legs, hang him upside down and smack him on the back until the piece is dislodged. Don't wait until he goes blue – start quickly.

Older children suffocate or choke on things

from time to time – in fact, this is a fairly common emergency in childhood. They may choke on beads and small toys as well as food. Put the child over your knee with his head down on the floor and smack him firmly on the back. This will usually dislodge the foreign body. There is another good way of getting a child to expel an inhaled foreign body, called the Heimlich manoeuvre. Get behind the child with your arms round him, make a fist with one of your hands, clasp it with the other and then press the two hands firmly and sharply inwards and upwards over the upper part of the child's abdomen. As you pull your clasped hands towards you, you force air out of the lungs and this often dislodges the object.

If your child inhales a foreign body which cannot be quickly removed by one of these methods, get medical help at once. Do not do the kiss of life or you may blow the object further down into the lungs.

Children can also be suffocated by putting their heads into polythene bags, record sleeve linings, or by climbing into old refrigerators,

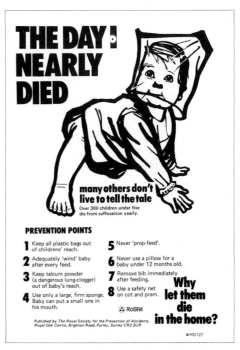

A warning about everyday dangers of suffocation published by The Royal Society for the Prevention of Accidents.

for example. These are obvious hazards, once you're aware of them, and can easily be avoided.

It's best not to give a baby a pillow in the first year – he doesn't need it and although the chances are that he wouldn't smother himself (especially if it's a proper baby pillow) it'll give you peace of mind.

Aspirin   *See* ANALGESIC

Asthma   A common and distressing condition in which a narrowing of the air passages (bronchi) makes breathing difficult. The child often finds breathing out more difficult than breathing in, and the distress that this disease causes makes him panic, which in turn makes the breathing worse. In one recent survey it was found that one in 20 schoolchildren suffered from asthma. Twice as many boys are affected as girls before puberty and thereafter the numbers equalize.

Asthma tends to improve spontaneously as the child grows older. Half of the children with asthma at seven years old have stopped getting attacks at eleven. The usual age of remission is 10 to 15, and less than 20 per cent of asthmatic children carry on wheezing into adulthood. Our understanding of asthma is increasing all the time and we now know much more accurately what happens in an asthmatic's LUNGS. The basic problem in asthma seems to be that the lining of the bronchi is especially

A child using a device developed to enable a drug for the treatment of asthma to be inhaled into the lungs.

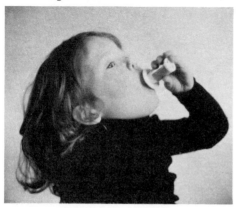

sensitive to certain stimuli, and the bronchial muscle reacts by going into spasm while the lining swells and produces lots of mucus. The narrowed air passages often make the child's breathing wheezy and cause a cough. The nasal discharge and phlegm coughed up by a child with asthma may look purulent and infected. This appearance is rarely due to infection however, but simply to collections of special cells produced by the inflamed mucous membranes.

The provoking factors are ALLERGY and infection. Asthma is often seen in children who are susceptible to eczema, hay fever and nettlerash, as these are all allergic conditions. It is not uncommon for this group of diseases to run in families, when they are known as atopic disorders. Allergic or atopic asthma is most likely to occur during the spring and summer. It is now well established that complete breast feeding (without even one feed of cows' milk) can reduce the expected incidence of allergic conditions in children from atopic families.

Perhaps the commonest sensitizing agent is the house dust mite. It lives on the scales of dead skin that we all shed and, as it is found especially in bedroom dust, it tends to provoke asthmatic attacks at night. The trouble is that it's almost impossible to get rid of mites from a house, but damp dusting, the use of synthetic bedding with foam pillows and mattress (or the enclosing of an ordinary mattress in a thick plastic cover), and scrupulous domestic cleanliness can help to keep the mite population down. Some experts believe, however, that this 'mite hygiene' is of doubtful value, and if exhaustive measures to reduce the house dust mite infestation don't improve the child's asthma, they can be stopped.

Other allergens provoking asthmatic attacks are grass pollen, pets and food. Some children with asthma have an allergy to certain foods, (commonly cows' milk and eggs but also nuts, fish and chocolate). The diagnosis of food allergy is difficult to make and skin tests don't always reflect the story of an attack following the eating of a particular food. Perhaps the best way of tracking down a suspected food allergy is by a trial of avoidance of that particular food for at least one month, to see if this prevents further asthmatic attacks. It is possible to measure specific food antibodies in the blood and if these decrease on avoidance of the particular food in question, this is a good sign that the food may have been causing the asthma.

While it is hard to insist on getting rid of a pet unless it is definitely responsible for the child's asthma, it is sensible to have a trial of any proposed new pet in the house to see if it causes asthma in the child.

Asthma provoked by viral infection (with the respiratory syncitial and parainfluenza viruses) is more common in the winter. It's important to distinguish between symptoms due to respiratory infection and symptoms due to hay fever (allergic rhinitis) – sneezing, nasal stuffiness and discharge, as hay fever may coexist with asthma. Many children with BRONCHIOLITIS or wheezy BRONCHITIS in the first two years go on to develop asthma in later childhood.

Emotional stress, either pleasant or unpleasant, can provoke asthma, though this is not an important cause. Some children respond better to treatment away from home, not because of the change of air, but because some of the domestic stresses are removed.

Exercise, extremes of temperature, fumes and other environmental pollution may also be provoking factors for a child prone to asthma.

During an attack of asthma a child may quite naturally feel very anxious because of his difficulty in breathing. Some children really believe that they're going to die. Despite the parents' own very real anxiety, they must try to comfort and reassure their child that his asthma can soon be relieved.

Asthma is so unpleasant for the sufferer that treatment must be quick and effective. Antibiotics have no effect on asthma or on wheezy bronchitis. However, if there is also a bacterial infection such as sinusitis, otitis media, or tonsillitis, they are useful. Basically, the drugs used relieve the bronchial muscle spasm. Corticosteroid drugs may be given both in an emergency and as a long-term preventive treatment. An anti-allergy drug, sodium cromoglycate, is especially helpful in preventing attacks. This, like many of the useful drugs for asthma, can be taken in an inhaler and even relatively young children can be taught to take it.

If a child with asthma is fighting for breath, restless, has a fast pulse or is blue, he needs emergency treatment and you should get him to a doctor or to hospital as soon as you can.

If the child is allergic to a specific substance (which may be discovered by skin testing), then the doctor can try to desensitize him by a series of injections. Some benefit may be obtained from desensitization to grass pollens but no convincing evidence is available that it is effective against the house dust mite or food allergies.

Improved modern drugs, together with breathing exercises and a more enlightened approach by both doctors and parents, mean that most asthmatic children can now lead a normal life. If the parents help their child accept the fact that he will continue getting attacks of asthma which can be treated, it will be easier for him not to worry about them in advance.

However, even when free from asthma, a child who is prone to it may be more susceptible to certain lung diseases because of an alteration in the reactivity of the muscles around his bronchi. Any respiratory infection in an asthmatic should for this reason always be treated promptly. Parents should avoid smoking and should have their child vaccinated against 'flu.

See WHEEZING

Astigmatism *See* VISUAL PROBLEMS

Athlete's foot A common fungal infection of the skin between the toes which may also occur, more rarely, on the soles of the feet. The fungus lives on skin that is soft and moist – hence the name athlete's foot, because people with hot, sweaty feet tend to suffer most from it. Children pick up the infection from public swimming baths, from parents at home, school showers and changing rooms, or by going barefoot anywhere where infected feet have been.

There are two main forms of the disease: the acute one in which there are weeping, inflamed blisters, and the chronic form with severe cracking and peeling of the skin with red raw areas beneath. Itching is usually the main symptom but scratching and picking only make the condition worse. The skin between the little toe and its neighbour is usually the most badly affected.

Treatment starts with prevention. Bare feet in public places encourage the spread from person to person, so feet should be kept covered if infected. Shoes with composition soles are especially bad for children who suffer from athlete's foot, as are socks made from synthetic materials. Both trap moisture and encourage the softening of the skin on which the fungus thrives.

The feet should be kept as dry as possible, making a special point of drying between the toes after washing. A dusting powder, a spray containing a fungicide or an anti-ringworm ointment are also helpful in killing the fungus.

Because athlete's foot is so contagious, the child who gets it should have his own towel and bathmat and should not use school changing rooms unless his feet are covered. Socks should be changed every day and boiled to kill the fungus. Athlete's foot can easily get a hold in a family or a class and it can be very difficult to eradicate unless treated promptly.

Audiometry The measurement of HEARING. This can be done in many ways (*see* HEARING TESTING) but can be carried out with a specially designed instrument called an audiometer. An audiometer produces pure tones of different frequencies and the sound at each frequency can be varied in loudness.

The testing can be done either with a 'free field' audiometer, when the child has to turn to the source of the sound, (suitable for younger children from about nine months) or with an audiometer suitable for a child old enough to be able to register what he has heard.

At each sound frequency the loudness of the sound is reduced to the lowest level the child can still hear, and this level is then plotted on a graph called an audiogram. The completed audiogram shows the hearing loss at each frequency and also gives clues as to the type of DEAFNESS that might be present.

A child thought to have any deafness should have his hearing tested unless he has recently had a cold or earache.

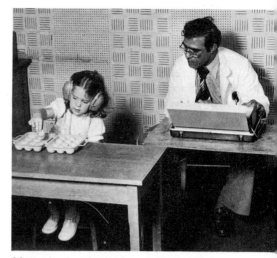

Measuring hearing with an audiometer. Sounds at various levels are produced, and the child is asked to move a ball from one box to the other each time she hears a sound.

Most children have a simplified form of this test in their first year at school and any hearing loss picked up is investigated further. Slight deafness is a very common problem in childhood and easily goes unnoticed by parents and teachers. It usually follows repeated infection of the middle ear. The child finds it difficult to hear the frequencies produced by speech and can readily drop behind at school. Often the child's own speech development is affected because he can't copy sounds he can't hear.

See EARS

Autism A condition affecting a small group of children – including more boys than girls – that is classified as a childhood psychosis. It is rare, affecting four to five children in 10,000.

Autistic children suffer from an inability to make sense of the information they receive through their eyes and ears from the outside world. They do not develop the ability to communicate with other people normally, either by speech, gesture, or in other ways, and become withdrawn and emotionally unresponsive, unable to form normal relationships with people and with a limited ability to differentiate between who is important to them and who is not.

Their parents usually suspect that something is wrong early in infancy, though the condition may present itself when the child is older. The baby fails to show signs of awareness of what is going on around him and may be difficult to feed. Later, in the second year, the toddler often has serious behaviour problems. He has a short attention span and may be especially sensitive to noise or light patterns. Later he comes to enjoy pointless repetitive movements such as spinning round and round. People are treated as furniture, with a few exceptions, and he rarely looks them in the eye. Other characteristics sometimes seen are delayed bowel and bladder control and over-(hyper-) active behaviour.

There is retarded language development and speech fails to develop altogether in about a third of these children. The rest learn to speak in a highly individual way, sometimes misusing pronouns and prepositions and repeating words over and over again, often without understanding. Understanding of speech is always delayed, though most learn that sounds have meanings. Autism is sometimes explained as a language communication problem, like the blind child's lack of sight.

Autistic children are of varying INTELLIGENCE but their measured intelligence as a group falls below average, and about half of them are severely mentally retarded. In contrast, their parents are often of higher than average intelligence.

Normal children may show features of autism during periods of physical or emotional illness but they lose these features eventually. Blind and deaf children may have autistic features and their true condition may be difficult to diagnose in the early stages.

The treatment of autism is as yet in its early stages, though research is adding to the pool of knowledge all the time. These children should ideally be taught by skilled teachers in special units, with back-up help from a psychiatrist, psychologist, child psychotherapist and social worker, and special counselling for their parents. Communication must take advantage of any signs of interest the child shows, doing without words altogether if necessary.

Many autistic children grow up with communication problems and need care and sheltered work all their lives, though the social withdrawal often lessens in adolescence. We do not know what causes the condition in the first place, though there are many theories. Often there are complications during pregnancy or childbirth, and about a third of them have some other problem such as epilepsy.

Autonomic nervous system There are two main parts of the body's nervous system. One controls the willed actions, our thinking, and the working of our muscles, and is called the CENTRAL NERVOUS SYSTEM. The rest of the system keeps the basic body functions going irrespective of any effort we might make and is called the autonomic or involuntary nervous system. All day, every day, our bodies carry out thousands of basic functions automatically. We do not have to tell our chests to breathe, our kidneys to produce urine or our hearts to beat. All these processes are controlled by autonomic nerves.

The autonomic nervous system consists of two divisions – the sympathetic and the parasympathetic. These tend to have opposing effects, for example, sympathetic nervous stimulation causes blood vessels to constrict, with whitening of the skin, while parasympathetic stimulation makes the vessels get bigger with flushing or reddening of the skin.

Functions as different as blood pressure control, breathing, heart beat, sweating, movements of the bowels, digestion, urine production and reproduction depend on the autonomic nervous system.

B

Baby battering Over the years every casualty department sees a number of children injured not by accident but by their parents, guardians or minders. The injury sustained is often called a 'non-accidental injury'.

Some babies cry a lot more than others. Research suggests that babies who have been separated from their mothers soon after birth cry more than others and that their mothers have more difficulty in coping with them.

Most mothers occasionally feel that their nerves are stretched to breaking point by their young children but, while the majority can cope with their exasperation, a few can't and end up hitting their child, burning it, shaking it, throwing it down, squeezing it hard or twisting its legs or arms. The damage caused varies from slight bruising to brain damage and actual fractures.

People who batter their children are no different from other people but instead of realizing that things are getting on top of them and asking for help, or leaving the child alone for a little while, they feel they have to stop the child doing whatever it was that was annoying them and so end up by battering it.

Often these people live under stressful social circumstances, though others may also batter their babies. The battering mother is likely to have had inadequate mothering herself and so has not had the chance to learn at an impressionable age how to be a good mother. She may feel that she is a poor mother because her child does things which annoy her, and so she either takes out her frustration on the child or decides to discipline him so severely that he will not do anything naughty again.

These days if a mother asks her health visitor, family doctor or social worker for help

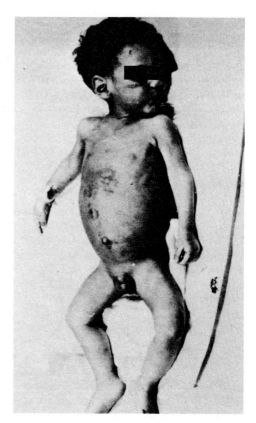

A battered baby : injuries of this type range from bruises to burns and fractures.

because she is scared of what she might do to her child, she is almost certain to get help and support. Self-help support groups (such as Parents Anonymous) will also help in an emergency. Regular attendance at baby clinics may reveal problems before they become serious. If a woman batters her child and the battering comes to light, she will also be helped, but how much better it would be to have the help before and not after. If you batter your child, don't put off getting help because you fear what the authorities will do. They will not take your baby away from you unless this would be better for you and the baby. Get help sooner rather than later and don't let the situation get too critical before asking a friend, relative, neighbour or professional for help.

See BONDING; CHILD ABUSE; CRYING; INCUBATOR; LOW BIRTH WEIGHT

Baby care Babies are totally dependent on the people looking after them and indeed would not last long if they were not looked after. During the first year a baby relies on his mother to feed him, move him from place to place, keep him at the right temperature, keep him clean, talk to him, give him interesting things to look at and to do and, most important of all, love him. Well-cared-for babies grow up to have far fewer problems later, and a well-cared-for child is in turn likely to look after his or her own children well.

The right FOOD will help a child thrive and so parents should try to learn a little about nutrition – which foods he should have and which are unnecessary and even possibly harmful. Experts are agreed that breast MILK is the best milk for babies and a mother owes it to herself and her baby to learn how to breast feed successfully. Babies are happier if fed on an unrestricted basis – as often and for as long as they like. Because they cry less if fed like this, life is easier for their mothers, and unrestricted BREAST FEEDING soon becomes a way of life. WEANING (introducing other foods) can be started at four to six months but there is no need to stop breast feeding until you or your baby want to. A baby cannot choose his own food, so he relies on his parents to choose the right things for him. (*See* BABY FEEDING; BOTTLE FEEDING.)

In our climate babies can easily get too cold if they are not dressed up and if their rooms are not heated in winter. It's all too easy to overheat a baby, and difficult to judge how warm he is if you're dashing around doing the housework. Temperature is more critical if the baby is very young, premature or small.

If a baby is ill and feverish, it is sensible to keep him relatively cool rather than smother him with blankets and extra clothes. (*See* FEVER; HEATSTROKE.)

Babies certainly don't need bathing every day but it is important to keep their skin clean in the nappy area and in the folds under their arms, round their necks and behind their ears. Both bathing and 'topping and tailing' (washing their faces and nappy areas) are good ways of keeping them clean and fresh. The water used should be warm (test it with your elbow) and the soap non-stinging.

Babies are likely to get several different sorts of spots which seldom need treatment. MILIA are little, whitish, pin-sized spots on the face, and go of their own accord. Many babies develop spotty faces in the first few weeks of life. These spots almost always subside and usually no cause is found. NAPPY RASH is a common problem, and many babies also suffer from CRADLE CAP.

Nails need cutting carefully because of the sudden movements babies often make. Use small scissors with blunt-ended blades or bite the soft nails of a young baby off with your teeth.

Cotton wool buds can be used if absolutely necessary to clean the outer ears and the nostrils; however, it's so easy to hurt the baby if he moves that you should hold him very firmly while doing this. Never poke anything up the ear canal, as a sudden movement may make you damage or even break the baby's eardrum.

A boy's foreskin doesn't need pulling back to wash beneath it until it retracts easily. Similarly, the vulva shouldn't be scrupulously washed but any large amount of matter gently wiped away.

We expect babies to SLEEP on their own in our society, but you may feel that it is kinder and more natural to let them sleep near you or in a sling during the day, and near you or even in your bed at night. People often worry about the correct position for their baby to sleep in. The best way is probably the way

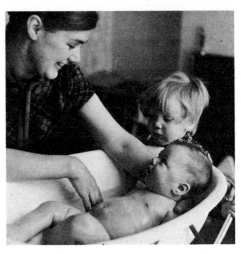

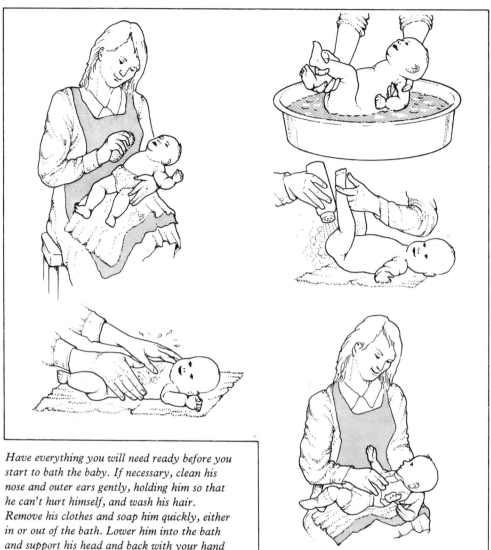

Have everything you will need ready before you start to bath the baby. If necessary, clean his nose and outer ears gently, holding him so that he can't hurt himself, and wash his hair. Remove his clothes and soap him quickly, either in or out of the bath. Lower him into the bath and support his head and back with your hand and arm all the time you are washing him. Make sure he is thoroughly dry, especially in the folds of his skin.

the child sleeps best, but if putting him to sleep on his tummy or side gives you peace of mind, do it this way. A pillow is unnecessary for a baby until he is at least a year old, but a pillow placed under the mattress is quite all right. The cot duvets now available carry the risk that the baby might pull them over his head and suffocate. In practice this is unlikely, but it is well worth anchoring a duvet to the sides of the cot to prevent it riding up, or using blankets instead. (*See* SAFETY.)

Equipment and toys for a baby must be safe. Toys needn't cost lots of money. A six-month-old baby is just as happy with a few brightly coloured plastic bowls and spoons as he is with 'proper' toys.

Caring for a baby means giving him interesting things to do, look at and listen to besides feeding and washing him and putting him to bed. He will be much happier watching you in the kitchen than left alone in his cot.

Well-cared for babies are also much-loved babies. It is never wrong to pick up a crying baby and cuddle him and it certainly won't lead to bad habits. A happy, relaxed, loving mother gets the most pleasure from her baby, and he from her.

See BODY CONTACT; BONDING

Baby feeding Advice on baby feeding has changed considerably in the light of recent research. The best way of feeding a baby is to breast feed him. The baby needs nothing but breast milk unless he is acutely ill. The healthy breast-fed baby thrives on milk *alone* for many months if BREAST FEEDING is successful, which it can be if the mother knows how to do it and doesn't automatically follow the schedules laid down by many hospitals. Solids need not be given before four months and preferably not until six months.

Increasing numbers of mothers in the West are allowing their breast-fed babies to carry on feeding as long as they and their babies want to. This 'baby-led' WEANING ensures that babies have the comfort and pleasure of the breast for as long as they need it – perhaps for several years. In the third world, prolonged breast feeding provides an essential part of the child's dietary needs if food is scarce.

Extra vitamins are unnecessary for the breast-fed baby provided the mother's diet is well balanced and the mother and baby have enough sun. Commercial baby milks are fortified with vitamin D, so bottle-fed babies don't actually need extra vitamin D, though this is recommended by some doctors and health visitors as an additional safeguard. Bottle-fed babies can be given vitamin C as orange, blackcurrant or tomato juice. Official advice about vitamins for babies is being reviewed, as the whole subject is controversial at present. However, from about six months (or when milk ceases to form the major part of the baby's diet), vitamin supplements are recommended as a safeguard for all children up to the age of five (and again during adolescence) in the winter, especially where there is comparatively little sunshine such as in the north of Britain and in cities where environmental pollution is bad. Though some vitamin D is retained in the body from sum-

mer sunshine, the raised levels only last a few months. If a well balanced diet is eaten and the child gets plenty of sun, vitamin supplements are unnecessary.

FLUORIDE supplementation in the form of drops or tablets can be given (if the drinking water is low in fluoride) to babies of over six months.

Breast-fed babies only need drinks of water or fluids other than milk if they are acutely ill or if the weather is extremely hot.

See BOTTLE FEEDING; FOOD; RICKETS

Back The midline of the back is marked by the spines of the vertebrae. The vertebrae form the flexible spinal column (the backbone) that supports the body. If the spine is curved forwards to produce a hump back, this is called a kyphosis. If the curvature is sideways (looking from behind) the condition is called a scoliosis.

A baby carried in a front sling – there is no evidence that carrying even tiny babies in this way is harmful to the baby's back.

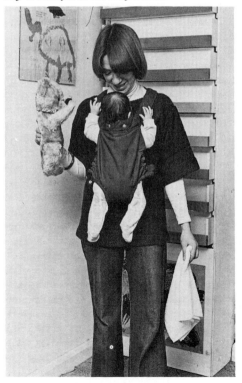

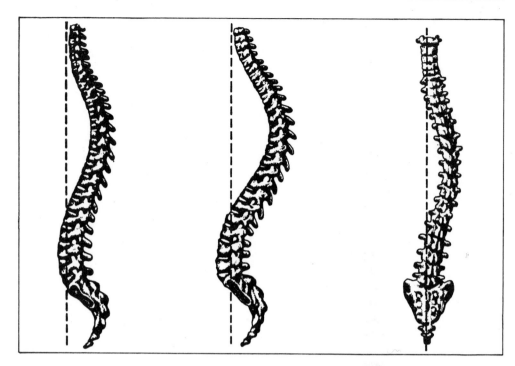

A normal spine, left, *and two types of spinal curvature. Kyphosis* (centre) *produces a hump back, and scoliosis* (right), *illustrated from behind, a sideways curvature.*

Sometimes these spinal curvatures are caused by poor POSTURE but there are many other causes ranging from chest disease, rickets and weakening of the spinal muscles to a difference in the length of the legs. Older children, often tall girls between the ages of 10 and 15, can get a postural curvature of the spine. This may be cured by exercise and attention to posture, though advice should be sought if there is any doubt about its cause.

These spinal deformities are uncommon in little children. A lot of parents worry whether they'll damage their child's back by encouraging him to sit up early. This can't happen. As soon as a baby wants to sit up, it's safe to encourage him to do so. Sitting will strengthen the neck and back muscles and can do no harm. Many parents also worry whether baby slings, baby bouncers, soft backed buggies and early standing will damage their babies' backs. There is no evidence that any of these is harmful.

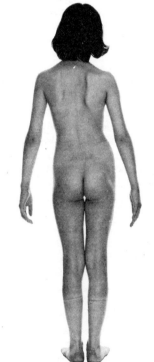

An example of scoliosis, most often seen in school-age children.

Bacteria Microscopic, single-celled organisms that cause many illnesses. Bacteria exist throughout nature and play a vitally important role in the normal function of things as different as soil in the garden and the large bowel of man.

They are all very tiny. A rod-shaped bacterium measures one micron (1/25,000 of an inch) in diameter by about four microns in length. Some bacteria are static but most move about spontaneously, especially those that have a tail such as the syphilis bacterium. Some bacteria form protective capsules and many can form spores. These spores are very resistant to heat, drying and the action of disinfectants and are usually formed by the bacteria when conditions are unfavourable and they need to preserve themselves. Not all bacteria are harmful (pathogenic) by any means; in fact our skin and bowels, for example, are populated by bacteria that are highly beneficial to us.

Pathogenic bacteria may be spread from person to person in droplets of saliva, by direct contact, or may be transmitted in infected urine and faeces.

When a doctor has taken a swab of a sore throat or a specimen of urine, for example, the bacteria-laden material is spread over a special plate of nutrient jelly in which the bacteria grow. The bacteria on the plates are then cultured in an incubator at body temperature for 24 hours, after which the plate is examined and the growth identified under a microscope. Other plates can be used which have several little discs in them, each impregnated with an antibiotic. As the bacteria grow, those that are killed by a particular antibiotic are absent from around that particular disc. This antibiotic is then chosen to cure the patient's infection.

Even without ANTIBIOTICS our bodies can cope very well with many bacteria because they are covered with skin and lined with mucous membranes which are the first line of defence against bacterial invasion. Tears, saliva, breast milk and other body fluids contain natural antiseptics. Inside the body there are even more sophisticated antibacterial barriers. The lining of the breathing system contains special 'hairy' cells that trap

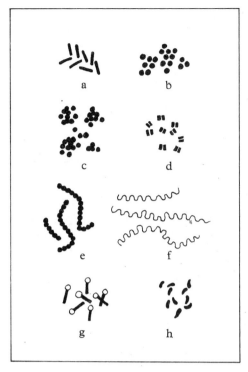

Bacteria classified by shape. a. Bacilli, b. Cocci, c. Staphylococci, d. Diplococci, e. Streptococci, f. Spirochaetes, g. Clostridia, h. Vibrios.

Below, *a culture of the bacterium Haemophilus welchii growing on a plate of blood agar.*

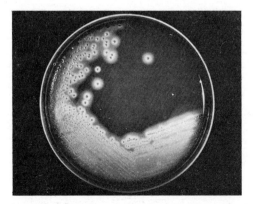

bacteria, and the stomach's acid kills many that we swallow. Bacteria or their toxins can be overcome by antibodies and special cells produced by the body's immune system. Antibodies also render bacteria susceptible to

27

being 'eaten' by specialized blood cells called phagocytes. The large bowel and the vagina have populations of specialized bacteria that actually stop others from growing (rather like ground cover plants stopping weeds in a flower bed). The bacteria normally present in the bowel may be killed by treatment with certain antibiotics resulting in diarrhoea. Eating live, natural yoghurt prevents or cures this problem.

Over the centuries bacteria have been the greatest killers of man. Today, pure water supplies, well organized public health and effective IMMUNIZATION have reduced their toll. Another useful weapon in combating the infections has been the antibiotics: as a result, we now have a potentially serious situation in which antibiotics are being over-used.

Bacteria are great survivors. If we use an antibiotic willy-nilly for trivial infections and for shorter periods than is recommended, resistant strains of bacteria emerge that cannot be killed by that antibiotic. So far, we've managed to keep one jump ahead of the bacteria by producing new drugs that will kill them even when they become resistant. The question is, how long can we keep one jump ahead? Problems are already arising with the treatment of certain types of VD, for example, which are becoming almost impossible to cure.

See IMMUNITY; VIRUSES

Bad breath   *See* HALITOSIS

Balanitis   An inflammation of the end of the PENIS (the glans penis). It occurs mainly in uncircumcised boys when matter is trapped under the foreskin. Sometimes the inflammation is so bad that the foreskin can't be retracted (pulled back) and there may also be a discharge.

Usually, the only treatment needed is improved attention to personal hygiene. A doctor will only advise CIRCUMCISION to prevent infections if they are repeated and troublesome. A tight foreskin by itself is not a reason for circumcision.

Baldness   Alopecia – partial or complete baldness – has a variety of causes, but in children by far the most common types are alopecia areata and baldness due to RINGWORM. Children sometimes pull their hair out as a nervous tic and this too can produce patches of baldness (*see* HABITS).

Alopecia areata affects the scalp primarily, although the eyebrows, eyelashes and beard area in adolescents may also be affected. It is first seen as one or more small, circular, well demarcated areas of baldness. The condition usually clears up spontaneously in a few weeks or months, although in rare cases the baldness may progress to become total.

The bald patches may be slightly red and small broken stumps of hair looking like exclamation marks are seen round the edges. Healing is heralded by the growth of fine, white, downy hair, followed by the growth of normal hair.

The cause of this condition is unknown. Many people have suggested that shock may be the culprit, but the evidence for this does not stand up to scrutiny.

Treatment, if necessary, is by local injection of a suspension of a steroid drug under the skin.

Ringworm causes patches of baldness similar in shape to those of alopecia areata. The skin, however, is pink and scaly, with stubbly broken hairs. The diagnosis (which can only be made with certainty by a doctor) is made by looking at the area under illumination with ultra-violet light filtered through a special filter (Wood's light), when the hair stumps fluoresce greenish-blue. Ringworm spores can also be seen under the microscope.

Treatment of ringworm of the scalp is with the drug griseofulvin.

Bandage   Bandages are mostly used for anchoring dressings over wounds or for giving support to sprained joints or weakened muscles. In general, those used for covering dressings are lightweight, gauze bandages and those for support are firm and elasticated.

A gauze bandage should be applied lightly, but firmly enough to keep the dressing underneath in place even when the person moves. An elastic bandage, in contrast, has to be applied tightly and often in special ways so as to have the desired effect on the underlying muscles or joints. You may have to learn the different ways of putting on an elastic bandage from a doctor or nurse because each area (be it hand, knee, ankle, etc) needs to be bandaged differently for the best effect and to ensure that the bandage doesn't fall off after the person has moved the limb a few times.

Bandages are not used today nearly as much as they were. Adhesive strapping and self-adhesive dressings have largely replaced old-fashioned dressings and bandages. Tubular gauze bandage comes in many different sizes and widths with metal applicators to match, and enables things as different as a finger or a head to be bandaged neatly, easily and quickly. Even the crêpe bandage which was used for support for so long has been superseded to a great extent by tubular support bandages.

Triangular bandages, usually made of calico or a similar material, are often used as slings for injured arms.

Some bandages are medicated, being impregnated with icthamol and hydrocortisone or zinc paste, and yet another type is impregnated with plaster of Paris. These plaster bandages are made of muslin and are kept airtight until needed when they are immersed in warm water and applied to the area of the body to be treated. The plaster in the bandage dries in a few minutes to give rigid support to the area.

Bandy legs   *See* BOW LEGS

BCG   *See* TUBERCULOSIS

Bedbugs   Small blood-sucking insects that live on human blood. They live hidden in cracks and dark places during the day and come out at night to feed. Their bites are usually small and trouble-free but some people are allergic to them and develop URTICARIA (nettlerash). The best way to get rid of bedbugs is to use DDT or a similar disinfectant in the room where they live by day. Your doctor will help you to get expert advice on their eradication.

Bed wetting   Most children become dry at night during their third or fourth years,

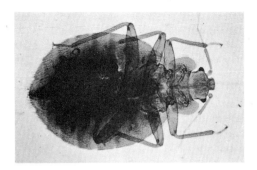

The bedbug.

though they may have occasional accidents after that. Other children are wet at night for much longer, usually because the signals sent to the brain by the full bladder are not strong enough to wake them up, especially if they are heavy sleepers. The voluntary and involuntary nervous control of the bladder develops at different rates in different children, explaining why some are dry at night much earlier than others. Some children suddenly become dry at night, whilst others gradually have increasing numbers of dry nights.

A few children have a physical abnormality which causes their wetting, such as a urine infection, diabetes or a congenital abnormality of their urinary system, so advice should be sought from the doctor if a four-year-old is still wet at night, or if he restarts wetting, having been dry before. However, it's important to keep a sense of proportion because 50 per cent of two-year-olds, 25 per cent of three-year-olds, and 10 per cent of five-year-olds are still wet at night, as are five per cent of 11-year-olds.

An older child who occasionally or usually wets the bed may suffer from a loss of self-esteem if his mother is over-concerned about it. A child who wets the bed may smell of stale urine and so be feared or shunned at school. Regular washing in the morning overcomes this.

Often a child may be too frightened to get up at night to pass water, especially if his room is dark and the lavatory is a long way away. A potty placed by his bed and his bedroom door left ajar to let in light will help. Emotional problems at home or at school may make a child wet the bed so, if possible, these should be cleared up or at least discussed.

All normal children eventually become dry, so provided there is no physical or emotional cause for bed wetting, it is best to keep calm about it and not worry the child. Some children are helped by putting stars on calendars when they are dry, by using a 'buzzer' to wake them when urine is first passed, or even by certain medicines (tricyclic antidepressants) though why these work is not known. Treatment with medicine only stops bed wetting completely in 30 per cent of children, many of whom are wet again in a few months. Many area health authorities run special enuresis (bed wetting) clinics, staffed by doctors trained in treating this condition.

A double nappy under plastic pants for the young child and a rubber sheet will help keep the mattress dry. There is little point in limiting normal fluid intake before the child goes to bed but you may like to wake him before going to bed yourself to sit him on the potty.

See ENURESIS; POTTY TRAINING

Bee-sting *See* BITES AND STINGS

Behaviour A child's behaviour is influenced by many things, including his age and state of maturation, his relationships with people, particularly his parents, and his environment in general, as well as his genetic inheritance from his parents.

On the whole it is considered that the inheritability of behaviour is low, though certain traits may be more strongly inherited than others. A child's behaviour will, however, be considerably influenced by the way in which he perceives the outside world, and this changes over time. Just as a child is able first to sit up, then crawl, walk on the flat and then up stairs, and then ride a tricycle, so his conception of the world as he sees it also changes and increases in scope. Therefore, just as it is no good expecting a three-month-old to start running after a ball, it is equally ridiculous to consider that at three months he will have any concept of what is good and what is bad or naughty. Expectations of behaviour in a baby must match what the child is able to do.

Jean Piaget, the well-known psychologist, outlined four stages in the development of intelligence. The first stage, from birth to one and a half years, is the period of development when the baby is all sensation and action, with very direct links between the two: the baby is hungry – he cries. The second stage is divided into two parts: the first, lasting from one and a half to four years is called the symbolic stage, where the symbol is an object or action which stands for other objects or actions (a pebble becomes a sweet; a cardboard box, a boat, for example). Words are signs or symbols and this is the period of LANGUAGE development. The second part of the second stage, to the age of seven, is when the child begins to think in language but the use of language and thinking remains totally centred around him. For example, he still thinks that the sun follows him around because it seems to be in the same place wherever he goes. The third stage, from seven till ten, is when the child can begin to vary two or more relationships simultaneously. If he is told that A is greater than B and B is greater than C then he also knows that C is less than B and less than A and that B is less than A. The last stage, not reached until puberty, is when the child becomes capable of solving problems by hypothesizing factors and deducing consequences.

Obviously these things will influence how the child will behave at different ages. In the face of abnormal expectations by the parents, behaviour problems may arise because of the child's inability to understand what the parents want, and his inability, unless he has reached the appropriate stage of maturity, to meet their expectations.

See INTELLIGENCE

Behaviour problems There is a large variation in normal BEHAVIOUR patterns and there is a similarly large variation in the extent to which parents and others are willing to accept various forms of children's behaviour as normal.

Behaviour only becomes a problem if it is unacceptable to the child's parents, school, friends or even to himself.

See AGGRESSION; BED WETTING; BREATH HOLDING; DIRT EATING; HABITS; JEALOUSY; LEAD

POISONING; MALADJUSTMENT; MASTURBATION;
NAIL BITING; OBSESSIONS; OVERBREATHING;
TEMPER TANTRUMS; THUMB SUCKING; TRUANCY

Bereavement In many societies death and mourning are public affairs in which whole families and even societies join. In the West, death and all that goes with it has become a more private business, yet even so children soon realize what death means. Many children have lost a pet or know of a friend or relative that has died. Children have to get used to the idea that death is the inevitable end to life and so should not be sheltered from it.

Most children ask about death in the same way that they ask about other things, but they don't think about it in the same way that adults do until they are about nine or ten years old. Until then, most children can't accept that dead things won't come back in some magical way. Some children feel that the death of a person close to them is partly their fault and they sometimes even try to make amends – as if to try to bring the person back. This is especially seen in those children who have had a cot death in the family – they often feel that they have been responsible for the death. Don't forget that when there's a death in the family there are usually lots of other disturbances, both mental and physical, and these alone can be upsetting to a child. After a death, your child may not appear to be very 'sorrowful', as little children especially don't grieve like adults.

Talking about death is rather like discussing sex. They're both taboo subjects, even in this so-called enlightened age, and many parents fight shy of them. This is scarcely surprising because death is especially hard to come to grips with in our society and people often feel guilty talking about death in advance. As many parents are confused about death, it's hardly surprising that their children are as well.

If a child knows he is dying, answering his questions about his own death is difficult. Be guided by the nurses and doctors looking after him – they'll have come across the situation before and will know how to cope. It's probably wise when talking to children about death to prepare them for the fact that it's not only the old who die.

Parents who have some concept of an after-life often find talking to their children about death much easier than those who have no such belief.

See CANCER

Bilirubin *See* JAUNDICE

Birthmark The good thing about most birthmarks is that they disappear with time, so they don't usually warrant the anxiety parents have about them. Several sorts of marks may be present on the skin of newborn babies and the very act of being born can give rise to all sorts of temporary skin discolorations. These all disappear within a few days, as do the marks made by obstetric forceps.

The so-called 'stork's beak marks' are small patches of red discoloration on the eyelids, on the forehead above the nose, or on the back of the neck at the hairline, and may take a year or more to disappear.

The next most common birthmark is the strawberry naevus (cavernous haemangioma) which may not be present at birth but appears several days later. This is raised from the surrounding skin, is soft and red and looks like the surface of a strawberry. These birthmarks usually disappear by the end of the second year (although some may take a lot longer), leaving no trace behind. They often enlarge (sometimes alarmingly) as the child grows before disappearing over the course of several weeks. Enlargement is thus a good sign because it heralds disappearance. Should they bleed, a light dressing or adhesive plaster will stop the flow. Although it can be upsetting to watch these particular birthmarks grow, it's better to let them subside of their own accord because any treatment will leave a scar the child won't thank you for.

The least common of the birthmarks is the worst – the port wine stain (capillary haemangioma). This mark doesn't go and is dark red or purple, with or without a knobbly surface. When it's on the face it can be very disturbing for both child and parents. Cosmetics are available to mask facial marks completely and are especially useful for adolescent girls. At one time doctors were prepared to perform plastic surgery for port wine stains, especially if they were in very prominent places. Today, however, most would not consider this approach because the results are not very good and because make-up has advanced so far, enabling even bad marks to be concealed.

See BLEEDING; MOLE

Bites and stings We are fortunate in Britain in not having many stinging animals and insects. Bees and wasps sting, a few insects bite and we have only one poisonous snake – the adder.

Most children suffer only temporary discomfort from stings and bites but real emergencies can occur if the sting involves the mouth or throat or if the child's body over-reacts to the injected poison. *In either case get medical help at once.*

Bee stings. A bee leaves its sting (barb) in the flesh but it can easily be removed with clean fingernails or tweezers. Be careful not to squeeze the poison sac that is often left along with the barb. If you grasp the sting low down near the skin, you should have no trouble. Apply a cold dressing or calamine lotion.

Wasp stings leave no barb in the skin. Put some lemon juice or vinegar on the sting.

Insect stings and mite bites usually aren't serious but soothing lotions or antihistamine tablets (or medicines) can be useful if there are lots of bites. Surgical spirit is also soothing.

There is only one poisonous *snake* in the UK, the adder, which is easily recognized. It is grey, yellow or reddish brown, about 30 inches long,

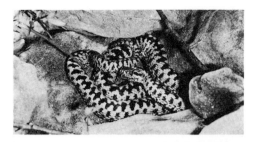
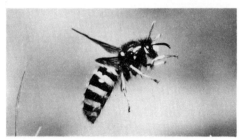
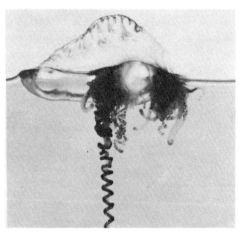

When a bee stings, its barb is left behind in the flesh. It should be carefully removed, by grasping it low down under the poison sac, so that the poison is not squeezed through the barb into the skin.

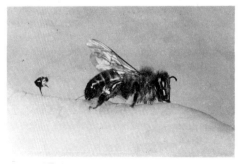

The wasp, above centre, unlike the bee, does not deposit its sting. Less common hazards are the adder (top) and the Portuguese man-of-war.

with a broad head. It has black zig-zag markings on its back. Adder bites are painful but rarely cause death. Rest the child, reassure him and give him full doses of painkilling tablets or medicine. Get medical help. Don't suck the venom out or apply a tourniquet.

Animal bites are rarely troublesome. Clean the area with disinfectant and put on a light dressing if necessary. Always get medical advice because the puncture wounds of animals' teeth can carry infection deep into the tissues.

Jelly-fish can also sting – the worst being the

Portuguese man-of-war. You can tell this one from others by the bladder it has sticking out on top like a sail. If your child is stung by a jelly-fish, get him to the shore, cover your hands with sand and pick off any adherent pieces of jelly-fish. Stings by the Portuguese man-of-war need medical treatment.

Plants, such as nettles, sting, but soothing lotions are usually all that is needed.

See BEDBUGS; FLEAS; NITS; PETS; SCABIES

Black eye *See* BRUISE

Blackhead *See* ACNE

Blackout *See* CONVULSIONS; EPILEPSY; FAINTING

Bladder control *See* BED WETTING; POTTY TRAINING

Bleeding Bleeding may occur from any of the three interlinked blood-containing channels: capillaries, veins and arteries. The arteries are thick-walled, elastic tubes that take blood from the heart to all parts of the body, and the veins are thin-walled collecting vessels that convey blood depleted of oxygen and nutrients back to the heart and lungs. The arterial and venous systems are linked in the tissues of the body by a network of tiny blood-carrying tubes called capillaries.

Capillary bleeding is usually slight and is seen, for example, when a graze bleeds. Tiny pinprick areas of blood appear from the capillaries in the skin. These usually stop bleeding if a sticking plaster is applied or if a light gauze dressing is held on with a bandage. If left undressed, a graze stops bleeding of its own accord. Bleeding from birthmarks comes from capillaries – in fact many birthmarks (especially the port wine stains) are made up of capillaries. Should a birthmark not stop bleeding after a few hours even with a dressing or plaster, a doctor may have to cauterize the bleeding point. This involves the application of heat to the bleeding area.

Bleeding from the veins is fairly uncommon but occurs when leg or arm veins are severed in accidents. Venous bleeding is easy to recognize because the blood is dark red and does not pulsate as arterial bleeding does. Bleeding veins can be more serious than most people think, mainly because the majority of the body's blood is in the veins at any one time.

Arterial bleeding is more dramatic. Most cuts and wounds sever arteries, which means that in a short time quite large amounts of blood can be lost.

Bleeding from whatever cause needs to be stopped. If the bleeding is reasonably slight (and remember a tablespoonful of blood goes a long way on a dressing or handkerchief) it can be stopped by firm pressure on the edges of the wound or by direct pressure over it.

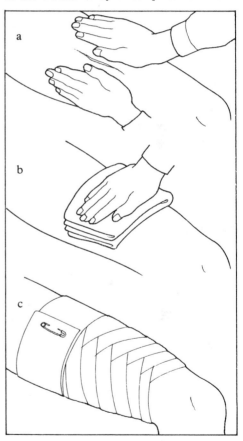

How to stop bleeding from a wound: a. press the sides of the wound together or b. apply firm pressure over the wound, over a clean dressing or handkerchief. When the bleeding has stopped, apply clean dressings and bandages (c) over the blood-soaked ones, so as not to disturb the newly formed blood clots.

This pressure should preferably be applied over a clean dressing or freshly laundered handkerchief. A few minutes' pressure alone will stop most minor bleeding.

For more serious bleeding, lay the child down, preferably with his feet raised. Loosen any tight, constricting clothing. Don't worry about washing your hands or sterilizing anything – the blood itself will wash away any bacteria, and stopping the bleeding with pressure as described above is more important.

Once the bleeding has stopped, don't disturb the area because clots will have formed and these are essential in the healing process. Apply more dressings and bandages over existing blood-soaked ones so as not to disturb clots. If you try to wash or disinfect the wound when it's fresh, you may dislodge clots and restart the bleeding. Apply a dressing and bandage firmly. Get medical help.

After an injury a child may lose blood internally. A broken bone may leak a lot of blood into the surrounding tissues yet no bleeding will be seen. Body organs may also be ruptured. If a child becomes pale, sweaty, feels faint and has a weak, fast pulse, get medical help at once. (*See* SHOCK.)

Children can bleed even if they haven't been injured. Bleeding from the gums can occur after the too vigorous use of a toothbrush. A child whose gums bleed easily and who bruises a lot should be seen by a doctor.

Children frequently fall and hit their heads and there are certain danger signs which shouldn't be ignored. Medical help should be sought if there is a head wound, if the child vomits, has any bleeding or blood-stained watery discharge from his nose, mouth or ears, or if he seems to be behaving strangely. Loss of consciousness for however short a time may also be serious. (*See* HEAD INJURY.)

NOSEBLEEDS are common in children, especially after colds, with accidents and if the child is in the habit of picking his nose.

Blood is the most essential body fluid and we can't afford to lose much of it. An adult can lose a pint or even two without serious side effects but children with their smaller blood volume can afford to lose much less.

See BLOOD DISORDERS; HAEMOPHILIA; MENSTRUATION

Blepharitis An inflammation of the edges of the eyelids involving the hair follicles, often caused by seborrhoea, with or without bacterial infection. (*See* DERMATITIS.) The child usually has a pussy discharge from the eyelids and the eyelashes may be matted together with dried pus. The edges of the eyelids are red and the child rubs the irritating eye. Sometimes ulceration, styes and even bleeding can occur. Other causes of blepharitis include allergy and exposure to dust, smoke and irritating chemicals.

If caused by infection, the condition is treated with antibiotic creams or drops and frequent bathing of the eyes to remove the discharge. It's important for the doctor to treat all affected members of the family because the infecting organisms spread easily. If the condition is left untreated, trivial though it may seem, it can become very long-lasting and may even cause permanent loss of the eyelashes and scarring of the eyelids.

See CRADLE CAP; STYE

Blindness Very few children are totally blind (about 220 in the UK) but there are large numbers of children with poor eyesight, who can however see well enough, with the aid of special magnifying lenses and other visual aids, to be able to read print. These children are officially known as partially sighted and there are special schools throughout the country equipped to help them lead an everyday life that is as normal as possible. If enough help is available in an ordinary school, a partially sighted child may manage without special schooling.

If a child's eyesight is so bad that there seems little chance of his being able to read print, then the decision may be made to educate him in a school for blind children.

The causes of blindness are many and varied and the diagnosis is often made very early in life. Sometimes, as with cataracts, the loss of vision is obvious at birth. Some blind babies have persistent wandering eye movements, or

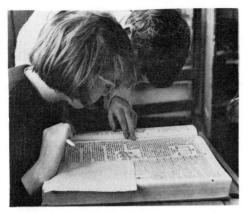

Using a large-print dictionary at a special school for the partially sighted. Children such as these are far more numerous than the totally blind.

nystagmus, which may alert the parents to the possibility that there is something wrong. Others rhythmically rub their eyes with the backs of their hands. Occasionally a mother seeks advice because her baby is not following moving objects with his eyes during the early months of life. The earlier a diagnosis is made, the better, as treatment (such as removal of a brain tumour or a CATARACT) can sometimes save vision and it is also important to make sure that a blind child receives enough stimulation from hearing, feeling and so on to make up for the loss of visual stimuli.

A high proportion of blind children have inherited a progressive degeneration of the retina. This is often first suspected from the age of about six weeks, when the baby fails to start fixing his gaze on things.

Cataracts may be caused by the GERMAN MEASLES (rubella) virus if the mother acquires the infection during the first three or four months of pregnancy. Cataracts can also be caused by poor nutrition and can be inherited.

Buphthalmos (congenital glaucoma) is a condition in which there is defective drainage of the fluid inside the eyes. The pressure inside the eyes builds up and makes them appear large, bulging and often rather beauti-

ful. About seven per cent of blind children have this condition and in the majority there is a good chance of regaining useful vision with expert treatment. Buphthalmos is usually noticed in the first year.

The most common tumour of the eye in children is a retinoblastoma. This is sometimes noticed at birth but may appear at any time in the first few years. It can affect both eyes and may run in families. If a baby is examined thoroughly after birth it is possible in many cases to make the diagnosis straight away and early operation to remove the eye may save the child's life. As this condition is so rare, only children with a family history of retinoblastoma have their eyes examined for this at birth – it is not a routine test in most places.

Other causes of blindness include injury to the eyes; retinal detachment; certain drugs (such as thalidomide) taken by the mother in pregnancy; other maternal infections during pregnancy such as toxoplasmosis; structural abnormalities of the eyes such as total absence or very small eyes; infestation with the worm Toxocara (caught from dogs or cats); and severe infections of the eyes. Blindness in one eye may result from neglect of a SQUINT or a short-sighted eye, the eye becoming progressively more 'lazy' until it finally ceases to see at all as the brain suppresses the image it forms.

Children at a school for the blind, typing and reading in Braille, and learning canework.

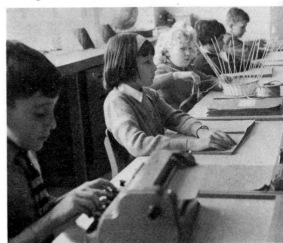

A preventable cause of blindness is retrolental fibroplasia, caused by giving too high a concentration of oxygen to babies during resuscitation after birth or during treatment for the RESPIRATORY DISTRESS SYNDROME. In 1969 this was the commonest cause of children being admitted to schools for the blind, but now it is very rare because a lower concentration of oxygen is used.

Some blind children have other handicaps and need specialized help from the start to ensure that they realize their full potential.

See COLOUR BLINDNESS; EYES; VISION TESTING

Blinking A harmless but annoying habit or tic (*see* HABITS). It can also be a sign of allergic conjunctivitis (as in hay fever). If your child's eyes are red, take him to a doctor. If the eyes are not red and the blinking disturbs either you or the child, get medical advice. Your child will not stop blinking simply because you tell him to.

Blister A raised area, filled with fluid, on the skin surface. Small blisters occur after persistent rubbing of an area, for instance on the finger after a lot of writing or on the feet after a long walk. Extremes of temperature – of boiling water especially – can cause blisters.

The treatment of small blisters is simple – a self-adhesive dressing to cover the area is enough while the blister fluid is reabsorbed by the body. Should the roof of the blister come off, leaving an area of new pink skin beneath, keep it covered for a day or two.

Large blisters from scalds or sunburn should be seen by a doctor who might burst them under sterile conditions. If you burst a blister yourself, be sure to use a sterilized needle. You can sterilize a needle by boiling it for ten minutes or by holding it in a flame until it is red and then letting it cool before using it. In either case the needle should not touch anything before it is used to pierce the blister.

Multiple blisters, wherever they occur on the body for no apparent reason, should be seen by a doctor.

Blood A vital body fluid consisting of straw-coloured plasma in which several kinds of cells and platelets are suspended. The cells are red or white and perform very special functions. An adult has about eleven pints of blood and a child has proportionately the same amount in relation to his body weight. The blood is pumped round the body by the heart, flowing in the arteries to the tissues, and back to the heart in the veins. Blood is the body's messenger system for carrying oxygen, nutrients and other substances to the cells, and carbon dioxide and waste products away from them.

The red blood cells give blood its colour and are responsible for absorbing oxygen from the lungs and giving it up in the tissues. Red blood cells containing oxygen are bright red (in the arteries) and dark purple-red when they have given up their oxygen (in the veins).

Forty-five per cent of the blood consists of red cells, one per cent of white cells and the other 54 per cent of plasma. When the percentage of red cells is diminished for any reason, when the cells are too small, or when they contain too little haemoglobin, the person is said to be anaemic. (*See* ANAEMIA.)

The white cells are one thousand times fewer in number than the red cells but are vitally important, having a very different function. Some of the white cells (phagocytes) engulf bacteria that find their way into the bloodstream and so help protect against infection. Other white cells (lymphocytes) are important in antibody formation – an essential part of immunity to disease.

Platelets work together with other clotting mechanisms in the blood to plug up damaged blood vessels and so stop BLEEDING. If there are too many platelets, the blood is more viscous than it should be and clots form more easily. These clots are called thrombi. (*See* BLOOD DISORDERS.) A blood vessel blocked by a clot is said to be thrombosed.

The plasma carries all these cells round the body to wherever they are needed, and also carries various chemicals round the body in solution. Sugar, drugs, hormones, food from the bowel and many other substances are transported around the body in the plasma. Waste products produced by the body's metabolism are removed by the liver and kidneys, purifying the plasma which is re-circulated round the body for further use.

See BLOOD GROUPS; HAEMOPHILIA

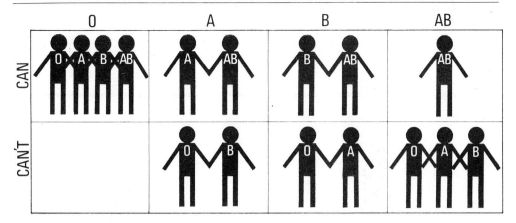

Those who can and cannot receive blood of each group.

Blood disorders The large number of possible disorders reflects the complexity of the BLOOD.

When the red cells are too few, when those present are too small, or when they contain too little haemoglobin, the child is said to be anaemic. ANAEMIA can also be caused by abnormal haemoglobin as in sickle cell anaemia and thalassaemia. Should there be too many the condition is known as polycythaemia.

The excessive production of white cells is a feature of LEUKAEMIA. The cells are also abnormal in structure.

A shortage of platelets can be part of a generalized disease of the bone marrow or it may be an isolated condition. Children with this condition tend to bruise and bleed easily and must be seen by a doctor.

A less common group of blood disorders is that in which clotting is a problem. Nature has given us a very good clotting mechanism that prevents us losing blood when we cut ourselves. Without this clotting process we'd bleed to death from the slightest cut. In diseases such as HAEMOPHILIA one or more of the proteins responsible for clotting is missing or present in only very small amounts.

See BLEEDING; BLOOD GROUPS; HENOCH SCHÖNLEIN PURPURA

Blood groups Since the discovery of the first blood groups in 1900, our knowledge of the subject has come a long way. At least 14 blood groups have been discovered since then,

and two are especially important in practical terms, the ABO and rhesus groups.

Present knowledge of blood grouping means that we can now safely give one person another's blood in an emergency by giving blood of a compatible group. If two people's bloods don't 'match', the two bloods are said to be incompatible. If one gave blood to the other, the red cells would clump together and break down, possibly even leading to death in certain cases.

Blood is grouped according to the antigens and antibodies present in the red cells and plasma. The best known groups are those of the ABO system. People may be group A, B, AB or O (40 per cent, 10 per cent, 5 per cent and 45 per cent of the population respectively). Type O blood can safely be given to anybody (provided the other antibody systems are compatible), while group AB blood can only be given to group AB people. The ABO blood group system is inherited just like other body characteristics and blood groups can be used to test for paternity in cases where there is doubt.

People of certain blood groups are more susceptible to particular diseases than others. Group A people, for example, have more stomach cancer and pernicious anaemia than people of other groups, while group O people have more duodenal ulcers than average.

The rhesus system was discovered when red cells from a rhesus monkey were injected into a rabbit. This system is important for two reasons. First, because transfusing rhesus positive blood (which contains the rhesus factor) into a rhesus negative person can cause that person to produce rhesus antibodies and,

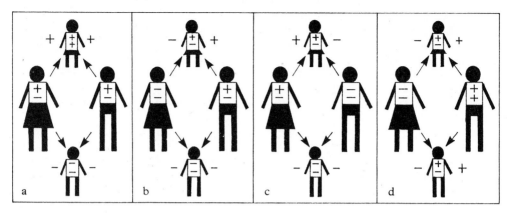

How the rhesus factor is passed down.
a. Both parents are rhesus positive, but with a negative factor. Their children will be either positive or negative, and there will be no danger during pregnancy.
b. The mother is rhesus negative, and the father positive, but with a negative factor. Danger arises only if a child is rhesus positive like his father.
c. The mother is mixed rhesus positive, and the father purely negative : there is no danger during pregnancy.
d. The mother is purely rhesus negative and the father purely rhesus positive. In this situation every child will be rhesus positive, and his rhesus factor will be incompatible with that of his mother.

second, because the presence of a rhesus positive baby in the womb of a rhesus negative mother can lead to the production of rhesus antibodies by the mother, which can pass into the baby via the placenta and damage or destroy its rhesus positive red cells. This gives rise to the disease known as haemolytic disease of the newborn or rhesus incompatibility. Because this can be so serious, (mainly because the breaking down of the baby's red cells causes JAUNDICE which, if severe enough, can lead to brain damage), mothers are always tested for their rhesus blood group early in pregnancy. Should the mother be rhesus negative, the level of rhesus antibodies in her blood is checked both then and later on in the pregnancy, and the mother and foetus carefully watched if the level rises.

Only 11 per cent of pregnancies occur as a result of the mating of a rhesus negative woman with a rhesus positive man and only a fraction of these will have any trouble. About 15 per cent of women in this country are rhesus negative.

The blood of a rhesus negative mother is tested for the presence of her baby's red cells soon after the baby is delivered, because a rhesus positive baby's red cells can 'leak' into the mother via the placenta during pregnancy and especially during labour. The baby's blood group is also established and, if necessary, the mother is given an injection of rhesus antibodies (anti-D immunoglobulin) which destroy the baby's red cells in her blood. This prevents her from sensitization to the baby's rhesus positive red cells which could endanger the life of a subsequent rhesus positive baby.

First rhesus positive babies of rhesus negative mothers are rarely affected seriously. The problems arise with second and subsequent rhesus positive babies unless the mother was immunized after the birth of the first rhesus positive baby.

Sensitization of a rhesus negative mother to rhesus positive blood from her baby can also occur after a miscarriage, an abortion, or a haemorrhage into the womb during pregnancy, so an injection of anti-D immunoglobulin should, if necessary, be given in these circumstances as well.

Immunization with anti-D immunoglobulin has now fortunately greatly reduced the incidence of rhesus haemolytic disease of the newborn. Few babies need an exchange transfusion nowadays.

A baby suffering from rhesus incompatibility may need medical treatment for anaemia and jaundice, depending on the severity of the condition. Treatment for the most severely affected involves exchanging the baby's blood for rhesus negative blood. This provides the baby with the vital red cells he needs until he can replace them himself. Exchanging the blood reduces the amount of jaundice and prevents the brain damage that can occur. Phototherapy (treatment with light) is very helpful in reducing the bilirubin levels in jaundiced babies. Very high levels of bilirubin in untreated jaundiced babies can cause mental retardation, deafness, or athetosis – a peculiar sort of writhing movement of the body (see CEREBRAL PALSY) in babies.

See BLOOD TRANSFUSION

Blood sugar   *See* DIABETES

Blood transfusion   The giving of one person's blood to another. Until the beginning of this century and the discovery of the BLOOD GROUPS, this was a dangerous undertaking. Once the major groups had been identified, blood of a compatible type could be given which would not cause the recipient's blood to break down after transfusion.

Knowing the right blood to give is only the first stage of being able to transfuse blood into a person who needs it. First, the blood has to be collected from donors. In Britain donors give their blood free of charge and there's a national blood transfusion service with regional blood banks so that blood can be distributed to the patient who needs it quickly and efficiently. As blood keeps for only a few days, even when refrigerated, it has to be collected, stored, and used quickly in strict rotation, and organizing this is a skilled job.

Today, blood can be broken down into useful fractions so that several recipients can be given particular components of any one pint of blood.

The problems of collection and storage, large as they are, are not the only ones. Circulating blood is, of course, usually free from dangerous bacteria but unless it is collected, stored and subsequently transfused under perfectly sterile conditions, the recipient will contract blood poisoning.

The second problem is that of clotting. Blood collected in a bottle clots within a few minutes but the addition of a harmless chemical called sodium citrate prevents this clotting process while the blood is stored.

Anyone can give blood who is not anaemic and who has not had infectious hepatitis or syphilis (both of which can be transmitted in blood). The blood transfusion service always needs more donors, especially today when serious operations can only be performed at all because of the availability of blood for transfusion.

Children can receive blood just like adults and some babies may even have to have most of their blood replaced by a process known as exchange transfusion if they are suffering from haemolytic disease of the newborn. (*See* BLOOD GROUPS.)

Children with bleeding diseases such as HAEMOPHILIA also benefit from whole blood transfusion or from special anti-haemophilia blood fractions.

Blue babies   Babies look blue because their blood is not sufficiently well oxygenated. Some newborn babies are temporarily blue immediately after birth and this is due to a relative shortage of oxygen reaching their blood from the placenta during labour. Most of these babies regain their colour and recover completely as soon as they start breathing.

A baby may look blue because the heart or main blood vessels coming from it have not developed properly. This allows blue, de-oxygenated blood to mix with red, oxygenated blood in the big arteries. This poorly oxygenated blood makes the lips, tongue and fingers look blue. The 'hole in the heart' blue baby is blue because de-oxygenated blood which has returned from the body passes into the arterial side of the circulation through the hole in the heart.

Recent advances in surgery mean that many of these blue babies can now undergo successful heart operations even in early infancy. Some are best left until they are older.

See APGAR SCORE; ASPHYXIA; HEART DISORDERS; RESPIRATORY DISTRESS SYNDROME

Blushing   A short-lived flushing of the skin,

especially of the face and neck. This is an almost universal phenomenon although most people think that women blush more than men. It's very common in young boys and girls soon after puberty, is most easily seen in fair skinned people, and is very difficult to see in negroes and dark skinned people.

Blushing is caused by a sudden widening of the small blood vessels in the area concerned. The resulting rush of blood is responsible for both the redness and the warmth of the skin. Embarrassment is the commonest cause of blushing both in children and adults.

Teenagers usually grow out of their blushing problem quickly. Should the condition be really troublesome and persistent, psycho-therapy, hypnosis, or a mild tranquillizer can be used with success.

Body contact The first few months are the time when the foundations for security are laid and a baby starts making contact with others. Correct care and nourishment are important but the baby's need for loving physical contact should also be satisfied so that his emotional and psychological development can proceed normally.

The first fully functioning sense organ is the skin. Even an eight week old embryo that has not yet developed eyes and ears reacts when

Physical contact between a mother and her baby is vital to his psychological development. The familiar warmth and movements of her body are comforting for him; she is more responsive to his needs for food; and the bonding of the mother to her baby happens easily and naturally.

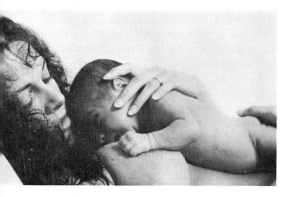

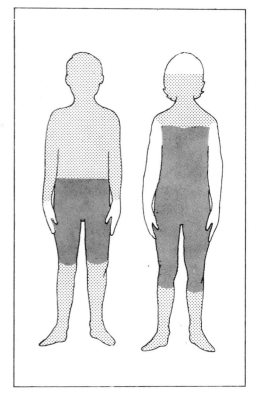

Where parents most often touch their children. Most parents tend to have more physical contact with their daughters, and will often only touch their sons' hands. Almost all touch their children in the mid-grey areas in the diagram, about 50% in the light areas. About 75% of parents never touch their children's bodies in the parts shaded dark grey in the diagram.

gently stroked on the upper lip. When a baby is born, the senses of touch, temperature, pressure and movement are already perfectly developed. This is why physical contact is so important for children. Whenever a mother lovingly touches her baby, when she feeds, nurses, strokes, carries or holds him in her arms, she is giving this essential contact. Holding babies is valuable for many reasons. First, the mother's familiar heartbeat and other body sounds may be comforting; second, her body actually keeps him warm; last, she'll be aware of his needs earlier and so be able to respond sooner. This makes for a happier and more contented baby and one that cries less. For these reasons many women throughout the world carry their babies in some sort of sling so that they are never far apart. This can work very well in the West too, as many mothers are finding to their pleasure today.

It is virtually impossible to show a baby too much love and tenderness and it would also be a good thing if parents showed their love to older children more freely and directly – not just with words but by physical contact too. Just how little physical contact occurs in our western world and to which parts of the body it is limited has been described by American scientists. This is shown in the accompanying diagram.

See BONDING

Boil A raised, reddened area of skin caused by infection. The body is covered with hair, and each one, however small, has a channel, or follicle, in which it comes through the skin. A boil starts at the root of the hair and usually occurs when bacteria (usually staphylococci) infect the follicle. The commonest places for boils are where the skin is rubbed by clothing, such as the neck and buttocks.

A pimple is a small boil but isn't usually serious. Boils are painful until they burst of their own accord, are lanced by a doctor, or simply heal spontaneously. Boils should never be squeezed to bring them to a head because as well as squeezing pus upwards and outwards, this also squeezes the infection into the surrounding tissues, so encouraging it to spread.

Boils are infectious and so may spread to the surrounding skin. Children recovering from an acute illness or suffering from a long-term severe illness or malnutrition can get crops of boils that are difficult to cure. A carbuncle is a group of closely connected, deep boils.

The treatment of a boil is simple. Cover it with a dressing and then leave it alone. Keep the skin clean by careful washing and let the boil come to a head and burst. This may happen spontaneously or can be encouraged by the application of heat in the form of a poultice or covered hot water bottle. When the boil has burst, keep the area covered until it heals; this only takes a few days.

Should the boil be really large or in a difficult place such as the face, in the ear, or the armpit, take the child to a doctor. If red streaks appear around the boil it could be a sign that the infection is spreading, so ask for your doctor's advice.

If your child has a boil, don't give him antibiotics. Unless it is a very bad one which has spread, a boil is a local infection that cures itself. The misuse of antibiotics can actually prolong the healing time of a boil and produce a sterile, pus-filled lump that won't go away.

Bonding A phenomenon whereby adults become committed (by a one-way flow of concern and affection) to children for whom they have cared during the first months and years of life. It is a much misused term that does *not* mean the mutual affection between a baby and an adult. Adult-child bonding is usually greatest in the mother, who almost always spends more time with her baby than anyone else.

Bonding takes time, but the more a mother does for her baby the more opportunity she has of being the person who answers his needs, and so the more quickly and strongly bonding will develop. If the conditions are right – if a mother and baby are able to stay together after birth, if natural, unrestricted BREAST FEEDING is practised, if a mother is allowed to meet her baby's needs, and if she has the love and support of the father – bonding to her baby happens easily and naturally.

However, conditions are often less than ideal for a mother and baby, and it has been shown that interference with bonding can lead to later problems both for the mother and the baby. This is not to say that an individual mother who has been separated from her baby after birth, for example, *cannot* develop a good relationship with her baby, but just that overall, in a group of mothers who have been separated from their babies, there will be more who do not become adequately bonded to their children than in a group who have not been separated. Inadequate opportunities for bonding may make a mother less able to cope with her baby later.

Bonding can be interfered with if a mother and newborn baby are separated, and also if a mother is separated from an older child, for instance if her child goes to a minder or a nursery, or is looked after by a nanny or an au pair. The natural place for a baby or a young child is with his mother, both for his sake and hers.

Bonding is not the same as 'feeling maternal' or 'falling in love with your baby'. Very many mothers describe how they didn't feel at all maternal or in love with their baby at first. However, while the process of bonding is going on and if it is not interfered with, almost all mothers experience a growing feeling of love for their babies. Some mothers experience this immediately after the birth, but some may not feel it until the baby is up to eight weeks old.

The mother-baby bond is the foundation for all the baby's future relationships. He learns that she is kind and loving and answers his needs at once, and so grows up with a sense of trust in people, and also with the feeling that he is considered important.

Worldwide studies have shown that babies who are premature and separated from their mothers, as well as full term babies who are kept in HOSPITAL without their mothers, are not only more likely to be battered by their parents but are also more likely to fail to thrive. Extreme examples of maternal deprivation such as these are accepted as being far from the ideal, and it has been recommended by the British Department of Health that there should be facilities for all mothers of children under five to live in the hospital with them. This, of course, includes newborn babies and their mothers, but snags soon arise because once a newly delivered mother is ready to go home, there are rarely enough hospital beds for her to stay in if her baby has to be detained for care and treatment. In the future, special care baby units will be planned with facilities for mothers to live in. Only in this way can a mother have the best chance of developing the natural bond between her and her baby.

Ideally, a mother should not routinely be separated from her baby from birth onwards at any time, day or night. Studies have shown that early and prolonged contact after birth leads not only to an increased likelihood that a mother will breast feed, but also to an increased success with breast feeding. Mothers allowed to see more of their babies are also seen to behave differently towards them even up to two years later, and their babies' language development is more advanced. It seems that there is a sensitive period immediately after birth which is a special time for the mother-baby relationship.

See BABY BATTERING; CHILDBIRTH; FAILURE TO THRIVE; INCUBATOR; LOW BIRTH WEIGHT

Booster   A follow-up dose of a vaccine or toxoid which boosts immunity to a disease. The commonest immunizations in this country are against diphtheria, whooping cough, tetanus and polio and the first three of these are usually combined in a triple vaccine given as a course of three injections in the first year. An oral dose of polio vaccine is given at the same time as each injection.

A booster dose of diphtheria, tetanus and polio vaccine is given when the child is about five. The whooping cough vaccine is not given at this age because the danger of whooping cough is by then relatively small. Further booster doses of tetanus and polio are given to school-leavers and after that as necessary.

See IMMUNIZATION

Bottle feeding   Many mothers either choose to give their babies modified cows' MILK instead of breast milk or fail to breast feed successfully.

Cows' milk differs from human milk in many respects – it contains more protein, sodium, potassium, calcium and phosphorus and fewer unsaturated fatty acids and anti-infective substances among other things. Some of these differences can adversely affect the baby's health and it's sensible during the early months of life to give a preparation of cows' milk which has been modified to resemble breast milk as closely as possible. The change to liquid 'doorstep' milk may be made later when the baby is better able to cope with it. Lists of recommended milks may be obtained from your health visitor, clinic doctor or general practitioner.

Provided a suitably modified milk is given, there is rarely any need to change the milk used, though special milks such as soya bean protein milk, lactose-free milk and low phenylalanine milks are available when necessary.

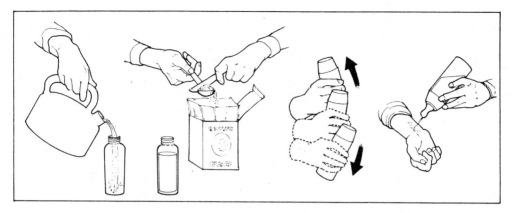

Making up a feed. Pour cooled, boiled water into the feeding bottle; measure the amount of milk powder carefully with the scoop supplied; screw on the cap and shake the bottle to mix the feed. Test the temperature of the milk before giving it to the baby.

The bottles and teats used for feeding must be adequately sterilized to prevent infection. Babies fed on preparations of cows' milk are more liable to suffer from GASTROENTERITIS than are breast-fed babies, so every care must be taken to keep the equipment clean. Sterilization can be done either by boiling the bottle and teat in water for about ten minutes (having first washed and brushed them to remove the milk residue), or by using one of the chemical sterilizing preparations available.

Feeds are prepared by adding dried milk to boiled, cooled water in the bottle (though in hospital the milk sometimes comes in pre-packed polythene feeder bags). The milk powder must be measured correctly because there are dangers in giving milk that is too strong. There are directions with each brand of milk and the scoop used should be the one supplied with the milk. The water and powder are shaken together in the bottle, the temperature adjusted by placing the bottle in a bowl of warm or cool water, and the feed is ready.

A number of feeds can be prepared at the beginning of the day and stored in the fridge, but milk should never be left at room temperature for long periods or kept warm in a thermos flask, because this provides the ideal situation for bacteria to thrive. For journeys, take a thermos flask of water at the right temperature that has previously been boiled and mix the feed as you need it.

The amount of milk given varies according to the baby's age and appetite. Bottle-fed babies are rarely underfed but if the baby puts on too much weight, cut down the number of scoops of milk powder by one scoop per feed, while still giving the same volume of water. Sugar should never be added to bottle feeds.

The bottle-feeding mother should try to copy the breast-feeding mother and always give her baby the feed herself, cuddling him close. It is dangerous to leave a baby alone lying down or propped up with a bottle in his mouth, because he might choke unnoticed on the milk, or on vomited or regurgitated milk.

Solids shouldn't be given before four to six months at the earliest and as the baby eats more solid food, the amount of milk given can be gradually cut down, either by making the feeds more dilute or by substituting other drinks such as plain water for some of the milk feeds. (*See* WEANING.)

Breast milk should ideally never be given by bottle as this accustoms the baby to a method of sucking which is not only different but also easier than that at the breast. Premature babies should be fed by tube, spoon or dropper until they are able to suck at the breast.

The bottle-fed baby's milk is fortified with vitamins A and D. However, some doctors and nurses recommend extra vitamins as a safeguard. Vitamin C should be given as unsweetened orange, blackcurrant or tomato juice.

See BABY FEEDING; BREAST FEEDING; CONSTIPATION; DIARRHOEA

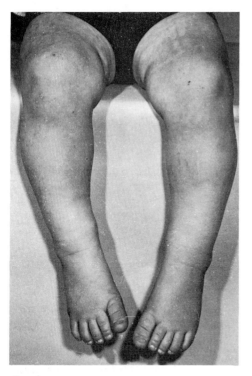

Bow legs.

Bow legs The outward curve of one or both legs in a child. A newborn baby whose legs were straight would look peculiar. Some curving of the bones is natural and becomes less as the child grows. When the curve remains, this is not caused by the child putting weight on the legs too early, as many mothers think. A child's body is constantly changing in the early years and the legs simply go through a phase of unusual curvature by adult standards. Almost all bow-legged children have normal looking legs by the age of five, although obese children appear to stay bow-legged for longer than others.

Severe bow legs are a feature of RICKETS, a disease of vitamin D deficiency.

Don't worry about letting your child play in a baby bouncer or walker – let him enjoy these things as soon as he wants to as they won't make him bow-legged.

A really bulky nappy between the legs can exaggerate a child's normal bow-leggedness. This is only important when the child is learning to walk and can easily be avoided by pinning the nappy so that there's as little bulk as possible between the legs.

If ever you are worried about your child's bow legs or if only one leg is bowed, see your doctor. Sometimes, when the bowing is severe enough to affect walking, treatment is needed.

Brace *See* ORTHODONTICS

Brain *See* CENTRAL NERVOUS SYSTEM

Brain damage A baby's brain can be damaged before, during, or after birth and the disorders produced depend upon the type of damage, its timing, its severity, and the part of the brain affected.

Before birth, the foetus can be infected with the GERMAN MEASLES (rubella) virus, the cytomegalovirus, toxoplasmosis (*see* PETS), or – very rarely now – syphilis. All these infections can damage the brain.

Prolonged shortage of oxygen (anoxia or ASPHYXIA) to the baby during or just after birth is the commonest cause of brain damage. Anoxia during labour is most likely if there is a difficult labour and if the placenta is not working as well as it should, for instance in some mothers who have suffered from pre-eclamptic toxaemia. One of the main benefits of good obstetric care is the prevention of brain damage due to birth asphyxia. The state of the baby during labour may be monitored and the delivery speeded up by, for example, rupturing the membranes, an oxytocin drip, using forceps, or doing an emergency caesarean section if there is cause for concern. Some mothers have their labours induced before term if there is a chance that the placenta isn't working well enough. (*See* FOETAL DISTRESS.)

A baby may be born with no problem but then have difficulty in starting to breathe. If a mother has been given pain-killing drugs in labour, difficulty in breathing is more likely, as it is if the baby was short of oxygen during labour. Blockage of the breathing passages by mucus, blood or amniotic debris can also interfere with breathing, which is why some babies need to be 'sucked out'. Some babies need oxygen, which may be given through a tube passed via the mouth down the trachea, via a mask, or in the form of air breathed into the baby by another person (the KISS OF LIFE) if there is no special equipment available.

The severity of birth asphyxia is often measured by the APGAR SCORE, which gives some indication of the likelihood of brain damage. However, there isn't a simple relationship between the Apgar score and brain damage, and some babies with apparently severe birth asphyxia recover completely soon after birth and develop quite normally thereafter.

Rhesus haemolytic disease is now well on the way to being controlled in this country (see BLOOD GROUPS). However, it is possible for a baby's brain to be affected if the disease is unrecognized or untreated. Very high levels of bilirubin in untreated jaundiced babies can cause MENTAL RETARDATION, deafness, or athetosis – a peculiar sort of writhing movement of the body (see CEREBRAL PALSY) in surviving babies. Severe untreated JAUNDICE as a result of other conditions can also damage the brain.

A newborn baby's brain is especially sensitive to a low blood sugar and this is one of the reasons why early and frequent feeding at the breast is so important. Similarly, the low birth weight baby who is unable to suck should have early and frequent feeds of expressed breast milk. Glucose water as a routine is quite unnecessary and is a poor substitute for breast milk, which contains plenty of sugar of its own. Severe, untreated hypoglycaemia (low blood sugar) can lead to convulsions and brain damage. If a baby cannot keep milk down, he will need to be given a glucose-containing fluid to maintain his blood sugar level.

In some very difficult labours there may be actual structural damage to the brain caused by the baby's head being forced too fast through the birth canal, producing tearing and bleeding into the brain with later scarring. This is one reason why good obstetric care is so essential.

Because the brain controls the working of all the parts of the body, brain damage can cause widely differing signs and symptoms but the most commonly seen are cerebral palsy, EPILEPSY, mental retardation, unusual clumsiness (see CLUMSY CHILDREN) and behaviour problems. The severity depends on the amount of underlying damage. However, it's important to remember that the outlook for a brain damaged child is modified considerably by his environment, which makes it difficult to forecast the degree of disability. Training and continual encouragement can greatly influence the outcome. Brain damage is often not apparent for some time and the diagnosis can be very difficult to make. A child is usually only diagnosed as being brain damaged if there is a positive story of a difficult birth, difficulty in breathing afterwards, or any other obvious cause, and if every other possible cause has been ruled out. Sometimes an EEG (electroencephalogram) will show that there are areas of the brain producing an abnormal electrical discharge which may represent areas of scar tissue, but often the EEG is normal.

Only the most severely brain damaged child needs to go to a special school – the type of school depends on the nature of the disability. (See EDUCATIONAL SUBNORMALITY.)

Brain tumour The nervous and urinary systems are the commonest places for cancers in children – in fact three-quarters of all childhood cancers affect one of these systems. Brain tumours are, however, very uncommon. The symptoms are varied and depend on the type of tumour, but vomiting and headache due to a rise of the pressure inside the skull are often present. In older children vomiting is a suggestive sign if no other cause is apparent and if it is present first thing in the morning. Headaches can also be an important symptom, especially in young children because they so rarely complain of headaches from other causes. Later, as the tumour grows, the child becomes lethargic and drowsy.

Many of these tumours are difficult to treat and this makes it important that any child complaining of persistent pain in the neck or head should be seen by a doctor as soon as possible. Early diagnosis can help the outlook.
See CANCER; HEADACHE

Breast feeding The ideal way of feeding babies is by breast feeding. The advantages of breast MILK compared with cows' milk (whether dried, evaporated or liquid 'doorstep' milk) are very real and have influenced the British Department of Health to recommend that all babies should be breast-fed for

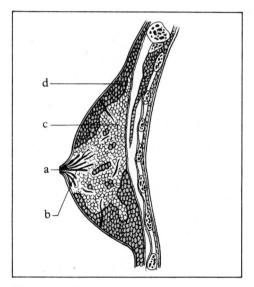

Diagram to show the human breast in cross-section. a. nipple, b. milk ducts, c. milk glands, d. fatty tissue.

think that many of the bottle-feeding mothers have simply never been given accurate information about the benefits of breast milk to their babies.

According to a 1978 report, among mothers surveyed who started breast feeding, less than one in four was still fully breast feeding at two weeks, one in 13 at six weeks and less than one in 100 at four months! The commonest reason for stopping or for introducing complements of cows' milk was an insufficiency of milk, and this is very sad because almost all of these mothers wanted to continue but thought they couldn't. In fact, 94 per cent of them were advised to stop or to give complements by their doctor, health visitor or midwife, though they should have been told how to increase their milk supply. This is a simple matter and involves feeding the baby very much more often and for as long as he wants to suck. The amount of milk available to the baby varies in different women but in any one woman is dependent upon the amount of time her baby spends at the breast. There is no upper limit

Breast milk, given on an unrestricted basis, forms the perfect food for a baby.

at least the first two weeks and preferably for four to six months. Breast-fed babies are less likely than bottle-fed babies to get gastro-enteritis, respiratory infections, dental decay, eczema and to die from cot deaths. There is as yet little evidence about the long-term advantages of breast feeding but there is a chance that the development of such conditions as coronary heart disease, ulcerative colitis and multiple sclerosis may be influenced by the way in which a baby is fed in the early months.

The fact remains that breast feeding has become unpopular and, on average, only one mother in two gives her baby any breast milk at all. The reasons for this are many and include mothers saying that breast feeding is too embarrassing, too time consuming, prevents them going out without the baby, is unfashionable, means they have to go into another room to feed the baby and that it is too 'animal like'. Interestingly, bottle-feeding mothers give as their reasons for bottle feeding negative reasons against breast feeding, not positive ones for bottle feeding. On the other hand, the reasons mothers give for breast feeding are all positively in favour of breast feeding. Their major reason is that breast milk is better and healthier for their babies and it's tempting to

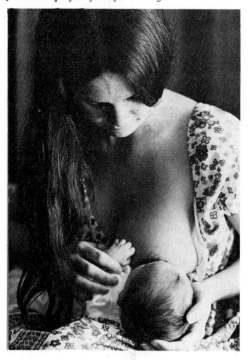

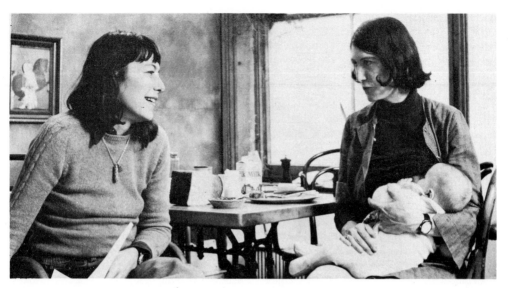

There is no reason why breast feeding should inconvenience the mother unduly : the baby's feed is always readily available, and there are very few places where she cannot take her baby.

to this time and virtually every woman can produce enough milk for her baby if she lets him suck often and for long enough and forgets all the advice she has been given about three- to five-hourly feeding for ten minutes a side. Some mothers can produce enough milk even if they feed according to a schedule, but most can't.

It's all too easy to let a baby cry because 'it's not time for a feed' and this is the prime reason for the failure of breast feeding, because the milk supply is not stimulated by the baby sucking when he wants to. A baby can't be spoiled by being fed when he's hungry, and the milk supply will soon be in danger if he is not fed when he is hungry.

Rural peoples in developing countries don't feed their babies by the clock but carry them around with them and let them feed whenever they want, and they have a much higher rate of successful breast feeding than we do. They tend to feed their babies whenever they are restless, because the commonest reason for restlessness is a need to suck at the breast (whether for food or comfort). If a western mother from the beginning feeds her baby on an unrestricted basis whenever he's restless (and

she'll be more aware of his state if he's with her all the time) instead of just when he cries (or worse, by the clock), she'll soon find she has plenty of milk and a contented baby who never cries because he never has to.

After the baby is born, a thick, creamy-coloured milk called colostrum is made by the breasts. If the mother is feeding her baby on an unrestricted basis, as outlined above, the 'mature' milk will come in very quickly – probably on the second day. The less time she spends feeding her baby, the longer the milk will be in coming in, and this is why in most mothers feeding their babies according to rigid schedules the milk doesn't come in until the fourth or fifth day. The baby does not need anything other than the colostrum and milk that his mother can give him. Instead of losing weight in the first week (which most schedule breast-fed babies do) the baby fed on an unrestricted basis may lose none or very little and soon starts putting weight on. Most hospital maternity departments offer breast-fed babies drinks of cows' milk or glucose water during the night and often during the day as well to top them up, and it will only be with public pressure that this practice will die out. A breast-fed baby needs breast feeds day and night from the day he is born. Frequent feeding throughout the 24 hours also helps prevent the breasts becoming engorged, reduces the chances of getting sore nipples, and makes a blocked duct, mastitis or a breast abscess very unlikely. Low birth weight or jaundiced babies, or those whose mothers had pethidine in labour, may be extra sleepy and not wake often enough for feeds. It's especially important to offer these babies the breast frequently.

If possible, the baby should be put to the breast immediately after birth while the mother is cuddling him before he is washed and weighed. The stimulation of the breasts by the baby sucking helps the womb expel the afterbirth and helps stop bleeding. Breast feeding also encourages the womb to return to its normal size.

Breast-fed babies have fewer nappy rashes and their nappies smell pleasant, unlike those of bottle-fed babies. They are less likely to vomit and, if they do, the vomit is less smelly than that of a bottle-fed baby. A breast-feeding mother will find that breast feeding is not at all restricting because there are few places where she cannot easily take her baby.

Any problems a mother may have with breast feeding are easily overcome if the mother knows what to do. If for any reason her baby cannot be put to the breast, her milk supply can be maintained by an electric pump or by manual expression, and her milk can then be given to the baby. This happens with very small premature babies (for whom breast milk is almost always the best food), for babies with severe cleft palates, if the mother wants to go out without her baby, or has to have an operation, for example.

Breast feeding should continue as long as the baby and mother want. Elsewhere in the world, breast feeding is often continued until the next child is born (or even longer), usually for around two or three years. More and more mothers in this country are realizing the very real pleasure of the close relationship between them and their breast-fed babies and are continuing to breast feed until the baby gives up of his own accord, sometimes after several years.

Provided the breast-feeding mother has a well-balanced diet, and she and her baby have enough sunshine, there is no need for vitamin supplements to be given to the baby. When breast milk ceases to form the major part of the baby's diet, vitamin supplements (in the form of vitamin drops) can be given in the winter as a safeguard.

See APPETITE; BABY FEEDING; BONDING; FOOD; MILK; RICKETS; WEANING

Breath holding Breath-holding attacks are alarming to parents and are seen mainly in toddlers. They are a form of temper tantrum and a very powerful one, as any parent who has been on the receiving end will know!

The attacks rarely occur when the child is alone because he needs an audience for his show. The child is usually intelligent and easily frustated and reacts in a dramatic way to gain attention. An attack often starts with the child taking a very deep breath in as if he were going to scream, but instead he holds his breath and his face goes redder and redder and eventually blue. The attacks aren't usually dangerous, although occasionally a very long attack can end with a convulsion or a short period of unconsciousness because the child's brain becomes short of oxygen.

Simple measures like slapping the child are usually ineffective but a good trick is to hook your finger over the back of his tongue and pull it forwards. This makes it impossible for him to hold his breath and the attack is cut short. The trouble is that the parent has to do this very early in the attack before the child clenches his teeth. If the attacks are controlled early, they seem to disappear.

With luck, a combination of preventing frustrating situations (not as easy as it sounds without continuously giving in and ending up with a spoiled, unmanageable child) and sensitive handling of each attack will control this problem. Most children will have grown out of these attacks by school age.

See TEMPER TANTRUMS

Breathlessness Difficult breathing. Apart from blocked nostrils, the two main reasons for a child having difficulty in breathing are heart disease and chest disease. In many forms of congenital heart disease the child has problems with breathing because changes in the circulation of blood make the lungs stiff and produce a lowered oxygen level in the blood. Because of the increased effort required to draw air into these stiffened lungs, the child finds him-

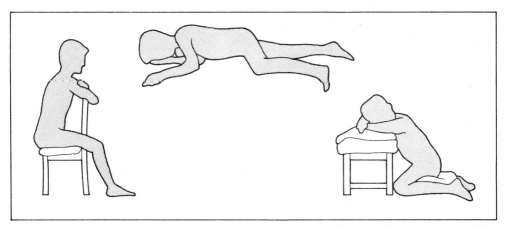

Ways of sitting to combat breathlessness and help a child to relax. He should try to breathe with the lower chest, keeping the upper chest still.

self using other muscles to pull the diaphragm down to enlarge the ribcage.

As a result of the action of these other muscles, babies who have difficulty in breathing often have dips or gullies between their ribs, and the neck muscles stand out. Feeding is difficult because the baby becomes even more breathless when sucking. If your baby seems to be exhausted when feeding, tell your doctor.

Chest conditions such as ASTHMA also make children breathless but the classical asthmatic attack is easily recognizable to the parent of an asthmatic child. Infections such as CROUP and BRONCHIOLITIS can also make a child short of breath and both of these must be seen and treated by a doctor. Severely anaemic children and those who have taken certain poisons can also be short of breath.

Unless your child is a known asthmatic (when you'll know what to do) always get medical help for any shortness of breath, especially in babies.

See PNEUMONIA; RESPIRATORY DISTRESS SYNDROME; WHEEZING

Bronchiolitis A viral infection of the bronchioles (the smallest respiratory passages in the LUNGS) seen most commonly in babies between two and six months of age in the winter and spring.

It may occur in epidemics. Most affected babies have a history of exposure to an older child or an adult with a minor respiratory disease. The viral invasion of the bronchioles causes their lining to swell and the bronchioles themselves to fill with mucus and other matter. The normal exchange of gases in the lungs is impaired, the baby becomes short of oxygen and starts to fight for his breath.

The baby with bronchiolitis may wheeze, cough, have obvious difficulty in breathing and go blue. Hospital treatment for babies too ill to be watched at home includes giving them oxygen in a tent or incubator, tilting them up into a position enabling them to breathe more easily, clearing the nose and throat by sucking them out before a feed, making sure they have enough fluids, whether by mouth, via a nasogastric tube (from the nose to the stomach) or intravenously (into a vein) and carefully watching for signs of deterioration.

The routine use of antibiotics is unnecessary except in certain situations (if there is also pneumonia, lung collapse, a high fever or a complicated medical history).

More than fifty per cent of babies with bronchiolitis due to the respiratory syncitial virus (the commonest virus in this condition) are likely to have recurrent episodes of mild WHEEZING with an asthmatic basis during childhood.

Bronchitis An inflammation of the delicate membranes lining the bronchial tubes (air passages in the LUNGS), often caused by viruses. The trachea is nearly always affected as well, so a more correct name is tracheobronchitis. It is usually associated with an upper respiratory tract infection such as a cold or sore throat.

Bronchitis usually affects older children, though it can affect children of any age and causes a slight fever and loss of appetite. The child has a dry, hacking COUGH at first which changes into a productive cough in one or two days. The green or yellow phlegm is coughed up and usually swallowed, and this, together with the cough, can cause vomiting. There may be some pain under the breastbone. The mucus in the bronchi together with spasm of the muscles lining them may lead to WHEEZING, which may be difficult to differentiate from ASTHMA, though the wheezing of bronchitis is always preceded by a cough and fever.

Some children are more prone to acute bronchitis than others: the reasons are unknown, though it is thought that climate and air pollution play a part. Bronchitis is also more likely to occur in a child with a sinus infection, tonsillitis, congenital heart disease, or a chronic condition such as cystic fibrosis. The 'bronchitis' of teething babies is most often simply a bubbly cough caused by an excess of saliva. Of course it is possible that teething (which after all goes on for a very long time) may be accompanied quite independently by bronchitis but this doesn't mean that teething causes bronchitis.

Not every child that wheezes with acute bronchitis is asthmatic. However, children with recurrent wheezy bronchitis almost always have a basic asthmatic disorder even if they are feverish. Wheezy bronchitis is more common in fat children and tends to disappear by the age of seven years.

Bronchitis is treated with physiotherapy to help the child cough up the phlegm. Once a mother has been shown how to do this she can easily put her child's head down over her knees and pat him vigorously on the back to loosen the phlegm and so help him get rid of it. Antibiotics are not usually necessary unless there is a secondary bacterial infection. No cough medicines have been shown to be helpful and indeed it is unwise to prevent the cough which is needed to clear the air passages.

Sometimes 'acute bronchitis', as it's thought to be at the time, actually turns out to be the early stages of measles, whooping cough, 'flu, or scarlet fever.

See BRONCHIOLITIS; CROUP; LARYNGITIS

Bruise A darkening of the skin usually caused by a knock which, although powerful enough to break small blood vessels beneath the surface, does not break the skin surface itself. Blood from the broken vessels leaks into the tissues and darkens as the pigments from the blood cells age.

A bruise slowly disappears as the blood cells are broken down and their constituents reabsorbed by the body. This process is accompanied by colour changes which are a sign of healing. This usually takes about a week for a medium-sized bruise.

Bruises are common in toddlers and adventurous children, but if a knock has been very hard, there may be concern that the underlying bone is broken. If there's any real doubt, an X-ray should be taken. A good rule of thumb is that bruises tend to get less painful as the days go by, whereas a fracture gets more painful if left untreated.

A black eye is, of course, just a bruise and disappears after a few days although the swelling can be very unpleasant at the time. Apart from putting something cold (such as a pad of wet cotton wool) over the eye to soothe it, there's very little else that helps. Should your child ever get a black eye for no reason, take him to your doctor.

An uncommon but important group of diseases that cause bruising are the bleeding disorders such as HAEMOPHILIA and LEUKAEMIA. If your child seems to bleed or bruise very easily or if he has lots of bruises for which there is no obvious explanation, it's essential to mention this to your doctor. (*See* BLEEDING.)

Burns The severity of a burn is gauged by several factors: 1) the percentage of the skin involved; 2) the depth of the destruction; 3) the age and state of health of the victim; and 4) the other effects of the heat or fumes on the body.

Needless to say, the longer the person has been in contact with the source of heat, the worse the burn will be.

The major problems from a burn are fluid

loss and infection. When the skin is severely burned, tissue fluids escape very easily and the body's volume of fluid is soon so low that SHOCK sets in.

Because a raw area of the body is exposed after a burn, infection can easily occur. For this reason burns are kept covered, sometimes even with antibiotic-impregnated dressings.

If your child burns himself, the burn should be put under cold water immediately and held there for several minutes. Although this is painful, it stops much of the blistering and keeps tissue damage to a minimum. Never put butter or fat on a burn. If the skin is damaged through its full thickness and the area is charred or raw, the child must be taken to a casualty department immediately. Never pull away charred clothing – leave that to the experts or you may do more harm than good. The burned area should be covered with a freshly laundered handkerchief on the way. Never cover a burn with any fluffy dressing such as lint. Soluble aspirin will help relieve the pain. It's important to keep as calm as possible as it can be a very frightening time for a child.

With minor burns the skin always grows back again but if the deepest parts of the skin are affected, skin grafting may be essential to make good the deficit. Until healthy skin has covered the whole of the burned area the child is still in danger of picking up a serious infection. Skin grafting is a long-term affair and it may be many months and sometimes even years before the whole of the burned area looks anything like new again. But marvellous things can be done with today's modern surgical techniques, and there's no reason for a child to remain disfigured for life.

Seek medical advice for all burns, however small, in children.

As with so many other accidents in children, prevention is better than cure. Teach your children to respect fires, electrical appliances and cookers, and keep fires guarded. Remember that it is an offence to leave a child under the age of 12 years alone in a room where there is a fire without a fire guard. (*See* SAFETY.)

Cancer Cancer is luckily rare in children, but because most other childhood illnesses are now either preventable or can be cured, it has become a leading cause of death. However, children tolerate the treatments of cancer much better than adults, and therefore the outlook is continually improving.

In spite of an enormous amount of research, the causes of most cancers remain unknown but they all have one thing in common – they are almost all due to the uncontrolled multiplication of one type of cell or another in the body which then gives rise to a lump. If this lump arises in a place which cannot expand, such as inside the head, it may produce trouble before it has grown very big. If it grows where it can expand easily, such as inside the abdomen, it may grow quite big before it is noticed that anything is wrong.

Children tend to have cancers different from those of adults – the common ones are those involving the blood-producing cells (LEUKAEMIA); those affecting the cells of the kidney (Wilms' tumour); and those affecting the brain cells and cells of the other parts of the central nervous system. Cancer of the bone cells mainly affects adolescents.

The main types of treatment involve surgery, radiation and drugs. Frequently such treatment is long and hard, not only for the child himself but for the whole family. Ten years ago even with treatment the outlook was still so bleak that many parents must have wondered whether it was all worth it. Nowadays, with intensive drug treatment (chemotherapy), more than 50 per cent of children who have developed acute leukaemia, for instance, are surviving for five years or longer and many appear to be actually 'cured'. Because of this, the weeks and months of discomfort and sickness for the child and agony for the parents are definitely worthwhile.

Dealing with the emotional needs of the child and his family during treatment has been almost as important an advance as the new drugs. There is nowadays far more inclination to tell the child all about his illness and the difficulties of treatment, as this appears actually to decrease the complications. As with any serious disease, there is always a case to be made for prolonging life if only because with so much research going on worldwide, a cure for certain conditions might be just around the corner.

See BLINDNESS; BRAIN TUMOUR; KIDNEYS

Candidiasis *See* MONILIASIS

Caput A swelling on a baby's head caused by the pressure of the presenting part of the baby against the birth canal during labour. It is formed by a leakage of tissue fluid into the tissues of the scalp and usually disappears, if not in hours, at least by the second or third day after birth.

There are no after-effects, even if the caput is on the baby's face, and no treatment is necessary.

See CEPHALHAEMATOMA

Carbuncle *See* BOIL

Cast *See* SQUINT

Cataract An opacity of part, or all, of the lens of the eye, present in one or both eyes. A cataract is often visible as a whiteness in the pupil, but small or early cataracts can sometimes only be seen with a special optical instrument.

A baby can be born with a cataract for many reasons, among which are GERMAN MEASLES (rubella) contracted by the mother in the early weeks of pregnancy; poor nutrition whilst still in the mother's womb, producing a baby that is small for dates; GALACTOSAEMIA; and chromosomal disorders such as DOWN'S SYNDROME.

Cataracts may develop later in life after such things as an eye injury or inflammation of the inside of the eye.

Treatment depends on the degree of vision remaining. Operation to remove the cataract is only advisable early if it is present in both eyes and is making the baby nearly blind, otherwise it can be left until the child is older.

See BLINDNESS

Catarrh An increase in the normal amount of mucus produced by the mucous membranes lining the nasal passages, throat, ears and sinuses. Usually the catarrh trickles down the back of the nose into the throat and is then either swallowed or coughed up. Children are often sick after swallowing a lot of catarrh and catarrh is one of the commonest causes of a chronic cough in people of all ages.

This increased secretion of mucus has a variety of causes, the commonest being COLDS, infection of the sinuses (*see* SINUSITIS), inflammation of the ADENOIDS and ALLERGY. Deviation of the nasal septum and nasal polyps can also produce catarrh. The clear mucus turns to yellow or green pus if a bacterial infection is present.

Catarrh can be associated with deafness (if the openings of the eustachian tubes in the nasopharynx are blocked), bronchitis, and vomiting and diarrhoea (if the viruses have spread to the stomach and intestine).

Treatment is aimed at removing the cause of the increased secretion if possible, (such as removing chronically inflamed adenoids or nasal polyps); or at reducing the amount of secretion by using nasal sprays or drops such as antihistamines (if allergy is present), decongestants, or antibiotics (if there is chronic infection). The prolonged use of decongestants should be avoided as this can eventually lead to an increase in the amount of mucus produced. Catarrh associated with the common cold usually disappears within a few days and there is no need for any treatment.

See GLUE EAR; HAY FEVER

Central nervous system The brain and spinal cord. The system is called 'central' to distinguish it from all the 'peripheral' parts of the nervous system which include all the nerves that run from the central nervous system to the rest of the body.

The central nervous system collects nervous impulses from the peripheral nervous system,

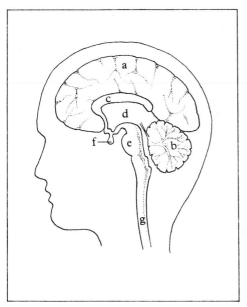

A cross-section through the brain. a. cerebral hemisphere, b. cerebellum, c. corpus callosum, d. third ventricle, e. pons, f. pituitary, g. spinal cord.

distributes them to special areas in the brain and thereby activates specific parts of the body. This system is so highly developed in man that it enables him to perceive, interpret and intellectualize on all the sensations available to him. It is considered that this last power of the central nervous system has given man power over the rest of the animal kingdom. (*See* AUTONOMIC NERVOUS SYSTEM.)

In order to survive in a hostile environment, animals must have a communication system that tells them about the world outside. As the animal gets larger and more complicated (like man himself), it not only needs to collect information from outside and act on it but also to convey messages around its own body.

Because these messages are so complex and so numerous there has to be a central co-ordinating system to initiate, interpret and control them. This centre is the *brain*, without which man's nervous system couldn't function the way it does. The brain is a firm organ the consistency of thick blancmange and is contained within the rigid bony skull. It is covered with three layers called the meninges and is bathed in a liquid called cerebrospinal fluid. There are four major parts to the brain, each with its own function. The *cerebral hemispheres* (or cerebral cortex) form the bulkiest part and are responsible for initiating body movements. Sensations of heat, cold, pain and so on are also sent here and interpreted. Stimulation of any part of the sensory cortex, by an electrical impulse, for example, gives rise to the particular sensation that would normally be processed there. For instance, if the 'smell' area is stimulated, then the person will be conscious of a smell. Stimulation of a part of the motor cortex causes muscles to contract.

If a slice of the brain is cut, the outer edges appear grey (the grey matter) and the inner parts white (the white matter). The grey matter gets its colour from the millions of tiny nerve cells that are present while the white parts consist of the miles of nervous pathways that connect all these cells together. The need for such a complex interconnection of nerve cells can be understood if we consider one part of the brain's activity, such as speech. The cells in the speech area of the brain don't initiate speaking as such. Speech is a highly complex activity involving the co-ordination of breathing muscles, mouth and tongue muscles, throat, soft palate and lips. The speech centre stores the 'memory' for the exact combinations of all these things so that we can produce the right sound exactly when we want to. It's because there are so many interlinking functions within the brain that the bulk of the organ is made up of interconnecting nerves.

The second major part of the brain is the *cerebellum* and this controls balance and muscle tone and co-ordinates body movements. The *pons* is the 'railway junction' of the brain and the *medulla oblongata* connects the brain to the spinal cord. In the medulla oblongata are also important centres controlling the vital functions of breathing, pulse rate and blood pressure.

Associated with the brain are two small glands. One, the pineal gland, is a mystery because no one knows what it does but the other, the pituitary gland, is the central control for the hormone system of the body. Through its nervous connections with the brain this small gland is influenced in such a

53

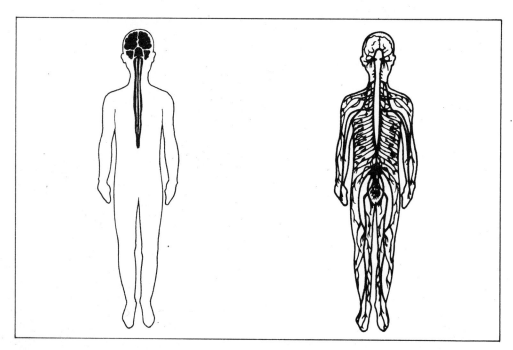

The central and peripheral nervous systems.

way as to produce hormones affecting every corner of the body.

The spinal cord is an oval column of nervous tissue, about 18 inches long in an adult, that runs from the medulla oblongata at the base of the brain down the back inside the bony spinal column. All the nerves to the trunk and limbs lead off the spinal cord and it also serves as a local reflex centre for quick (reflex) reactions. The spinal cord doesn't fill the space inside the spinal column – it is surrounded by cerebro-spinal fluid which is in continuity with that surrounding the brain. The nerve cells are not on the outside (as in the brain) but on the inside in the form of an H-shaped mass that runs the entire length of the cord. Parts of the H connect the brain to the cord and various parts of the cord to itself. In a condition called SPINA BIFIDA part of the bone surrounding the spinal canal is missing. There may also be a loss of skin and a defect of the exposed spinal cord.

Cephalhaematoma A large collection of blood (something like a severe bruise) which lies between the scalp and skull bones of a new-

born baby. As the blood is outside the skull, there is no need to worry about the baby's brain inside. The normal forces of labour acting on the scalp are what cause a cephalhaematoma. It may not be present at birth and can appear after two or three days. Unlike a CAPUT which can appear anywhere on the head and is caused by tissue swelling, a cephalhaematoma is much more localized and never extends across the midline of the scalp to the other side of the head. It usually subsides within a few weeks and gives no further trouble.

Cerebral palsy A term used to describe a variety of disorders in children, including spasticity, PARALYSIS, involuntary movements, and inco-ordination of movement. It occurs in about two in every thousand liveborn children, is a manifestation of damage to or deficient development of the brain itself and is not due to damage or disease in the muscles or nerves. This damage to the brain does not get better or worse – it is static, and can be associated with low intelligence (though about half the children with cerebral palsy have normal or near normal intelligence) and also with hearing, visual, speech and emotional difficulties. There may also be impairment of touch and position sense, and of appreciation of relationships in space.

The causes of this BRAIN DAMAGE are many and may operate before birth (for example, because of maternal infection with toxoplasmosis, the cytomegalovirus, or rubella, or poor nutrition to the foetus); during birth (for example a lack of oxygen, or a bleed into the brain); or after the birth (for example, a lack of oxygen, infection or bleeding into the brain). (*See* ASPHYXIA; FOETAL DISTRESS.) Cerebral palsy is relatively common in low birth weight babies, in multiple pregnancies (twins, etc.), in babies of older mothers, and in those born after an unduly long pregnancy, but in a number of cases no cause can be found.

The commonest type of cerebral palsy (50 to 60 per cent) is spasticity and some people mistakenly refer to all children with cerebral palsy as 'spastics'. Muscles of the affected limbs are stiff, though only in one direction of movement, and this stiffness persists while the child is asleep. Sometimes another form of the disorder – rigidity – is added to the spasticity of the muscles; this makes them stiff in all directions of movement. A spastic child may be affected in one side of the body (hemiplegia), the legs alone (paraplegia), or all four limbs (diplegia, quadriplegia or double hemiplegia, depending on the distribution of the stiffness). CONVULSIONS may occur in some of these children and sometimes the condition is first noticed after a convulsion in the first year of life.

Other forms of cerebral palsy are athetosis (15 per cent of cerebral palsied children), ataxia, loss of balance, and combinations of the three. Athetosis (involuntary, rhythmical movements which the child cannot control) may be caused by very severe, untreated JAUNDICE in a newborn baby and may not be apparent for at least the first year. High tone

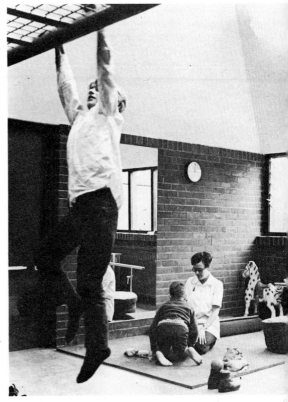

Cerebral palsied children having physiotherapy at a special school for handicapped children.

deafness is often present, and the bizarre movement of the limbs and the usual speech impediment may give people the impression that the athetoid child is of low intelligence, though his intelligence is often quite normal.

It is often very difficult to tell whether or not a baby has cerebral palsy until it is about nine months or a year old. This is because the abnormal signs such as spasticity do not usually appear until the end of the first year. However, more sensitive tests are being developed that may be much better at predicting earlier which babies will be normal and which will have cerebral palsy.

Early diagnosis is important, for although people are still arguing about the benefits of physiotherapy, all agree that intensive support for both the child and the parents at an early stage, and help for the parents in learning about their child's special needs, are essential. Once the trouble is suspected, the child needs to be assessed by a team of specialists, usually in an assessment centre. Other associated problems may also be recognized and the best help can be arranged. The damage to the brain cannot be cured, but a great deal of help can be given to prevent further problems, both physical and educational.

When a normal person bends his arm, not only do the bending muscles contract, but the 'opposing' extending muscles relax. This balance is usually lost in cerebral palsy, and the result may be joints that become fixed, deformed or even dislocated. Keeping the full movements of the joints is one way of preventing this serious secondary effect. The child and his parents have to understand and accept the true situation, otherwise the emotional stress can be unbearable. Moral support and full explanation for the family can also prevent secondary effects.

Many cases of cerebral palsy might be prevented by improving social conditions, decreasing poverty, and improving nutrition, but before these things happen we have to establish whether advances in obstetric and paediatric care might minimize the incidence of this handicap.

Cheilosis *See* LIPS

Chickenpox (varicella) A highly infectious illness that causes mild symptoms in children. It is probably one of the commonest infections in the world and usually affects children under ten. It is spread by personal contact or in the tiny droplets of saliva that spray out of the infected person's mouth when he speaks, coughs or sneezes. A child with chickenpox is infectious from 24 hours before the spots appear until they're all covered with scabs, usually six or seven days after the rash appears. The dried scabs are not contagious.

Chickenpox is caused by a virus very similar to the one that causes shingles. Children who come into contact with a case of shingles quite often get chickenpox as a result, but it is rare for an adult to get shingles from a child with chickenpox.

After an average incubation period of 13 to 17 days, the illness starts with a headache, a general feeling of being unwell, a fever,

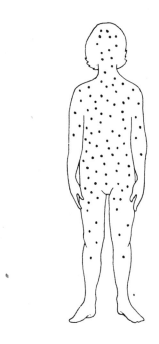

The distribution of the chickenpox rash.

swollen lymph nodes and a blotchy rash, which goes as the typical chickenpox rash appears.

The spots look like pimples at first, then change into small, oval blisters containing clear fluid. After 24 hours the fluid becomes cloudy. The blisters dry and heal by forming scabs which fall off in about ten days. Little scars may be left but these ususally disappear.

The spots are most numerous on the body and often involve the scalp and the palate but the arms and legs are usually relatively spared. The rash may be itchy and can cause such severe scratching that the child is left with permanent scars. Ask your doctor to help if your child is scratching a lot. The spots come out in crops for three to four days, which means that there are spots in many different stages at any one time.

There are two possible complications. The first, infection of the rash, occurs quite frequently, especially after severe scratching. This may lead to impetigo, conjunctivitis or boils, which need treatment. Very rarely, the virus causes encephalitis (inflammation of the brain) between the fourth and tenth day after the rash appears. If the child becomes drowsy, has a headache or vomits, call the doctor.

There's no special treatment for chickenpox. The majority of children are up and about because they don't feel ill enough to be in bed. Calamine or other soothing, bland lotions help control the itching. It's sensible to keep your child's nails cut short at this time so that even if he scratches his rash, he won't damage the skin surface.

Child abuse A term covering not only physical assault to babies (*see* BABY BATTERING) and older children, but also emotional abuse, sexual abuse, neglect of the child's dietary needs and neglect of medical care.

Physical punishment is acceptable in our society, and it is often difficult for outsiders to be sure that a child is being excessively punished. Health and social service workers are now well aware of the existence of physical child abuse and do their best to spot it and step in if necessary for the sake of the child.

Sexual exploitation of children probably occurs more often than is generally realized and mainly involves girls. If the adult involved is the girl's father, the girl and her mother may try to protect him from discovery (*see* INCEST).

Obvious emotional neglect can be dealt with by the social service agencies but a more serious problem is the children who are subtly rejected, continually blamed and told off, always made the scapegoat in the family, and even sometimes frankly terrorized. It may be impossible for an outsider to help the family at all, either because no one realizes anything is wrong or because help is rejected outright. Such children grow up with lasting damage to their personalities in almost all cases.

See DEPRESSION; FAILURE TO THRIVE

Childbirth Although it seems to many parents that childbirth is an entirely natural process needing no interference from the medical and nursing professions, this is not the case if they are to be as sure as possible of producing a healthy, normal baby. Certainly it's true that millions of mothers the world over give birth to perfectly healthy babies without the help of doctors and nurses, but without intervention there are many needless tragedies.

The care of the pregnant woman is an

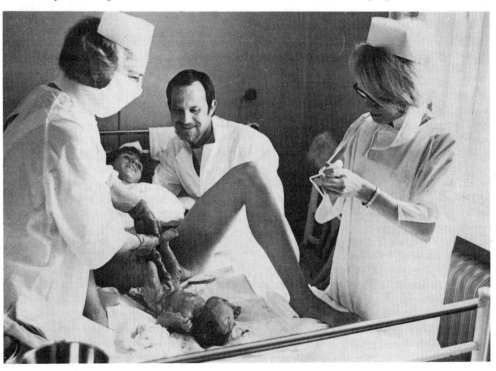

essential foundation stone in the production of a healthy baby. Preparing for childbirth starts the day you know you're pregnant and however much you think you know you'll still benefit from visiting your doctor or antenatal clinic regularly. (*See* ANTENATAL CARE.)

Childbirth itself, assuming the pregnancy has been normal, usually starts spontaneously after about forty weeks of pregnancy. There are three ways in which it may start: the waters may break; there may be a 'show' of blood; or the womb may start to contract. If any of these things happens the woman should contact her doctor or midwife or go directly to the hospital where she has been booked in.

It's helpful to describe birth in three stages. The first stage is the longest and lasts about 10 to 14 hours in a woman having her first baby. During this time the baby is being pushed down on to the cervix (the neck of the womb) by the contracting womb, and the cervix is dilating. Doctors don't let this part of the birth go on for very long today because it's known that the mother and baby can easily become exhausted. During this stage the mother may be in bed, sitting down or walking about. She may have an enema and be shaved. It's during this first stage that a woman needs company, especially because it can be very lonely waiting for the second stage to start.

Gradually the intervals between contractions shorten and the contractions become stronger. A vaginal examination shows that the cervix has dilated enough to let the baby out and soon the woman feels that she wants to push. This second stage is usually complete within an hour. The mother is encouraged to use each contraction and to relax between them to regain her strength. This stage is very hard work and once more the father can be helpful, both with his encouragement and by actually comforting her physically.

Slowly the baby emerges and the mother can stop pushing. The doctor or midwife guides the baby's head out and once the baby is born, makes sure it is breathing properly. Most babies start breathing spontaneously and can be given to their mothers to hold straight away. The umbilical cord can be cut and tied when convenient.

The third and last stage of the birth is the delivery of the placenta (afterbirth) which kept the baby alive and healthy inside the womb during pregnancy. It usually comes out easily and painlessly.

A woman may find painkilling drugs helpful, especially in the first stage, though many women find relaxation and breathing exercises alone sufficient. Others choose epidural analgesia, which is increasingly available in obstetric units.

Though most women have a normal birth and their babies are healthy throughout their pregnancy and labour, some women or their babies develop signs or symptoms which mean that some sort of obstetric intervention is necessary. Induction of labour before term, caesarean section before or at term, and the use of obstetric forceps are just a few examples of potentially lifesaving procedures. Many hospitals routinely use electronic equipment to monitor the baby's heartbeat during labour so as to detect problems early.

See ASPHYXIA; APGAR SCORE; FOETAL DISTRESS; INCUBATOR; LOW BIRTH WEIGHT; PERINATAL MORTALITY

Choking *See* ASPHYXIA

Chorea Continuous, rapid, jerky movements performed involuntarily. Adults may suffer from Huntington's chorea but this is entirely different from childhood chorea which is called St Vitus's Dance or Sydenham's chorea.

Chorea in children is usually a symptom of RHEUMATIC FEVER and is very rare today. Even rheumatic fever itself is rare in Britain and St Vitus's Dance occurs in only a tiny fraction of children with rheumatic fever. The disease (which is more common in girls) usually starts as a jerkiness or clumsiness in the limbs and gets more severe. It lasts about two months and then goes. There is no specific treatment.

Chromosomes The parts of the human cell that carry the inherited characteristics from one generation to the next. All human cells contain 46 chromosomes arranged in 23 pairs except ova and sperms which have only half this number (23 single chromosomes) so that when a sperm and an ovum join, they re-form the total of 46 needed for a cell.

Of the 23 pairs of chromosomes in each cell, one pair determines the sex of the individual. There are two sex chromosomes, an X and a Y, which are different in both size and function. Every egg contains an X but a sperm may have an X or a Y. If the egg is fertilized by an X sperm, it will produce a girl (XX). Fertilization with a Y sperm produces a boy (XY). So the father's sperm determines the sex of the child.

Each chromosome consists of a large number of genes. Genes control such diverse features of an individual as eye colour, blood group, and size of feet. In fact, they determine the form and development of every part of the body. It's scarcely surprising that babies grow up to be like their parents since they get half of their genes from each parent.

Usually the chromosomes transfer information from generation to generation in a trouble-free way but sometimes an abnormality occurs and the resulting baby is damaged in some way. DOWN'S SYNDROME is a well known example of a chromosomal abnormality. Inherited disorders due to genetic abnormalities also include HAEMOPHILIA, MUSCULAR DYSTROPHY, various metabolic disorders and COLOUR BLINDNESS.

Our modern knowledge of chromosomes and their function means that we can prevent mothers from having certain types of deformed or abnormal babies. There are doctors in most areas who specialize in this field of medicine and offer a GENETIC COUNSELLING service to help parents who are worried about the passing on of diseases from one generation to the next.

This would allow them to decide whether to take the risk and have a child if their chances of having an abnormal one were increased. Tests are done on foetal cells in the amniotic fluid surrounding the baby in the womb to predict certain types of chromosomal abnormality in the baby (*see* AMNIOCENTESIS) but these tests cannot foretell every abnormality. At the moment such tests are too expensive to be done on every pregnant woman but can be offered to any woman likely to have a baby with an inherited abnormality so that the pregnancy can be terminated if the risk is recognized

early enough. Certain other genetic abnormalities can be detected by special tests performed either before or after birth (e.g. PHENYL-KETONURIA).

See INHERITED DISEASES

Circumcision   The removal of the foreskin – the loose fold of skin that covers the end of the PENIS (the glans). Circumcision is not often carried out today but may still be done for religious or, more rarely, medical reasons. Whereas the operation used to be favoured both by parents and the medical profession, doctors are now loath to do it unless there is a good reason. They are reluctant because circumcision can lead to infection, bleeding and scar tissue formation and there are always dangers, however small, associated with a general anaesthetic.

Circumcision at birth is usually carried out without an anaesthetic but many doctors think that this is unreasonable because it is obviously very painful.

In Jewish families, baby boys are circumcised on the eighth day after birth. Muslim boys are circumcised between their third and fifteenth year.

A newborn boy's foreskin is united to the tip of the penis and only becomes separated later. The separation usually occurs by the third or fourth year but can be later than this, so there is no need to consult your doctor unless your son's foreskin can't be pulled back when he is five. The first school medical is an appropriate time to mention any problems.

Medical indications for circumcision include repeated infection of the tip of the penis (BALANITIS) and a foreskin that looks like being permanently non-retractile at the age of five, though this is difficult to predict. A tight foreskin can balloon out as the child passes water and can sometimes interfere with the stream.

The best way to look after your baby son's foreskin is to leave it alone. However, when it becomes easily retractile, you can gently pull it back at bathtime and wash the collection of white matter (smegma) away. If any force is used to pull it back, you may scar the delicate skin of the penis tip and make subsequent circumcision inevitable.

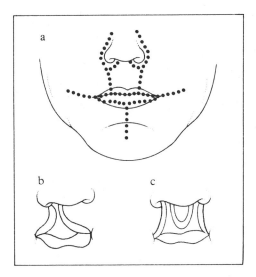

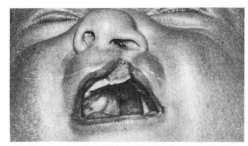

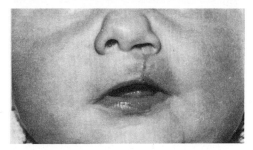

Cleft lip (hare lip) : a. normal lines of fusion in the development of the face ; b. incomplete fusion on one side ; c. complete failure of fusion.

Top, *a baby with a cleft lip and,* above, *the lip after repair.*

A cleft palate before and after repair by bringing the two free sides of the cleft together.

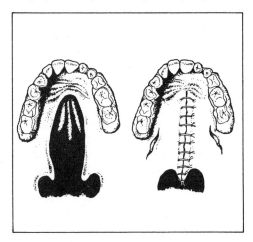

Cleft lip (hare lip) and cleft palate A defect in the lip and roof of the mouth caused by imperfect development before birth. The lip and palate both develop during the ninth week of foetal life but certain genetic or possibly environmental factors can prevent them from developing normally. Cleft lip and cleft palate can each occur alone or in combination.

Cleft lip occurs in about one in a thousand babies and cleft palate in about one in 2,500. Twelve per cent have a relative with a cleft palate but it's not an inherited condition as such. No one knows the cause, though X-rays, steroid drugs, German measles during pregnancy and other factors have all been incriminated at some time.

Often a cleft palate is first noticed at the first examination after birth but some are not discovered until the child has a feeding problem. These babies often can't suck well, but sitting them in an upright position to be fed helps. Breast feeding may be possible but if the baby can't suck well enough, the breast milk can be expressed or pumped and given (as can cows' milk) by bottle with a soft or specially shaped teat, or with a spoon. A special plastic plate can be fitted (by an orthodontic surgeon) over a cleft palate to allow the baby to suck properly. Cleft lip rarely causes a feeding problem.

A cleft lip can be repaired surgically in a healthy baby before he is three months old. Another operation may be necessary when the child is four or five years old for cosmetic reasons. The timing of a cleft palate repair depends upon the individual case.

Although about 80 per cent of children who have had a cleft palate repaired end up with perfectly clear speech, some have problems later with certain sounds, especially the consonants 'k', 'p', 't', 'g', 'b' and 'd' and need long-term speech therapy. There may also be dental problems and some degree of hearing loss. Teamwork between all the specialists looking after the child is essential for optimal treatment.

About ten per cent of children with a cleft palate have other developmental abnormalities such as BLINDNESS, MENTAL RETARDATION, or HYDROCEPHALUS.

Club foot A congenital deformity of the foot which may point unnaturally downwards or upwards and may be twisted so that the sole faces inwards or outwards.

Many babies are born with feet which look peculiar because of their position. When, as is usually the case, the bad position can easily be corrected, the condition rights itself (perhaps with the help of simple exercises). If only one foot is affected, or if correction is difficult or impossible, medical care is essential.

Club foot proper can be caused by mechanical pressures in the uterus before the baby is born, because of restricted foetal movement or an abnormal position in the uterus. Hereditary factors may also play a part and some children with club foot have spina

Club feet.

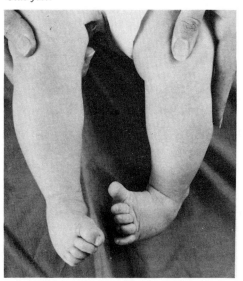

bifida. Occasionally, club feet are acquired later on in life, for example with cerebral palsy or poliomyelitis.

Club foot is an important problem because the child can't put his feet down flat when walking. If the condition is untreated, the child can develop irreversible deformities of the bones in the feet and may never walk properly.

Club feet are usually seen in otherwise completely healthy babies and it's essential to correct the deformity so that they can lead normal lives. Early diagnosis and treatment are advisable, so parents who are worried about their child's feet, should not hesitate to go to their doctor.

See CONGENITAL ABNORMALITIES; FEET

Clumsiness Children vary in their natural ability to do things with their hands and feet and in their general agility and co-ordination. We have probably all known at least one person who constantly drops things or falls over, and at the same time we have probably all known one really outstanding athlete or person with great manual dexterity. Some children develop manual skills later than others, appearing clumsy at first but catching up later, while others remain hamfisted all their lives.

The child who is remarkably clumsy may have some degree of damage to his brain. (*See* BRAIN DAMAGE.) If this is suspected by a doctor then it is easier to excuse the child for his constant mishaps. Sometimes such a child also has difficulty in distinguishing right from left and in assessing the distance between things accurately. There is not necessarily any relationship between clumsiness and the level of intelligence of a child.

If your child's clumsiness worries you, ask for your doctor's advice.

Coeliac disease A disease in which there is a sensitivity of the child's gut to the protein gluten which is found in wheat, rye, barley and oat flour. The child is normal until flour products (usually in the form of cereals) are added to his diet on weaning, and this is one reason why mothers are now advised not to give their babies cereals before four to six

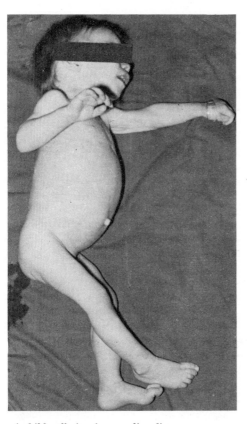

A child suffering from coeliac disease.

months. The condition is very common in some parts of the world, for instance in Western Ireland, where one in three hundred people is affected.

The first thing a parent notices is that the child loses his appetite, becomes irritable and passes pale, bulky, smelly stools. Because he may also vomit, the mother may think he has gastroenteritis. The basis of the trouble is poor absorption from the gut. After a while the baby loses weight (or fails to gain it) and his abdomen becomes blown out. Anaemia and other nutritional deficiencies follow because of the poor absorption of iron and vitamins, and growth is delayed if the condition isn't treated. A child with coeliac disease is more likely to get eczema than a normal child.

Doctors have to differentiate coeliac disease from many other conditions causing poor absorption from the gut but once the diagnosis has been made, all foods containing gluten are cut out of the child's diet and the dietary deficiences corrected. Treatment allows better absorption and growth proceeds.

The child may always have to stay on this diet because several related diseases may develop in people with untreated coeliac disease.

Colds The common cold is a viral illness mainly affecting the upper parts of the respiratory system. The viruses cause the membranes lining the upper respiratory tract (the nose, throat, ears and sinuses) to produce a discharge. The viruses can also produce a sore throat. Symptoms of a cold include sneezing, a sudden fever (especially in children between three months and three years), nasal discharge beginning within a few hours, and irritability and restlessness in babies. Some babies vomit and some have diarrhoea. Older children often complain of aching muscles, a cough, headache, loss of appetite and of feeling generally unwell. The high temperature may subside within a few hours or last for up to three days. The cold itself lasts from four to ten days unless there are complications. If the child's resistance to the viral infection is low, a secondary infection (caused by bacteria) may set in. This causes the yellow-green pus that comes from the nose and can also affect the throat, ears, sinuses, respiratory passages or lungs.

Although lots of reasearch has been carried out on cold viruses, we're still not much nearer to being able to prevent colds or even treat them effectively. This is mainly because there are so many cold viruses that suffering from an infection caused by one of them doesn't seem to build up an immunity to the others. This can be especially frustrating to mothers with young children because a child at school can bring back one cold after another, so spreading colds to all the family. Some mothers say that their children never seem to be free from colds for almost the whole of the winter.

No one knows why some children seem to get so many colds, while others get so few. On average, children have between three and six colds a year. People have tried vitamins, vaccines and removing the tonsils and adenoids but none of these measures is really effective.

Some experts believe that really large doses of vitamin C can prevent colds if taken as a protective measure, but this is not yet proven. Whatever you do, your children will probably get just as many colds, so it's hardly worth worrying too much. Folklore has it that wet feet, chilling, dampness or excessive central heating make children more likely to pick up colds, but there is no direct proof of this.

Young babies seem to be more upset by colds than older children, mainly because they find it difficult to breathe, especially when feeding. Babies can become very ill with conditions that may follow a cold such as pneumonia, so a cold should be taken seriously in a baby. A really young baby should if possible be protected from other children and adults with colds. Babies can be given special decongestant nose drops just before a feed to enable them to suck.

It's always difficult to know how seriously to take a cold. It's usually reasonable to let your child go to school unless he has a temperature or seems really unwell. If every child with a cold stayed away from school, classrooms would be almost empty for much of the winter. Colds are infectious from a few hours before the appearance of symptoms up to one or two days after they begin. If your child has a high temperature, vomits persistently, becomes deaf or has painful ears, has a sore throat or looks really ill, he must see the doctor. No doctor will mind seeing a child with any of these things if they're associated with a cold.

Even though we know what causes colds, we don't know how to cure them. Viruses aren't killed by antibiotics, so these drugs are a waste of time and even possibly harmful unless there's a secondary infection present. Never give your child leftover antibiotics from the medicine chest. If he has a high temperature (see FEVER), cool drinks are very soothing and the child should anyway have plenty to drink. Remember that a feverish child can lose lots of body fluid as sweat and this must be replaced. This is especially true for babies (see DEHYDRATION). If your baby is being breast-fed, simply feed him more often. If your child goes off his food with a cold, don't force him to eat but do encourage him to drink.

A child only needs to stay in bed if he feels like it. Decongestant medicines by mouth are widely used but are of little value, and cough medicines should not be used because the coughing prevents catarrh from running into the lower respiratory tract and should not be suppressed.

The common cold need not be more than a nuisance to you and your child. Usually it's a trivial illness that doesn't need medical attention. But if you are worried or if any of the problems outlined above occur, don't hesitate to see the doctor.

Cold sores *See* HERPES SIMPLEX

Colic A loose term frequently used to describe bouts of CRYING in babies under the age of three months. This is why it's known as 'three-month colic'. These bouts of crying often (but not always) occur in the early evening after a feed and may last for an hour or more. The baby is often not improved by being given more milk to drink, more attention, nappy changing or being put to bed to sleep, and the sight of her baby red-faced and yelling, with his knees drawn up, may worry the mother so much that she can think of nothing else until the baby is quiet.

A baby can't explain why he is crying and we adults have taken it upon ourselves to explain this sort of crying as being due to colic – spasmodic pains in the colon (large bowel) due to wind. There is no scientific basis for this explanation and it's highly likely that many babies with colic haven't got wind at all but are crying for some other reason. Babies often pass wind from their back passage while they are crying but this doesn't mean that the wind made them cry – it's normal for the bowel to contain wind after a feed and crying itself can make a baby swallow air. By all means try to 'burp' the baby immediately after a feed by sitting him upright, but don't worry if nothing comes up. Many babies elsewhere in the world are never 'burped' and don't seem to suffer for it.

Crying may be caused by several things. The baby may be hungry, so the first thing to try is some more milk. Second, the baby may have had enough to drink but may still want to suck – this can happen in both breast- and

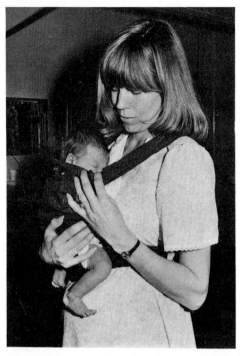

Many babies stop crying when they are carried – a front sling enables the mother to do this and to get on with other things at the same time.

bottle-fed babies. For a bottle-fed baby it's worth trying a teat with a smaller hole so that the baby has to suck longer to get the same amount of milk, or a dummy can be given. A breast-feeding mother can simply let her baby suck at her empty breasts on and off for as long as he wants, and this will not only comfort him but will also increase her milk supply within a few days.

The crying baby that has had enough time at the breast and doesn't have any wind may be lonely or bored if he has been put straight to sleep after his feed, so get him up and see if he will quieten if he is amused. Many mothers find that babies stop crying when they are carried about – the snag here is of course that the commonest crying time is just when you are trying to cook the supper, get other children to bed and tidy up the house. It's easier to work if the baby is quiet though, so you may find that you quickly master the art of preparing food and laying the table one-handed, with the baby in your other arm. A

baby sling makes this much easier and leaves both hands free. A foolproof way of quietening many babies is to take them for a pram or car ride, but again this may be difficult at this time of the day.

Some people have suggested that babies cry in the evenings because they somehow realize that their mothers are in a hurry and so become unsettled. Try keeping as calm as possible to see if this makes a difference – bath the baby in the morning when you have more time, try and prepare as much of the evening meal as possible earlier in the day, and persuade the baby's father to help as much as he can. Gripe water and other medicines to disperse wind and cure colic are of little value. They probably work by relaxing the mother's tension and so help calm the baby!

Babies may cry from more serious underlying causes but there are nearly always other signs present in these cases. A baby crying for a long time who also has diarrhoea, vomiting, goes very pale or has anything else wrong should be seen by a doctor, as should any crying baby who has been off his feeds.

Recent research indicates that a large proportion of breast fed babies can be cured of colic if their mothers cut out cows' milk and cows' milk products from their own diet. These babies are thought to be allergic to even the very tiny amounts of cows' milk protein that get through unchanged into breast milk.

Colour blindness A condition in which colours cannot be distinguished normally. It's about twenty times more common in boys than in girls, and can be a real problem at school. In fact, about eight per cent of boys are colour-blind. The colour-blind child may be mistakenly labelled as stubborn or backward at school, so recognition is important.

Special test cards made up of coloured dots are used to test children with suspected colour blindness. Normally sighted children can see pictures, numbers or letters on these cards but the colour-blind ones can't.

The commonest confusion is between red and green, but even this seemingly great problem doesn't mean that such children won't be able to cope in everyday life. After all, even children with really severe colour blindness can usually learn to distinguish shades of the colours in question but would not match colours as if they were normally sighted.

Apart from working as an airline pilot, in certain parts of the armed services, as a train driver or in a print or paint factory, most other jobs will be open to these children when they grow up.

Coma There are several different levels of unconsciousness. If a child is drowsy (as, for example, when he is dropping off to sleep), he is easily aroused and can even answer simple questions, yet relapses into unconsciousness. A stupor is the next stage, when the child can only be aroused with difficulty. He will be aware of painful stimuli (if you pinch him he'll move or moan) but won't be aware of being spoken to. In a coma a child cannot be aroused at all. This is serious and needs medical attention at once.

Children can become unconscious after asphyxia, a fall involving a bang on the head, a severe shock, after taking an overdose of drugs, during an epileptic fit, after convulsions with a fever, or if they're diabetic.

Unconsciousness must be taken seriously. If your child loses consciousness for any reason (apart, of course, from normal sleep) you must call the doctor. If there's an obvious cause, he'll sort it out very quickly but he may think it wiser to admit the child overnight to the local hospital so that he can be watched.

If a child becomes unconscious, lie him down, preferably on the floor on his side with the uppermost leg drawn up to stop him from rolling over. This is essential because unconsciousness is sometimes accompanied by vomiting and the unconscious child lying on his back can all too easily inhale his own vomit with serious results. If he's not breathing, make sure that there's nothing obstructing the mouth or throat – children inhale the strangest things which can then get stuck in the throat. (*See* ASPHYXIA.) If there's no obvious obstruction and the child still isn't breathing, start artificial respiration. (*See* KISS OF LIFE.)

Artificial respiration should be carried out with the child on his back, but once breathing has restarted, lie him on his side as described above. Never give an unconscious child anything to drink. If there is no sign of a heartbeat or pulse, use HEART MASSAGE.

Parents of children with a condition such as EPILEPSY will be well used to seeing their child flat out on the ground, but to most parents it's a new and distressing affair. It's essential to keep calm and get someone else to summon medical help.

Concussion *See* COMA; HEAD INJURY

Congenital abnormalities If you consider that a baby develops from just two cells, the sperm and the ovum, into a complicated, self-supporting system made up of millions and millions of cells, each of which has to function perfectly in relation to all the others, then you'll see that it's a miracle that everything goes right so often.

However, development is not always normal, either because there is something wrong with the messages carried by the inherited genes in the ovum and sperm, or because something goes wrong with the development of the baby in the womb. If something goes very seriously wrong then the foetus may be naturally aborted very early in pregnancy – sometimes even before the first missed period. This happens in at least one in every ten pregnancies.

Out of every hundred children born, about 96 will be perfectly normal and about four will have some abnormality. This may be bad enough to be recognized immediately, such as a cleft lip and palate, club foot or a serious

An extra thumb, a mild congenital abnormality which can easily be treated.

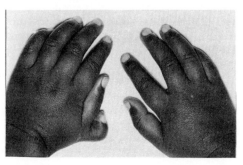

heart defect, but may be so mild that it is only recognized years later or even not at all, if it causes no trouble. Mild abnormalities include extra fingers or toes, birthmarks and umbilical hernias.

The inherited disorders are dealt with elsewhere (see INHERITED DISEASES) and a number of things may occur during pregnancy which interfere with the normal development of a baby. We do not know the cause for some congenital abnormalities, such as spina bifida and anencephaly, but we do know that certain infections in pregnancy can harm the foetus, as can some X-rays and drugs.

GERMAN MEASLES in the mother is thought to be the infection most likely to affect the foetus. The most dangerous time to catch it is in the first three months of pregnancy, and there's an extremely high chance of abnormality in the baby if the infection is in the first four weeks. The defects which may be produced include blindness, deafness, mental retardation and heart abnormalities.

Toxoplasmosis is another infection which can be passed by the pregnant mother to her baby. The small, single-celled organism responsible rarely produces any symptoms in the mother, but can cause prematurity, HYDROCEPHALUS, microcephaly (a small head), mental retardation, eye abnormalities (including blindness), CONVULSIONS, jaundice in the baby, or even stillbirth. However, according to one survey, nine out of ten babies whose mothers contracted toxoplasmosis while pregnant were quite normal.

Congenital abnormalities can also be caused by maternal infection with the HERPES SIMPLEX virus or the cytomegalovirus. Preventive measures against a mother acquiring this latter infection during pregnancy include not eating undercooked meat, as the parasite can be carried in the flesh of mammals and birds but is destroyed by high temperatures, and avoiding handling the litter of cats, which can carry the infection (see PETS).

X-rays used for diagnosis are used in such a low dose that they don't harm any of the tissues of the body except perhaps those of the testis and ovary. The developing testes or ovaries of a foetus are particularly sensitive and this is why X-rays should be avoided if

possible during pregnancy. If there is any chance that a woman might be pregnant, she should also avoid X-rays. Damage to the ovaries or testes doesn't affect the baby itself, but affects the baby's sex cells and so may produce abnormalities in any future offspring of that baby. This sort of genetic damage is known as a mutation.

There is a suggestion that X-rays in pregnancy may lead to the development of leukaemia in the child later, but this is not certain.

If an X-ray during pregnancy is advised, then the foetus is protected from the rays by a lead screen. A lead apron should also be used during dental X-rays.

During the first three months of pregnancy no drugs should be taken unless they're life-saving. The story of thalidomide is so well known that it doesn't need re-telling. All drugs are tested for safety before they are released into general use, but mistakes can still happen. Many drugs have been used by large numbers of pregnant women for years without ill effect, but more and more obstetricians are advising caution today.

Some congenital disorders are influenced by factors such as the age of the parents, the time of year, geographical location and the social environment into which the baby is born. In time continuing research will perhaps explain the significance of these factors.

In the meantime, the best way of preventing foetal abnormality is to avoid drugs and X-rays during pregnancy unless advised by your doctor, to make sure you are in good health before getting pregnant, and to contact your doctor if you are ill during your pregnancy. If you have already had an abnormal child, ask for expert GENETIC COUNSELLING if you are considering another pregnancy.

Some congenital abnormalities such as congenital dislocation of the hip, a hole in the heart, or a blockage of the intestine, can be cured. In others, there is no means of curing the condition, but treatment may enable the child to cope quite well in spite of the abnormality. An absent limb, for example, can be replaced with a mechanical one at some stage.

Congenital dislocation of the hip A condition seen in one in about seven hundred

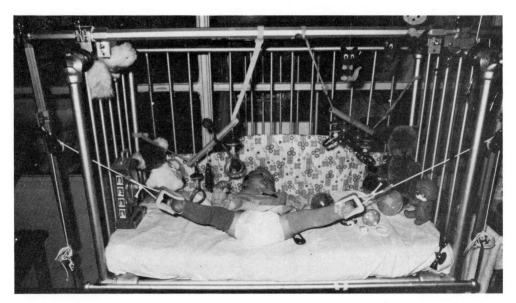

Treatment of congenital dislocation may involve immobilizing the legs.

A dislocated hip joint in an older child (below) *compared with the normal position of the bones.*

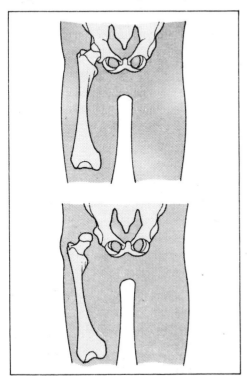

babies born in whom the head of the thigh bone (femur) is not in its socket in the pelvic bone. Six times as many girls are affected as boys; it is relatively more common in firstborn children; and there are more children born with it in the winter months than in the summer. The cause is unknown.

The child with an untreated dislocation may grow up with one leg shorter than the other and this will make him limp and later in life get osteo-arthritis of the hip. Often the hip is not actually dislocated so that the head of the femur is out of the socket, but is unstable, so that the head of the femur can be made to dislocate from the socket and then return to its normal position by the examining doctor. Because an unstable hip may dislocate when the child starts to walk, preventive treatment is just as necessary as for a truly dislocated hip.

The need to test all babies for dislocation of the hip is one of the many reasons for a thorough examination of the newborn child. As a hip may not dislocate or become unstable until later, repeated examinations of the hips should be carried out during the first year of life and these can easily be done by the doctor in the baby clinic or by the family doctor.

Treatment usually consists of splinting the legs in a frog position for the first six to twelve weeks followed by regular X-ray checks until the child is about five years old. Congenital dislocation of the hip is treatable if caught early enough. Some children, however, are missed till they are much older, when treatment is more complicated but still possible. When the diagnosis is only made because the child is slow to walk or later still, corrective treatment is still possible using manipulation and splinting or sometimes by an operation.

Conjunctivitis Irritation of the conjunctiva, the delicate membrane that lines the insides of the eyelids, and the exposed part of the eye. The usual causes are local infection or generalized illness such as measles. Irritation of this membrane also occurs if a FOREIGN BODY gets into the eye, if the eye is injured, and with certain allergies.

A STICKY EYE in the first 48 hours of life is very common.

The older child with conjunctivitis due to infection complains that the eye feels 'gritty' and sticky, especially when waking in the morning. The grittiness is worst when blinking. Many children cannot stand the light, and tears and a pussy discharge are produced.

The treatment of conjunctivitis due to infection is simple, quick and effective, with antibiotic drops, cream or ointment from your doctor. If sensitivity to light is a real problem, sunglasses may help. Simple measures such as washing the hands after touching the eye will help prevent the infection being passed to other people.

Allergic conjunctivitis is often a part of HAY FEVER, particularly if this is due to pollen. The eyes itch and water and the conjunctivae are reddened and even swollen. Special eye drops or ointments ease the symptoms. Desensitization to the provoking allergen may be useful if the child also has hay fever.

Constipation Difficulty or delay in passing motions which are usually firm and sticky. The bowels may be opened once a week or even less often. Constipation is the commonest disorder of the bowel in the western world. There have been many theories over the centuries as to the cause of constipation but the biggest single factor in the western world is now believed to be our faulty diet. The majority of the rural populations of the world are never constipated and pass large, soft stools several times a day. They do this because they eat foods rich in dietary fibre or roughage which is the way nature meant us to eat. By refining our foods in the West, we remove most of the roughage so essential for the normal working of the bowel.

To replace the fibre in our diet we should eat more fruit and vegetables, change from white to wholemeal bread, cut out all white flour products in our diet and replace them with wholemeal flour products; and cut out or cut down sugar which provides us with 'empty' calories and makes us fat.

Many children are constipated because they're eating the wrong foods. The trouble with being constipated is that it creates abnormal pressures in the bowel which can cause permanent damage such as diverticulosis. Many older children and young adults already have signs of long term bowel disease, piles and varicose veins, as they have been constipated for most of their lives and always have to strain to pass a stool.

Constipation can also cause an ANAL FISSURE as the hard, craggy, large stool is passed. A fissure may bleed on to the surface of the motion or the pants, and causes acute pain on opening the bowel...

It's important to remember that if a child has eaten little, for instance if he has been ill, there will be little food residue in his bowel for him to pass.

Parents should not give their children laxatives regularly to ensure that they go to the lavatory daily as this can permanently damage the bowel by encouraging it to become 'lazy'. All the bowel needs to work properly is plenty of bulk to contract on. Laxatives can be addictive because the bowel becomes so used to them that it won't work without them.

There's nothing magic about children opening their bowels once a day. People eating diets high in fibre may well open their bowels twice a day or more. However, it is helpful, especially in young children, to get them into the habit of going to the lavatory at a set time each day – for example after breakfast – and to make sure they have enough time. Lavatories in schools are often off-putting to a child, especially if they are crowded, nonprivate, dirty, smelly, or cold. A child may try hard to avoid opening his bowels at school, eventually becoming constipated, especially if there is always a mad rush at home in the morning to get everyone ready to go out.

Parents who are too insistent on POTTY TRAINING their toddler may have problems with a child who refuses to open his bowels even in his nappy and so becomes constipated.

Some children are chronically constipated, and loose or even fluid bowel motions can escape round the large, craggy mass of hard motion in the rectum to cause SOILING. Treatment should be of the underlying constipation. Such a child may have emotional problems and may actively withhold his motions. Your doctor's help in sorting out and treating this problem will be necessary.

A breast-fed baby older than a few weeks may pass only one motion a day or even every few days. This is because breast milk is the perfect food for babies and is so well digested that there is scarcely any residue. Proper constipation with hard, difficult-to-pass motions does not occur with fully breast-fed babies, provided they are not underfed.

A bottle-fed baby, however, usually passes a motion every day because there is more waste from cows' milk. If his motions become difficult to pass, see that he is having enough milk and ask your doctor if you are worried.

There is no need to wean babies on to refined foods any more than there is for older children to eat refined foods, as these make constipation more likely. (*See* WEANING.)

To sum up, constipation will be a disease of the past if children eat foods rich in dietary fibre or roughage. This is a very simple way of curing one of the commonest health disorders and will help prevent your children from developing certain bowel diseases later in life. *See* FOOD.

Convulsions (fits) A convulsion or fit is a sudden spasm of the muscles, possibly repeated several times, caused by a burst of abnormal electrical activity in the brain. Convulsions are common, especially in babies and infants. Epilepsy, which causes one kind of fit, is rare. There is no need to be frightened of epilepsy when a young child has a fit.

Children can have a convulsion for the first time at any age but the commonest type of convulsion – the febrile convulsion – occurs most often in children between six months and three years old and is rare after five years of age. A febrile convulsion is caused by a substantial rise in body temperature because of an infection such as tonsillitis, an acute ear infection (otitis media), a urinary infection or measles. There is often a family history of febrile convulsions in infancy. The child who is obviously very hot needs to be cooled down by tepid sponging, undressing and opening the windows. (*See* FEVER.)

A convulsion classically has four stages but sometimes is over so quickly that it's not easy for an onlooker to remember exactly what happened. The first stage is before the muscle spasms begin and consists of an aura: the child feels frightened or has a headache. In young children this stage is often not noticed. The second and third stages consist of the muscle spasms proper, the limbs first being held stiff and then jerking uncontrollably. This stage seldom lasts longer than ten minutes if the convulsion is due to fever. Finally the child becomes very sleepy and confused and often goes to sleep. Fits like this, especially the first, can be very upsetting for the parents. In one recent survey 30 per cent of the parents thought their child was dying or dead when he was fitting. If your child starts fitting, get him quickly to the floor, lie him on his side and simply prevent him from hurting himself on anything. There's nothing else you can do until he stops fitting, so don't panic. He won't come to any harm: he may wet himself, but he certainly won't die.

Someone should always stay with the child during the fit to prevent him from hurting himself during the jerking phase. Putting an object such as a spoon covered with a handkerchief between the teeth during the jerky phase may prevent the child biting his tongue or lips but this is not a good practice because it is so easy to break teeth. Bitten tongues heal – broken teeth don't. Once the fit is over and the child soothed, call the doctor unless someone else can get the doctor while you stay with the child.

The doctor will try to find the cause of the

fit. For fits due to a high temperature caused by infection, the child needs watching carefully but there is no need for further treatment of the convulsion itself. However, the cause of the the fever will need treatment, and if the temperature continues to stay up then the measures described above to keep the child cool must be continued. It is common practice for admission to hospital to be advised.

Some children have febrile convulsions for no obvious reason. The convulsions themselves can increase body temperature so in this case the fever is caused by the convulsion. Such convulsions should always be fully investigated. Tests used include an examination of the fluid bathing the brain and spinal cord (the cerebro-spinal fluid) obtained by lumbar puncture, an electroencephalogram (EEG), a skull X-ray and a brain scan. Convulsions with and without fever can be a symptom of many diseases and disorders.

In a baby the only sign of a convulsion may be that he stares fixedly ahead, stops breathing for a short time, or has spells of rapid breathing.

Treatment of a convulsion depends on the cause, several of the rarer types being treatable by specific remedies. The experts do not agree about the use of anti-convulsant medicines to treat febrile convulsions, some suggesting their use as a preventive measure, others disagreeing because only 5 to 10 per cent of these children have another fit. Some doctors recommend that phenobarbitone should be given as a preventive measure to a child with a fever who has had a febrile convulsion before. The treatment of true EPILEPSY is different.

Cot death   One in every five hundred children born in this country dies within the first few months of life from an unexplained cause. Cot deaths make up the biggest group of deaths after the first week and under two years of age. The commonest age for this tragedy to occur is between three and eight months with most of the deaths occuring at four months. For this reason it's probably sensible to be especially careful and get medical help if your baby is unwell at this age.

A lot of research is going on into possible causes of cot death and so far several associated factors have been implicated. The respiratory syncitial virus has been found in one in three children at post mortem, suggesting that a virus infection may have been responsible. However, in almost 50 per cent of the babies that die there are no preceding symptoms of illness – the death comes as a complete surprise. Cot deaths are known to be more common in families of low socio-economic status, especially if the mother is young and has several children. Low birth weight babies – both babies born before term and those born at term but weighing less than normal – are also more susceptible, as are those born after a short labour. The fully breast-fed baby seems to be less at risk of a cot death than the bottle-fed baby. Research is also beginning to show that these babies sometimes have congenital abnormalities in the conducting system of the heart which makes their hearts suddenly beat abnormally. There are signs that these babies react abnormally to infections and that some have breathing mechanism disorders. A link between smoking during pregnancy and cot death has recently been suggested as the result of a large British study.

In countries with a relatively high standard of health care, the number of cot deaths is lower, so it would seem wise for a mother to use the health facilities available before and after the birth of her baby as fully as she can. Unfortunately, the very mothers most likely to lose their babies from this condition are often the ones least likely to take advantage of the health care offered.

Parents who have lost a baby in this way feel mystified, upset and guilty and need lots of support from all concerned. A voluntary association has been formed to help them over their immediate problems and to help initiate and finance research programmes.

See BEREAVEMENT

Cough   A common symptom with many causes. In children colds and catarrh most frequently cause coughs, either because of the 'post-nasal' discharge of mucus which trickles down the back of the throat and irritates it; because of an associated sore throat or LARYNGITIS; or because of an associated infection of the windpipe and larger air passages of the lung (tracheobronchitis).

Coughing is nature's' way of removing irritating material from the respiratory tubes so that they don't become blocked or inflamed. Children, unlike adults, rarely cough up and spit phlegm when they have a respiratory infection. They usually swallow the coughed-up phlegm and this phlegm in the stomach may make them vomit. Children with allergic conditions such as ASTHMA and wheezy bronchitis also cough, as do children with CYSTIC FIBROSIS, an inhaled FOREIGN BODY, CROUP, BRONCHITIS, BRONCHIOLITIS and PNEUMONIA. A chronic cough may be due to one or both parents smoking, as children with parents who are smokers have more bronchitis and pneumonia than do children of non-smokers. It may also be an attention-seeking device or a habit.

Because coughing is a protective mechanism, it's not a good idea to use medicines to suppress it unless the cough is so bad that the child cannot sleep. Cough linctus can be useful as a soothing syrup in such cases but home remedies such as hot honey and lemon are probably just as effective. Antibiotics are of no value for coughs due to viral infections such as a cold or measles and shouldn't be given unless there are complications from a secondary bacterial infection. Similarly the cough of asthma associated with an infection is not usually helped by antibiotics as the infection is usually viral. WHOOPING COUGH has very special characteristics and needs special treatment.

See ASPHYXIA; TUBERCULOSIS; WHEEZING

Cradle cap A layer of brownish-yellow crusts over part or all of the scalp. Cradle cap is common in babies but can also affect children of one, two or even three years. Affected babies produce a lot of sebum, though the reason for this is unknown.

Cradle cap is often worst over the soft spot (fontanelle), perhaps because the mother is afraid to wash this soft part too hard. However, cradle cap is seen in the cleanest babies, even those whose heads are washed in the bath every day, and is no reflection of the cleanliness of the child.

Children with cradle cap may also have seborrhoeic DERMATITIS on their ears, forehead, behind their ears, on the nose, eyebrows, eyelids and folds at the tops of their thighs. This may be difficult to distinguish from eczema but responds quickly to treatment, unlike most cases of eczema.

The crusts of cradle cap can be removed in several ways or you can leave them alone if their appearance doesn't worry you. The simplest way of removing them is to rub olive oil or liquid paraffin into the scalp before the baby goes to bed and to try to remove the softened crusts gently the next morning with a comb. Alternatively, if they are not very thick, a solution of one teaspoonful of sodium bicarbonate in a pint of water can be used to wash the scalp. Shampooing alone is relatively ineffective at getting rid of cradle cap, but there are special shampoos available (containing coal tar, sulphur and salicylic acid) which help, and these are rubbed on as an ointment at night and used as a shampoo the next morning. Finally, a solution of cetrimide (one per cent), used as a shampoo on its own, without soap, is also effective. If you are worried because you can't get rid of your baby's cradle cap, and if the baby also has seborrhoeic dermatitis elsewhere, see your doctor.

Older children with seborrhoea tend to have dandruff or scurf instead of cradle cap, perhaps also with seborrhoeic dermatitis of their face, ears, shoulders, chest and folds at the tops of their thighs.

Cretinism The type of cretinism most often seen in Britain is caused by the congenital partial or complete absence of the THYROID gland. During pregnancy the mother supplies the foetus with thyroxine from her thyroid gland and it is only after birth that the baby is cut off from this supply of thyroid hormones. However, even though the mother can supply some thyroxine, it is not always enough, possibly because of poor transfer across the placenta to the foetus or because she is on anti-thyroid drugs herself, and the baby may already be damaged by a lack of thyroid hormone when it is born.

It is often difficult to diagnose cretinism at birth because the deficiency of thyroid hormones may not yet have caused the usual

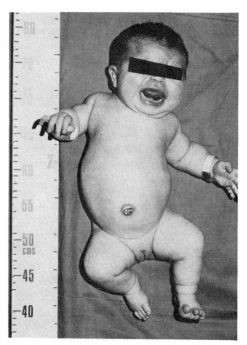

A cretin. The condition is due to lack of thyroid hormone before or after birth. Treatment restores a normal appearance, but may not cure the accompanying mental retardation.

appearance and other signs of the condition, especially if the mother supplied enough of the hormone. Because this is so difficult, doctors are developing a test to make the diagnosis at birth with certainty.

Within the first few weeks, cretinism usually becomes obvious: the baby is sluggish; has severe constipation; a hoarse, deep cry; dry, thick, puffy skin which is also sallow and cold; a protruding tongue; dry, thin, brittle hair with thin eyebrows; a pot belly, often with an umbilical hernia; and, later, delayed appearance of the teeth and retarded bone growth.

The most distressing feature of cretinism is the MENTAL RETARDATION which invariably accompanies it – retardation that is progressive unless the condition is treated.

Once the diagnosis has been made, treatment with thyroxine is begun and should continue for life. The dose varies with the individual child and must be increased until the right amount for that child is given. On no account should the child be taken off the medicine just because he looks better. Treatment restores the normal appearance of the child but unfortunately does not always correct the mental retardation, especially if he was affected before birth.

Cretinism may also be caused by a deficiency of iodine in the diet of the pregnant mother, or by a deficiency in the diet of the newborn child. Deafness, unco-ordinated movements, spasticity and mental retardation are seen in one type of this disorder, and mental retardation, growth delay, myxoedema (underactivity of the thyroid gland) and a GOITRE in the neck in the other. This sort of cretinism is now rare but is still seen in such areas as New Guinea and certain mountainous parts of the world where the inhabitants don't get enough dietary iodine. It is preventable by the addition of iodine to food.

Finally, some children have a genetically inherited form of cretinism and are born with a goitre as well. Treatment with thyroxine is best started at once but detailed studies must be done at some stage so that genetic counselling can be offered to the parents.

Crohn's disease (regional enteritis) A chronic condition with recurrent attacks of inflammation and ulceration of the bowel. It is as common in children as ULCERATIVE COLITIS, though the small bowel is the site most often affected by Crohn's disease whereas in ulcerative colitis it is the large bowel or colon that is affected.

Children with this disease have bouts of fever, perhaps with abdominal pain, diarrhoea or constipation and a loss of appetite leading to a severe loss of weight.

The cause of Crohn's disease is unknown but it is now thought by some experts to represent an immune response to some insult to the bowel. It has been suggested that breastfed babies are less likely to suffer from this disease in later life than are bottle-fed babies. Once the diagnosis has been made, treatment is with drugs. An operation to remove part of the bowel may be necessary at some stage.

Croup A type of acute LARYNGITIS seen in young children, which makes breathing difficult and gives rise to a high-pitched, croaky wheeze on breathing in. Croup may be due to infection (bacterial or, more usually, viral) of the respiratory tract; allergy; or an inhaled foreign body. The commonest type of croup is a catarrhal kind without fever. The child may have had a slight cold previously and often wakes coughing in the night. Breathing is difficult and the crowing noise alarms the parents especially when the child is blue.

Simple croup is not serious but you should call the doctor if your child's breathing is difficult, if his chest moves up and down with visible effort on his part, if the lower end of the breast bone is pulled in on breathing and if there are valleys in between the ribs.

In the meantime, try to comfort the child and don't show your anxiety as this may make his condition worse. Sit him up and have a kettle boiling in a safe corner of the room, as steam helps the croup subside. Cold vapour from a humidifier is even better if one can be obtained. Within a short time the distressing breathing should be relieved by these simple measures. Antibiotics are only necessary if there is a secondary bacterial infection. Severe cases may have to go to hospital but this is uncommon. Occasionally a child with a foreign body in the throat will make croup-like noises. If you think this could be the cause, take him to hospital immediately if you are near one, or else call your doctor urgently, because the chances are that you won't be able to do anything yourself. If the child is having *serious* breathing difficulties because of something he has inhaled, *see* ASPHYXIA.

See WHEEZING

Crying A loud vocal response to a stimulus with or without the production of tears. In a newborn baby the tears don't flow until the fourth week of life.

Over the last 150 years there have been nearly 130 authenticated cases of crying being heard from a baby still in the uterus. Mohamet and St Bartholomew were both said to have cried *in utero*. Clearly this can only occur once the membranes have ruptured, otherwise there would be no air in the foetal lungs.

Tears are produced by the tear glands which lie just above the outer side of the eye in the socket and are collected by an outflow duct just visible in the nasal corner of the eye which drains into the nose. Tears keep the eye free from bacteria and dust but just why they should be produced in unpleasant or emotional situations, no one knows.

In very young babies, crying is the only way they can communicate their needs to their mothers. Babies may cry because they are hungry, lonely, bored and wanting attention, tired, uncomfortable, wet, in pain, ill, teething, or about to pass water or a motion. Don't leave your baby to cry – he's crying for a reason and needs to be helped by you. You can't spoil a baby because he's not sophisticated enough to be leading you on or fooling you – it's simply the only way he can get attention. The breast-feeding mother's first job when her baby cries is to offer him the breast because that's probably what he wants.

Getting cross with a crying baby is no answer but we all find a baby's crying frustrating at times. If you can't find out what is wrong and you're getting frustrated and irritated, try and take the baby to someone else while you calm down a bit. Sometimes you'll have to let the baby cry but don't leave him for long periods because he'll get frustrated and you won't relax with him crying in the background. Comfort your child early and find out what's wrong rather than let the situation come to the boil. The crying of babies with three month COLIC can be especially worrying, particularly as it often happens at a busy time of day.

Children who cry at night are usually lonely or afraid and their crying is a reflection of our strange western habits of separating our children from us at night. (*See* SLEEP.) Babies especially like to be with their mothers all the time and many mothers have found a baby sling an ideal way of keeping their baby happy as they get on with their work.

Children with certain diseases cry in special ways. The cries of children with meningitis and hydrocephalus are usually shrill and high pitched. The infant with poor thyroid function (a cretin) has a coarse, gruff cry; a child with laryngitis is hoarse and one with pneumonia grunts. It's remarkable that cries are so different even in healthy babies. Research has shown that within 48 hours mothers are able to pick out the sound of their own baby's cry from all the others in the obstetric unit.

As a child grows older, different things make him cry. The boredom and loneliness of babyhood are replaced by the frustrations of the toddler and young child. He has to learn all the new skills of the adult world and this is often hard work and frustrating.

In older children, infections and other illnesses, tiredness, earache and tummy-ache may all end in tears. Any older child who cries a lot should be seen by a doctor. Don't forget that children can be depressed, disappointed, angry, or simply sad sometimes just like adults and when they are they'll want to cry.

See AGGRESSION; DEPRESSION; TEMPER TANTRUMS

Cyclical vomiting *See* RECURRENT ABDOMINAL PAIN

Cystic fibrosis An inherited disorder which affects one or two babies in every two thousand, and usually becomes obvious in the first few months of life, though sometimes not till much later.

The underlying problem in cystic fibrosis is an over-production of mucus from many of the mucus-producing glands in the body, among them those of the pancreas, lungs and bowel and the sweat and salivary glands. These large amounts of mucus are also more sticky than normal and tend to block the ducts of the glands, leading to overfilling and many problems.

A small proportion of affected babies have a condition called meconium ileus soon after birth. This is a blockage of the intestine (caused by abnormally sticky meconium in the bowel contents of the newborn) and can be cured by an operation. The majority of babies with cystic fibrosis, however, slowly develop a distended abdomen, have large, pale, revolting-smelling stools and fail to gain weight because of malabsorption of their food, though their appetite is good.

The rectum may prolapse from the back passage, turning itself inside out like a sock – in fact cystic fibrosis is the commonest cause of rectal prolapse in children. (*See* PROLAPSE

OF THE RECTUM.) Volvulus (a twisting of the bowel) and INTUSSUSCEPTION can also occur in babies with cystic fibrosis.

As the illness progresses, the lungs become more seriously involved, the blocked mucous glands leading to patches of infection and collapse. Many different lung disorders are seen and are the main cause of long-term illness. In very hot weather the child with cystic fibrosis is often seriously ill because the sweat glands lose large amounts of salt-rich sweat.

The diagnosis of cystic fibrosis is sometimes difficult but basically depends on finding low levels of pancreatic enzymes in the stools, a family history of the disorder, a history of repeated chest infections and high levels of salt in the sweat.

The treatment of the condition is complicated and includes a special diet with extracts of pancreatic enzymes; antibiotics; and inhalations to make the lung secretions less sticky. Parents should be careful not to let people with colds or chest infections near their child and should ensure that a full course of immunizations, including measles vaccination, is given.

A child with cystic fibrosis is likely to have repeated illnesses over a long period but for his own sake should be treated as normally as possible, trying not to make the life of the family revolve around him. With increasing knowledge and better treatment, affected children are now surviving into adult life and should be encouraged to join in everyday schooling and other activities, provided reasonable precautions are taken to prevent infection.

Cystic fibrosis is inherited via recessive genes, one from each parent, so if both parents carry the gene, one in four of their children will be affected. As yet there is no satisfactory way of detecting the carrier state or of detecting the condition before the baby is born.

Cystitis An inflammation of the bladder usually seen as part of a generalized infection of the whole urinary tract. Girls suffer more from urinary infections than do boys, perhaps because the urethra (the tube connecting the bladder to the outside world) is much shorter, so allowing bacteria up more easily. Children with any obstruction to the flow of the urine are more likely to get cystitis, and one in three with a proven urinary tract infection has an underlying abnormality of the urinary tract.

The main symptoms in older children may include burning pain on passing water, frequency of passing water, the feeling of wanting to go to the lavatory again even immediately afterwards, an urgent desire to go, foul, fishy smelling urine, and incontinence in a previously dry child. Urinary infection is sometimes found on urine testing when there are no symptoms. A child with frequency and pain on passing water does not necessarily have a urinary infection, although this should always be suspected.

The diagnosis is very difficult to make in young children and babies because they can't tell you it hurts to urinate and anyway frequency and urgency are normal in toddlers. Babies in nappies are wet much of the time, so it's difficult to know if they're passing water more often. An inflammation of the VULVA or PENIS is a more common cause of pain on urination than is infection of the urine. Signs of urinary tract infection in babies include a loss of appetite, poor weight gain, marked paleness of the face, misery and occasional vomiting.

The only certain way of making the diagnosis of urine infection in a child is for the urine to be examined for microscopic pus and by bacterial culture. This should always be part of the routine examination of a child with generalized symptoms that can't be explained. Your doctor will explain how to collect a sample of urine.

Although cystitis can be helped in women by all kinds of first-aid and self-help measures, it is wise to get medical help at once with children. Give your child plenty of fluids to drink to make him pass urine often and to 'flush' the infection through, and put a hot water bottle on the lower abdomen to relieve the pain while waiting to see the doctor.

Basic hygiene is the main preventive measure in babies and girls. Girls should be taught to wipe their bottoms from front to back so as not to drag bacteria from the area around the anus to the urethral opening just in front of the vagina. Mothers should also wipe in the same direction when changing their babies' nappies.

Urinary tract infection causes some babies to fail to thrive, others to have recurrent fevers, and a few to suffer from damage to the KIDNEYS, due to chronic or recurrent infections, so it's worth taking the trouble to get proper treatment.

Treatment of a urinary tract infection involves an adequate course of medicine from the doctor, and follow-up testing of the urine to detect recurrence of the infection. One in three children has another urinary infection within the next year. Recurrent urine infection may need very long-term drug treatment.

Most doctors believe that one proven urine infection is a good enough reason for carrying out a special X-ray of the urinary system (an IVP: intravenous pyelogram) to see if there is any abnormality.

See NEPHRITIS

Cytomegalovirus *See* CONGENITAL ABNORMALITIES; HEPATITIS; VIRUS

D

Deafness There are many causes of deafness in children, including a congenital malform- ation of the auditory nerve (running from the inner ear to the brain) or the middle ear; maternal infection with GERMAN MEASLES (ru- bella) during pregnancy when the risk of deafness in the foetus from infection in the first three months of pregnancy is about 30 per cent; severe JAUNDICE in the newborn; BRAIN DAMAGE due to a shortage of oxygen or injury during birth; OTITIS MEDIA; MUMPS; MENIN- GITIS; ENCEPHALITIS; and blockage of the ear canal by a FOREIGN BODY or WAX.

The most common cause of deafness in children past the newborn period is otitis media, which usually causes only temporary deafness. A complication of otitis media (GLUE EAR) can, however, lead to a more severe and even sometimes permanent hearing loss. It has been estimated that one in ten children in Britain is partially deaf as a result of glue ear. Children with otitis media must sit near the front of the class at school, especially since the temporary deafness may take some time to go after the initial earache.

The sooner deafness in a baby is discovered, the more likely is treatment to allow normal, or relatively normal, language development. The deaf baby doesn't start to babble in the second half of his first year. He doesn't turn or look towards sounds and he will only know you are in the room when he can see you. Various hearing tests are available for children of varying ages (*see* AUDIOMETRY and HEARING TESTING) and it's sensible to take advantage of the routine hearing tests carried out by the clinic doctor, family doctor, or health visitor.

It's important to remember that even slight degrees of deafness can interfere with the child's ability to hear speech and so can interfere with his language development. While severe hearing loss is obvious, minor loss may not be noticed by parents, especially if it is one-sided only. Only one or two in every hundred deaf children have no hearing at all. Hearing loss is not always just a question of not hearing sounds as loudly as they should be heard, because the ear may hear certain sound frequencies better than others, resulting in a distortion of the sounds heard. This makes the understanding of speech very difficult for the child, especially with a high tone hearing loss, which is relatively frequent and means that the child has difficulty in hearing high-pitched consonants. This is very disturbing because he hears only a string of disconnected vowel sounds.

The vast majority of deaf children can be helped to use what hearing they have by an ear, nose and throat specialist and by a teacher of the deaf, if necessary. Parents of children with a hearing loss will be advised to speak into their child's ear, repeating sounds so that he can learn to distinguish them. Anyone who comes into contact with the child should be taught how to speak so that the child is most likely to hear. A hearing aid can be fitted at a very early age and lip reading can be taught if necessary.

Many normal schools now have special units for partially deaf children who are integrated into normal school activities as much as possible. More severely deaf children may need special schooling at schools for the deaf.

See EARS

Dehydration A relative lack of water in the body caused by too great a loss, too small an intake, or both. Because water carries with it many salts essential for the working of the body, the loss of water is a serious matter.

About two-thirds of the body weight is made up of water both inside and outside the cells. Children usually become dehydrated because they've lost a lot of fluid by VOMITING, with DIARRHOEA or as sweat. Very loose motions contain large volumes of water and essential salts and a child easily becomes dehydrated and weak after severe diarrhoea.

A child with a FEVER of over 100°F (37.7°C),

can lose pints of fluid a day and this must be replaced if dehydration is to be avoided. Diabetes is a rare cause of dehydration and here the water loss is produced by the high blood sugar which encourages the kidneys to put out excessive amounts of urine.

The way the body deals with dehydration is to make us feel thirsty. This thirst is satisfied by drinking and so the water balance is returned to normal. In some conditions, however, especially with acute fevers, children don't feel like drinking and it takes perseverance by the parents to ensure that enough fluid gets down. It's worth the effort because simply restoring lost fluid makes the child feel better in spite of the illness. Severe dehydration causes the skin to feel dry and to crease, nappies to be unexpectedly dry or stained by concentrated urine, the eyes to appear sunken and the soft spot on the skull (the fontanelle) to be depressed, if open. If your baby is putting out more fluid than he is taking in, he is suffering from fluid lack and needs urgent medical treatment.

It's particularly important that a baby with vomiting, diarrhoea, or a fever is given a suitably modified brand of cows' milk to drink. (Ask your doctor or health visitor for advice). Some brands contain too much salt and in combination with dehydration can cause severe problems. A baby also eating solids must have plenty to drink at all times. If your child won't or can't drink and is becoming dehydrated, with the typical glazed, sunken eyes and dry mouth, call the doctor.

Delicate children An old-fashioned term used to describe children who, because of repeated illness, become disadvantaged socially and educationally. Many of the debilitating childhood illnesses that used to cause such trouble (such as whooping cough, tuberculosis, rheumatic fever and polio) have been dramatically reduced in incidence in the West and this means that there are correspondingly fewer children who could be called 'delicate'. The state of nutrition of the vast majority of children is also excellent, so we rarely see an undernourished, anaemic, vitamin-deficient child these days.

However, some ten thousand children attend special schools for delicate children in Britain, so the problem has obviously not been completely solved.

The biggest group of delicate children consists of those with ASTHMA. Most children with asthma manage perfectly well living at home and attending ordinary schools. Some are unable to manage in ordinary schools because of their wheezing and need for regular medication and many go away from home to boarding schools in an area thought to be relatively free from airborne allergens such as tree pollen. Delicate asthmatics are often severely affected by their disease and benefit from living outside their home environment, especially if there is friction at home that is triggering their asthma.

There are still a few children who have tuberculosis or who are TB contacts who are classed as delicate. Similarly, there are still some children who have had rheumatic fever or even CHOREA (St Vitus's Dance) who are not fit enough to cope with the rough and tumble of ordinary schools.

Other groups include children with DIABETES which is too difficult to manage at school; those with certain severe skin diseases who would be teased unmercifully; those with certain diseases of bones and joints; and those recovering from polio, for instance, who need watching over or who would not be safe in an ordinary school. Many delicate children are physically handicapped in some way, so several schools exist which cater for children who are both physically handicapped and delicate.

The standard of education of delicate children is good and the schools prepare the children for exams as necessary.

Dental Caries Dental caries (dental decay) is predominantly a disease of western civilisation. Only three in a thousand people in the West have TEETH free from caries. We still don't know the exact cause but one definite factor is eating refined carbohydrate foods (sugar, white flour and all the foods containing sugar and white flour).

The trouble starts with a thin layer of protein material which is deposited on the teeth within minutes of cleaning them. This thin layer is called pellicle and soon becomes

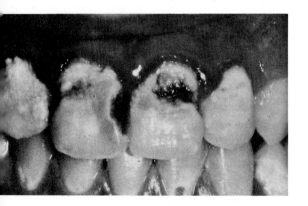

Severe dental decay, as a result of poor oral hygiene.

impregnated with micro-organisms from the saliva to form a thick, sticky slime called plaque. Plaque teems with millions of organisms that live off the refined foods we eat and these bacteria produce acids that dissolve the hard enamel coating of our teeth. This is how dental decay begins. When the decay has gone right through the enamel it reaches the dentine which forms the soft inner core of the tooth. This is well supplied with nerves and soon lets you know when it's being eroded by acids! So a tooth is already severely damaged by the time pain is felt. Once a child's second teeth have been damaged or decayed they don't grow back – they've gone for life.

The level of tooth decay in almost every country in the world is linked with its sugar consumption. Sweets and sugary foods should ideally be avoided altogether as should foods containing white flour. If your children can't stop eating sweets, it's been shown that it's much better for them to have them all at once, rather than spread throughout the day, or, even better, once a week.

Here are some horrifying facts:

- By the age of five, children in Britain have on average five decayed, filled or missing teeth.
- More than 22 million people in Britain have false teeth and even children sometimes have to have full DENTURES.
- Tooth decay causes millions of lost school days.
- Dental decay causes more pain and suffering to children than any other condition.
- Tooth decay costs the country more than any other disease except mental illness.

There are three ways of fighting dental decay. First, the fluoridation of public water supplies in low FLUORIDE areas has been shown to halve dental decay in children all over the world. In the USA a third of the population drinks fluoridated water yet in the UK some dentists and many local authorities still think it inadvisable. Dental decay is falling in the USA yet rising steadily in Britain. Fluoride can also be given to children in toothpaste, tablets or drops if the water supply is low in fluoride. Older children can have fluoride applied to their teeth directly by their dentists.

Second, dentists play an important part in finding caries early and then restoring the teeth to normal. However, there's no point in filling teeth that will just rot again. The cure must be aimed at stopping dental decay in the first place. This involves not only changing your child's eating habits but ensuring that he goes regularly to the dentist after the age of three and a half to be sure to catch any decay early and save his teeth. Even first teeth are well worth saving because they ensure that the second teeth come through properly.

Third, the best tool for fighting decay costs

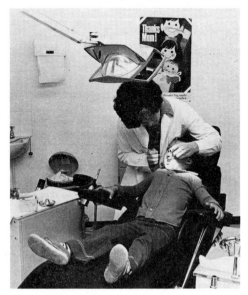

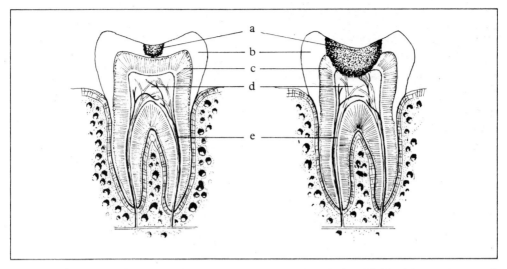

Dental caries at an early stage, and severe decay which has penetrated to the nerve of the tooth, producing toothache. a. decay, b. enamel, c. dentine, d. pulp chamber, e. nerve.

only a few pennies and is called a toothbrush. Most children (if they have a toothbrush at all) have one that is worn or soft – they should have a good, firm nylon brush. Talk to your dentist about how to teach your child to use the brush in the most effective way. In general, the teeth should be brushed using a stroking, rolling movement, always stroking from gum to tooth tip. If the gums are scrubbed, they'll bleed and can even be permanently damaged. Toothbrushing should never produce bleeding. If your child's gums bleed, see your dentist.

Dental disease of all kinds needs early recognition and treatment and you can't start too young. You should start cleaning your baby's teeth as soon as each one is fully out. Clean the first teeth gently with a cloth wrapped around the fingertip· and then, when he has all his milk teeth, clean them gently with a small nylon toothbrush. Encourage your child to play with his brush and soon tooth cleaning will become fun. Most children forget the back teeth, so make sure these are done properly. He'll probably need some help cleaning the inside surfaces. You may find that your child will get more fun (and therefore clean better) if he uses an electric toothbrush, but this obviously can't

be used until the child is old enough to use it properly.

Always use a fluoride toothpaste, except in tiny children who swallow it, and encourage your children to clean their teeth in the mornings after breakfast and at night before bed.

There are lots of other ways your dentist can help your child keep his teeth. Today, children don't have to lose their teeth – it's up to you.

Dental disease *See* DENTAL CARIES; GINGIVITIS; ORTHODONTICS

Dentures A set of artificial teeth made to take the place of lost natural ones. Usually the teeth are made of a special white plastic embedded in pink, gum-coloured plastic. There are many different types of denture and the type used depends on your child's dental problem.

There are over 22 million denture wearers in Great Britain today and many thousands of these are children. Even some pre-school children have dentures and this is scarcely something to be proud of as a country. The secret of keeping your child denture-free is to look after his natural teeth very carefully right from the start. Additional FLUORIDE as drops or tablets (if your drinking water is low in fluoride), meticulous daily brushing and complete avoidance or regulation of sweets and sugary things will help your child keep his natural teeth for life. We've become used to accepting tooth loss as normal but children who care for their teeth properly need never lose a permanent tooth.

See DENTAL CARIES; GINGIVITIS

Depression Many people confuse feeling low or having a touch of the blues with true depression. We all feel down from time to time when something or someone seems not to come up to our expectations. Depression is more serious because the sufferer can't snap out of it (contrary to the belief of many surrounding him).

Even babies may suffer from depression and an extreme example of this is seen in babies of over four months who are separated completely from their mothers. Their initial reaction is of apprehension and crying and this is followed by a withdrawal of interest in people. Over a period of time the child's psychological development is retarded and he becomes apathetic.

A similar picture of apathy, boredom, being fed up, unhappiness, retarded development or even regression can be seen in children of any age in response to circumstances that make them miserable.

Symptoms of depression may be masked by activity or unusual behaviour. Some children become extremely frustrated with their inability to live up to their expectations of themselves (and others' expectations of them) and may become aggressive or delinquent as a result. Such aggressive children are often so inward-looking that they become accident prone or develop aches and pains.

Suicidal thoughts are very rare in young children but are more common in adolescents and should be taken seriously. In England and Wales between 1962 and 1968, 31 children between the ages of 12 and 14 committed suicide. No child under the age of 12 killed himself. Suicide notes indicated intense feelings of anger and a desire to avoid punishment or humiliation for disciplinary problems at school.

If your child is often or persistently miserable, see your doctor, because he himself may be able to help or he may suggest referral to a child psychiatrist for individual or family therapy.

See HOSPITAL

Dermatitis A broad term used to describe inflammation of the skin due to many causes. Affected areas are usually reddened, swollen and itchy. Blisters may be present and scratching can make the skin thicken and can also introduce infection.

Dermatitis is basically caused by irritating chemicals which come into contact with the skin – a chemical is by definition a 'primary irritant' if it causes dermatitis in 50 per cent of people exposed to it. Irritants that children meet are relatively few: adults tend to come across them more often at work, for instance acids, alkalis, oil, cement and detergents. NAPPY RASH in its most usual form is a type of primary irritant dermatitis, the chemical involved being ammonia. This is released from the baby's urine by organisms from the bowel as urine and faeces come into close, warm contact in a wet nappy. Ammonia makes the eyes water and has a distinctive smell.

Treatment of primary irritant dermatitis is to keep the offending chemical away from the skin; with nappy rash, for example, the skin should be washed with soap and water at each nappy change to remove traces of ammonia and the nappy should be changed frequently.

Dermatitis may also be caused by an ALLERGY to certain chemicals. Only sensitive or allergic people react in this way. This sort of dermatitis is called allergic contact dermatitis (contact ECZEMA). It may not show up after the first exposure to the chemical involved – repeated exposure may be necessary to sensitize the child. Once sensitized, inflammation begins after ten days from the contact. The sensitivity is very specific, which is why patch testing can be very helpful in diagnosing which chemicals are to blame. (*See* PATCH TEST.) Allergic contact dermatitis in children may be caused by exposure to primula plants; certain chemicals in toys, shoes and clothing; and some drugs used in creams and ointments, such as local anaesthetics and antihistamines.

Another type of allergic dermatitis (eczema) is caused by eating certain foods or drugs.

It is usually very difficult to find out exactly which food is the culprit but when it is known, that food should be eliminated from the diet for good.

CRADLE CAP is often seen with a form of dermatitis called seborrhoeic dermatitis. This is a condition seen in people of all ages and takes the form of a greasy, scaly, brownish-yellowish rash on the scalp, face, behind the ears or, in babies, on the nappy area. Affected children may suffer from BLEPHARITIS or styes (see STYE). Treatment is with ointment containing hydrocortisone.

The sort of dermatitis most worrying to parents is atopic dermatitis (atopic eczema).

Desensitization   A form of treatment aimed at preventing the symptoms of children who suffer from HAY FEVER or ASTHMA.

The child is usually first patch tested to determine the allergens to which he or she is sensitive. The parents may have noticed that certain things produce the symptoms. If the patch tests confirm what has been noticed, a vaccine can be given corresponding to the child's individual sensitivities. (*See* PATCH TEST.)

Densitization takes the form of a course of injections of the vaccine over a period of several weeks or months. Very occasionally a hypersensitivity reaction occurs as a result of an injection, so the doctor giving the injection

will watch carefully for any immediate reaction in particular. Young children do not take kindly to injections and a balance must be struck between the severity of the symptoms and the emotional upset of the treatment.

Though this method of treating allergic conditions has been used for many years, it is only recently that the mechanism behind the method has been understood to any degree. Though useful, desensitization is by no means infallible and is not to be recommended unless the symptoms are really troublesome.

See ALLERGY

Development   From conception, through foetal life and childhood to adulthood, the body not only grows in size but also develops in complexity so that the maturing child gradually becomes capable of doing more and more. Development can be measured by assessing physical and mental prowess but, basically, all the changes in the body's workings are due to the maturing of various metabolic and cellular systems.

As a child grows, he develops the ability to move by himself—first by rolling, then perhaps by crawling or shuffling on his bottom, and, finally, by walking. At the same time he learns to keep his head steady so he can watch things easily, to turn it towards sound and also to grasp and manipulate objects accurately with his fingers.

Check-ups at child health clinics make certain that babies and young children are developing well both physically and mentally.

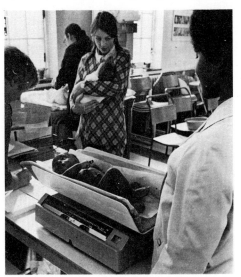

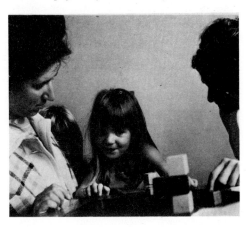

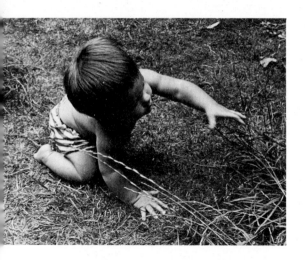

As a baby learns to crawl, he also becomes increasingly aware of the world around him. He can focus on small objects and manipulate them easily.

Later physical development is not so startling. The child becomes increasingly confident on his feet and develops skilled abilities such as being able to skip, kick a ball, write and knit. Fine manual dexterity varies a lot in different people and some children become dextrous more quickly than others, often remaining so all their lives.

There is a tremendously wide variation in the ages at which children sit, crawl and walk and, in fact, do most things, so although it is wise to take your child for routine developmental checks, there is rarely any need to worry if your child is relatively slow. Comparisons between different children may be interesting, but are rarely helpful. Speech development also varies greatly in timing in different children. However, a child who is late in talking is all the time listening and remembering and this is good preparation for the acquisition of 'proper' speech.

Mental development is just as exciting as physical development in children. From conception onwards the child learns how to deal with incoming information from his eyes, ears, nose, mouth and skin and how to react to the information. His brain is a complicated storehouse of memories which is also able to create new ideas and work out problems. Some

children are better able to use their brains in the accepted academic sense of the term than others. Although each child should be encouraged to reach his or her full academic potential, a clever child will not necessarily enjoy life any more than a dull one, so there is no point in becoming too concerned about school results.

Healthy emotional development is vital to the overall wellbeing of the person. Unless he develops a stable relationship with the person or persons – usually his parents – closest to him, a child will be in danger of being emotionally insecure for the rest of his life. Parental love is perhaps the biggest single gift that a child can receive. The ability to release a child from close family ties and to encourage his independence as he grows up is also important. A child will find it difficult to develop adult emotional maturity if he is never released from being his parents' baby.

For many people, spiritual development is important. It's often said that it's wrong to force religion down a child, but many millions of children the world over are brought up in societies in which God is a very important figure indeed to each individual. Perhaps the best way of encouraging a child's spiritual development is by letting him grow up in an environment in which God is obviously important to the people surrounding him so that he grows up aware of a spiritual dimension to life.

Parents in this country need more reassurance than ever before about their children's developmental progress. This is partly because their own parents often live far away and can't always give the benefit of their own experience in bringing up children. Also few families nowadays have more than two or three children, so parents themselves lack the experience that parents of much larger families in the past acquired. The system of child health clinics in Britain provides a good source of help and advice about the growth and development of children, and every child in the country is entitled to receive regular routine developmental checks until the age of starting school. After that the school medical service takes over. A fault with the system however is that the children most in need of help are often the ones not brought in by their parents. The remedy for this may come – as in Scandinavia – with more developmental checks being done by qualified workers in people's homes.

See GROWTH; LANGUAGE

Diabetes mellitus A complicated disease of metabolism in which the pancreas doesn't produce enough of the hormone insulin. The disease tends to run in families. Diabetes results in a high level of blood sugar (usually kept low by insulin) and a spill-over of sugar into the urine. There are lots of theories as to the cause of diabetes and it can be controlled by diet, tablets or injections. However, it is still a serious condition because, if it's not properly controlled, the high blood sugar level can permanently damage the arteries.

Four out of five diabetics in the UK suffer from a type of the disease called 'maturity onset' diabetes, caused by relatively too little insulin in the body because the person is too fat. When the sufferer slims, the body mass is reduced and the insulin can cope again. The other one-fifth of diabetics suffers from the 'juvenile' or childhood onset of the disease, which is more serious.

Diabetes isn't common in childhood and only about one in twenty of the diabetics in this country are children. When it does occur in a child, it's serious because the child can so suddenly become acutely ill. Most adult diabetics respond to tablets or even just to diet or slimming but this is not the case in children who must be treated with injections of insulin.

The first evidence of diabetes is sometimes COMA, the child becoming increasingly drowsy from the very high level of sugar in the blood – a condition that needs urgent medical attention. Usually the child has become thinner with increased thirst and the frequent need to pass urine. These symptoms are not always noticed. They should always lead to the testing of urine for sugar. You need not worry about occasional bouts of thirst or odd days when urine is passed more often if the child is well, energetic and maintaining his weight. Sometimes there is abdominal pain and vomiting in the acute stage of the disease. But don't worry if your child

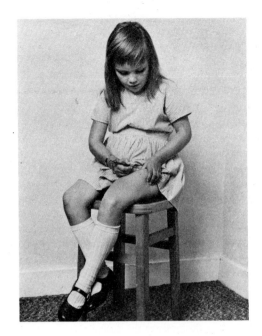

Many diabetic children are quite happy to take responsibility for administering their insulin injections themselves.

passes more urine than usual or indeed if he gets especially thirsty from time to time: it's unlikely that he's becoming diabetic and there is usually a simple explanation.

Your doctor will be able to tell you if your child is diabetic by simple tests. First, he'll test the urine and, if it contains sugar, he'll want to do a blood test.

Until the mid 1920s, childhood diabetes was a universally fatal condition but today it's a very different story. Insulin, the missing hormone, can now be produced from animals so that it can be injected into humans. Unfortunately, insulin cannot be taken by mouth because it would be digested in the gut along with other food, so this means it has to be injected subcutaneously. Try to overcome your distaste for injecting your child. Set him a good example because he will have to inject himself one day. The age at which children are ready to inject themselves varies. Many like to feel independent and take responsibility for themselves but no pressure should be put on them to hurry. Mothers can learn to manage their child's diabetes with only infrequent trips to the specialist. The amount of insulin needed is originally decided by the specialist but must be varied according to how much sugar there is in the urine. This means that the urine has to be tested regularly but this is easily done with home kits in a minute or two and can eventually be done by the child.

Insulin doesn't cure diabetes but prevents the unpleasant and dangerous symptoms from developing. There is as yet no permanent cure. However, some top politicians, doctors and even sportsmen are diabetic yet live perfectly normal lives. Parents of diabetic children should treat them as normally as possible, yet remain on the lookout for any potential problems and carefully watch their insulin and food balance. A 'blow-out' at a party will mean that more insulin is needed and the school sports day will mean that the child will need less. All these variations become a part of life that the interested mother learns to manage.

Diabetic children are expected to lead normal lives but they can get into trouble if insulin, exercise and food intake get out of balance. Almost always the trouble they get into is caused by too low a blood sugar. Should a diabetic child ever exhibit a combination of any of the following signs he should take sugar by mouth to make him better. Sometimes the very condition itself will make him confused so your prompt action could save his life. Signs to look for are: sweating, trembling, tingling around the tongue and lips, paleness, weakness, palpitations, hunger with nausea, staggering as if drunk, uncharacteristic behaviour, bad temper, and yawning.

Diabetic children ought to carry sugar lumps around with them for just such an emergency. If a child is conscious, get him to take a couple of sugar lumps or a teaspoonful of jam. *Never force an unconscious diabetic to eat or drink anything* as you may choke him. Only give him drinks and things to eat when he is conscious enough to hold the cup or spoon himself. *If he is unconscious – call an ambulance.* Once you have given him the first sweet food or drink, stay with him and give more if he isn't better within two or three minutes.

Diarrhoea The frequent passage of loose or fluid motions. The motions are loose because of the fast passage of bowel contents through the bowel.

Children get diarrhoea for many reasons. One of the commonest non-infective types in babies is simply caused by too much sugar or fruit juice in the diet. Breast-fed babies normally have frequent, orange-yellow, liquid stools during the first few weeks of life, usually passed after a feed. Every nappy may be stained yellow, and this is quite normal. Many young children, from the age of weaning to four years, have frequent soft stools containing bits of vegetables (especially carrots, peas, beans and tomato skins) which have passed through the digestive tract unchanged, but there is no need to do anything about this and the child will certainly come to no harm.

Intolerance to the lactose (milk sugar) in milk can cause loose stools (*see* SUGAR INTOLERANCE), especially in children of certain races. Lactose intolerance or intolerance of other sugars can cause continuing diarrhoea following an attack of acute GASTROENTERITIS in any child, and is due to damage to the lining of the small bowel which normally produces lactase and other enzymes which digest sugars. The avoidance of milk (and its replacement in a baby with a suitable substitute) for two to three weeks allows the small bowel lining to recover.

Some children get diarrhoea as a symptom of 'allergy' (intolerance) to cows' milk protein. Improvement in symptoms following the removal of, or reduction in, the amount of cows' milk and cows' milk products from the diet confirms the diagnosis. If breast milk is not available, there are suitable soya bean protein based milks available for babies as a substitute for cows' milk. Goat's milk can be used but may in turn cause allergy (*see* MILK).

Older children sometimes get diarrhoea if they are worrying about something such as an exam. Children of all ages may have diarrhoea during treatment of an infection with ANTIBIOTICS, though some doctors report that giving fresh, live yoghourt every day to children on penicillin prevents diarrhoea. An infection itself (usually of the respiratory tract or ears) can actually cause diarrhoea because the viruses responsible for the infection also affect the gut.

Older children may have loose stools containing blood and mucus if they are suffering from ULCERATIVE COLITIS.

Until recently it was unusual to find any evidence of infection when culturing stools from a child with diarrhoea, but we now know that a virus which was previously unrecognized (the rotavirus) causes much of this diarrhoea in children under the age of six years. The disease has an incubation period of 48 hours. Bottle-fed babies are much more likely to suffer from gastroenteritis due to infection with viruses or bacteria (especially E. coli) than breast-fed babies, because they don't have the protective immunity from their mothers' milk. When they come into contact with bacteria, for example from badly sterilized bottles and teats, they are less able to resist infection than breast-fed babies, because modified cows' milk doesn't contain the specific antibodies and the many non-specific anti-infective factors that are present in breast milk.

FOOD POISONING can cause severe diarrhoea and can be caused either by swallowing the toxins produced in food by certain bacteria or by eating the bacteria themselves. Dysentery, a disease caused by swallowing infected food, can be highly infectious and can spread like wildfire round schoolchildren unless scrupulous hygiene is observed.

When a child has diarrhoea, he loses a great deal of fluid as watery motions. If he also vomits, the fluid loss is more serious unless he is able to replace the loss by keeping down drinks. For an older child with mild diarrhoea only it is wise to give him plenty to drink and not to worry if he doesn't want to eat. A child with diarrhoea and VOMITING is more difficult to cope with, especially if he will keep nothing down. You should ask for your doctor's advice without delay. If the only fluid he has kept down for 24 hours is water, again you should ask for your doctor's advice.

In babies, diarrhoea is potentially more serious than in older children because of the relatively greater risks of DEHYDRATION. The breast-fed baby with diarrhoea alone should be breast fed more frequently to provide more fluid. The bottle-fed baby should be given

extra drinks of water if his diarrhoea is mild but if it is severe, or if he is also vomiting, your doctor may advise giving him a special glucose-salt solution instead of his milk. Milk is not only less likely to be kept down but can also (if too strong) increase the risks of dehydration and should be stopped for 24 to 36 hours. When the diarrhoea has stopped, milk and solids can be gradually reintroduced and the baby should be back on his full diet by the end of the fourth day. The breast-fed baby with both diarrhoea and vomiting may keep down a glucose-salt solution (prescribed by the doctor) better than breast milk, and his mother can maintain her milk supply by expressing her milk until he can again keep it down.

Any child of whatever age with diarrhoea and vomiting who can't keep enough fluid down may need to be given intravenous fluids in hospital.

A baby with mild diarrhoea should not be given unmodified cows' milk or too many solids as the strength of these feeds may make any dehydration much more severe. Use any one of the recommended modified dried milks available made up in the correct dilution.

A child with persistent, large loose stools who is failing to gain weight may be suffering from a disease such as cystic fibrosis or coeliac disease, so ask for your doctor's advice if your child has persistent diarrhoea.

Sometimes diarrhoea can be a sign of CONSTIPATION. In this case, the hard stools lie in the rectum and loose motions leak around the blockage. The child may soil his pants (see SOILING), and treatment includes altering his diet to avoid constipation in the future.

Digestion Every part of our body is made up from the food we eat but most of our foods are complicated chemical substances that first have to be broken down by enzymes before they can be absorbed by the gut (intestine). This breaking down of food into simple building blocks is called digestion.

Digestion starts in the mouth where enzyme-containing juices produced by the salivary glands start to break down starches. Chewing food helps digestion by making the particles

85

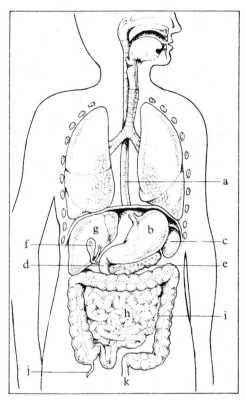

Diagram of the digestive system. a. gullet,
b. stomach, c. spleen, d. duodenum, e. pancreas,
f. gall bladder, g. liver (in section), h. small
intestine, i. large intestine, j. appendix, k. rectum.

Foods rich in roughage, once thought to be harmful, are now known to be a positive aid to digestion and actually help prevent certain bowel diseases.

Indigestion, a pain or discomfort in the upper abdomen, usually follows eating too much of certain foods, or a combination of foods that disagree with one another. If children are taught to chew their food properly and to avoid excesses of foods that upset them, indigestion shouldn't be a problem. However, any child who persistently complains of tummy pain or indigestion should see a doctor.

Certain disease conditions of the bowel prevent normal digestion. (*See* MALABSORPTION.)

Diphtheria A serious disease caused by bacteria spread from person to person, mainly by droplet infection from the mouth or nose.

Since the introduction of IMMUNIZATION against diphtheria for all children in this country, the disease has virtually disappeared. However, it is thought that if the proportion of people in the community who are immunized drops below about 70 per cent, then the disease may again become a hazard to both adults and children. The basic course of three immunizations for a baby starts in the first six months. Diphtheria immunization is usually combined with that of tetanus and whooping cough in a 'triple' vaccine, given at the same time as the oral polio vaccine. At the age of five years children are given a booster dose of diphtheria vaccine, together with tetanus toxoid and oral polio.

Diphtheria is still occasionally seen and it needs urgent treatment to prevent complications. The bacteria usually multiply in the throat, producing a greyish membrane over the tonsils and a characteristic smell. The child is very often ill but does not have a fever. Sometimes the nose is the main site involved, causing a blood-stained discharge from a nostril. When the larynx is affected, breathing becomes difficult from obstruction by the membrane and emergency hospital treatment is needed.

The bacteria don't spread throughout the body but produce a potent poison or toxin which attaches itself to tissues in the heart and

of food smaller and mixing them well with saliva. In the stomach, other enzymes (breakdown chemicals) split the food. The small intestine also produces enzyme-containing juices. Eventually, all food is broken down into very simple sugars, fats and amino acids which are then absorbed through the wall of the intestine. From here they travel in the bloodstream to the liver where they are stored or altered for special uses in the body.

The process of digestion goes on every minute of the day and night. Food stays for several hours in the stomach, where it's acted upon by acids and enzymes and it may take several days to go right through the bowel and emerge as stools. Lots of things influence the speed at which food passes through the gut but probably the greatest single thing is the amount of roughage (dietary fibre) that we eat.

nervous system especially. The involvement of the heart can cause heart failure and that of the nerves can cause, among other things, paralysis of the muscles of breathing, so it is imperative that treatment should be given before the toxin has a chance to do its damage. The problem is that the diagnosis of diphtheria may easily be overlooked because there are so few doctors today who have actually seen the disease. Once the diagnosis is suspected, early treatment can still save the child's life.

Treatment consists of giving the patient a dose of diphtheria anti-toxin together with antibiotics. As the child recovers, his activity is very gradually increased and when he is better he should have a proper course of immunization, as the disease itself does not produce lasting immunity.

Dirt eating (pica) Many quite normal babies and toddlers put dirt into their mouths or even eat unsuitable substances, such as earth, sand, grass, coal, flaking paint or plaster. This is all a part of the general exploration of their surroundings and they also do it for the enjoyment they get from sucking objects and exploring them with their tongues and mouths. However, neurotic or mentally retarded children are more likely to do it repeatedly.

There is a danger that by eating lead-impregnated matter the child may have too high a level of lead in his body and so suffer from the effects of LEAD POISONING.

Some children who eat unsuitable things have an iron deficiency ANAEMIA and, once this is treated, lose their abnormal appetites.

Yet others swallow hair from their heads or from dolls or brushes, or fur, wool or cotton from their clothes or blankets. This material usually passes through the bowels but it has been known for a hairball in the stomach to cause indigestion, or for one in the intestine to cause an actual blockage needing surgical treatment.

Down's syndrome The name for mongolism, a condition affecting about one child in every six hundred.

Down's children are handicapped to some extent in their mental development, and form a large proportion of the children in special

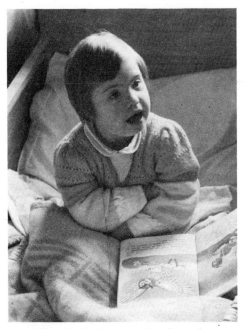

A small girl suffering from Down's syndrome (mongolism), with the characteristic small round head and slanting eyes.

schools for the educationally subnormal (ESN). Some are able to cope in ordinary schools or in schools for mildly ESN children, while others need the extra staff and care provided in those schools for the severely ESN. Their intelligence varies widely and while many of them will later be able to lead relatively independent lives, perhaps living in sheltered hostels, some will need the protection offered by parents or hospitals all their lives.

Physically they are fairly easily recognizable as a group: their eyes are small and slant up at the outer corners; there is a fold of skin at the inner corner of each eye; the nasal bridge is low; the head is small and round; the mouth is small and straight; and the hands usually show abnormalities of the crease lines, together with a small little finger, curved inwards.

The incidence of leukaemia is about three times the average and mongol children are prone to respiratory infections. They used to have a relatively short life expectancy but with modern treatment of respiratory infections they may now often live on into middle and old age.

The cause of Down's syndrome is a chromosomal abnormality in the baby. There are four basic types of abnormality of the chromosomes but the commonest type (90 per cent) is that in which there are 47 chromosomes instead of the usual 46 in each of the baby's cells. Older mothers are more likely to have a child with mongolism of this type and the risk of a woman having a mongol child increases sharply in the mid to late thirties, so that at 40 her risk is of the order of one in 40.

The basic cause of this type of mongolism is as yet unknown and such a mother is no more likely than anyone else of her age to have another affected child. AMNIOCENTESIS during pregnancy in older mothers determines whether the foetus is normal or not and an abortion can be performed (if the mother so desires) should the baby be a mongol. Amniocentesis is widely available and is especially helpful for pregnant women over the age of 35.

A few mongol children have inherited the condition from one or other parent, who may look normal but in fact has a chromosomal abnormality. Chromosomal studies are done on each mongol baby to determine which sort of mongolism is present: genetic counselling can then be offered to the parents so that they have some idea of the risks of having another child with the condition.

A Down's child changes a family's life. Many parents accept the challenge to do their best for the baby and hence give it the best possible start. Sometimes, caring for these children is so difficult and time consuming that the parents are unable to cope and need occasional or even permanent institutional care for the child. The health visitor, family doctor or social worker should be able to let parents know what services are available to help the family with a mongol child.

See EDUCATIONAL SUBNORMALITY; MENTAL RETARDATION

Drinking We live in a society in which the social drinking of alcohol is extremely common. Unfortunately millions of people's lives are ruined by alcohol and the patterns, as with smoking and other social behaviour, are set at home in the family.

Most children have their first alcoholic drink at home and one survey of 7,500 young people aged between 13 and 16 found that only 8 per cent of girls and 6 per cent of boys were non-drinkers (had only ever had one drink of alcohol or none). Although we hear about young people drinking more than they did in the past (it's certainly a fact that more youngsters are starting younger), probably fewer than 10 per cent of all children who drink are socially affected by it. When trouble does start it's usually in the form of truancy, hangovers, violence and falling foul of the police.

Small amounts of alcohol do no harm (unlike small numbers of cigarettes) so don't be prohibitive about drinking. Start your children off with watered-down drinks and teach them that alcoholic drinks are of different strengths. Many children think sherry, wine and spirits are all equally 'alcoholic' but of course this is not true. Your good example should set them off on the right tracks.

Drowning The most important thing to remember is that children can drown in only a few inches of water. A child can drown in his bath as easily as at the seaside or in a lake, so when bathing a young baby or small child, never leave him alone. Ignore the telephone or front door bell or take the baby with you, wrapped up warmly in a towel.

Drowning occurs more commonly at the

If a child has taken water into his lungs and stopped breathing, start artificial respiration (the kiss of life) as soon as possible – as soon as you can get a foot on the bottom.

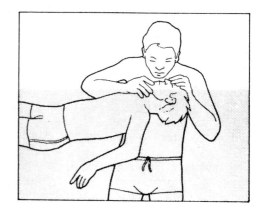

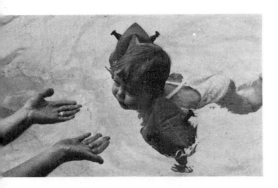

Ideally, children should be taught to swim as early as possible. Floatation aids allow them to get used to the water when very young.

seaside or when afloat. Always make sure that your children wear properly designed and tested life jackets if they are going to be on a boat, or well fitting 'floatation aids' if they can't swim. They may think you're being very fuddy-duddy and will want to be grown-up and leave them off. Do persist though because one wrong step can spell disaster for a small child even if he can swim and is used to water. Another preventive measure is to get children used to water as young as possible. A baby under a year may like playing in water with his parents, and older children should learn to swim as soon as possible.

If a child takes enough water into his lungs to cause breathing problems, there's only one thing to do in an emergency and that is to perform the KISS OF LIFE. Don't worry about emptying water out of his lungs because there's really very little water in a drowned person's lungs. Simply get on with mouth-to-mouth resuscitation as soon as you can, even before you get to dry land. As soon as you can get a foot on the bottom yourself get a few breaths into the child's lungs. Remember, if he is small, not to blow too hard.

Once breathing restarts, lie the child on his side in the recovery position so that he can't roll on to his back – this will prevent him from inhaling vomit and is important because people often vomit after being unconscious. Once the child has regained consciousness (or even sooner if there are people you can send off for help) get a doctor to see the child. It's worth persevering for a long time when resuscitating a drowned child because recovery can occur after a surprisingly long time.

See HEART MASSAGE

Drowsiness *See* COMA

Dummy Arguments have raged for years over the use of dummies, and many parents are confused as to whether to let their children have them or not. It used to be said that dummies were bad because if they got dirty they could transfer infections. Older babies often put dirty things in their mouths with no ill effects so this argument is scarcely valid. However, it's sensible to wash a dummy every time it's dropped on the ground or floor, or to tie it on to the pram with a short string.

There are three things wrong with dummies. First, they don't have a sense of feel like a finger or thumb. If a child has to suck anything – and it may be very comforting for him to do so – encourage him to suck his thumb or fingers. In this way he at least gets some 'feedback' from the feel of his own fingers and explores his mouth at the same time. Incidentally, a child can't lose his thumb, whereas the loss of a dummy by a dummy-dependent child can upset him greatly. Second, dummies can be coated or filled with sweet fluids and this is a real problem. Many mothers dip dummies in honey or treacle or give their babies a comforter filled with orange juice or rose hip syrup. This is very bad indeed for the child's growing teeth because we now know that it is in the first few months after they appear that children's teeth are at their most vulnerable to tooth decay. A constant bath of sugary fluid in the mouth is the surest way to rot valuable first teeth. Third, a dummy may discourage a sufficient supply of breast milk if the baby doesn't stimulate the breast because he prefers to suck the dummy.

There is no conclusive evidence that dummies or thumb sucking of themselves cause crooked teeth. A child whose teeth grow crooked would have had this problem whether or not he had ever sucked his thumb or a dummy although thumb sucking can bring an underlying predisposition to crooked teeth to light.

Dwarfism *See* SMALL CHILDREN

Dyslexia A term surrounded by confusion which has led many parents to worry that their child with poor reading ability in fact has unrecognized dyslexia. The term dyslexia is mainly used to refer to a specific reading retardation, as opposed to general reading backwardness often found in children with other learning problems. Three times as many boys as girls have a specific reading retardation.

Children with a specific reading retardation may be very bright or very dim, but the thing they have in common is that while other areas of learning present no problem (within the limits of their intelligence), reading is extremely difficult. They are unable to recognize words even if they can pick out individual letters, and they cannot spell words even if they can write down individual letters. The letters are also often wrongly written.

The reading difficulty may create emotional problems which are often more noticeable in the bright child who is expected, both by his parents and teachers, to succeed. The child may become withdrawn or aggressive, drawing attention away from his basic problem and making diagnosis more difficult. He may have symptoms of stress such as abdominal pain, asthma or cyclical vomiting.

Reading is a valuable skill in our society and most of us need to be able to read, even if only to fill in forms. It is therefore of great importance that children with a reading disability of any kind – and particularly a specific reading retardation – should be picked out and given appropriate help. With skilled help, they can learn to read, though they may always have problems, especially with spelling. Remedial reading lessons are in short supply at many schools, and parents will be advised in some cases to get extra lessons outside.

Before the diagnosis of dyslexia is made, it is essential to consider whether there are problems with deafness, visual problems, emotional troubles other than those caused by the difficulty in education, an unstimulating home background, or poor general intelligence, all of which may produce a similar picture.

Dysmenorrhoea *See* MENSTRUATION

E

Earache Most earache in children is caused by OTITIS MEDIA. Infection of the ear canal, especially if there is a boil in it, may also cause pain, as may GLUE EAR and inflammation of the eardrum, commonly seen in measles and German measles.

However, earache can also be caused by several conditions which have nothing to do with the ear but affect areas which have a nerve supply in common with the ear. Pain from these areas is then referred to the ear. Such conditions include dental decay (especially in the lower molar teeth but also from an unerupted wisdom tooth); a disorder of the jaw joint; mumps; and a sore throat. Children who have had their tonsils out often have ear pain between the third and sixth day after the operation. Some children get earache after swallowing something rough such as a hard crust which scratches the back of the throat. Earache can also be caused by extremely cold weather, including a cold wind.

If your child has earache, warmth next to the ear, for instance from a hot water bottle, may help relieve the pain while you are awaiting medical advice. Analgesics in the correct dose are also useful.

If ever your child is miserable, rubs his ear, or screams with pain for no apparent reason, always get medical advice.

See DEAFNESS; EARS; OTITIS EXTERNA; PHARYNGITIS; TONSILLITIS

Ears The ear is made up of three parts – the outer fleshy piece, the pinna, the second part called the middle ear, and the inner ear which is embedded in the bones of the skull. The outer ear is separated from the middle ear by the eardrum.

The human ear is remarkable. It can pick

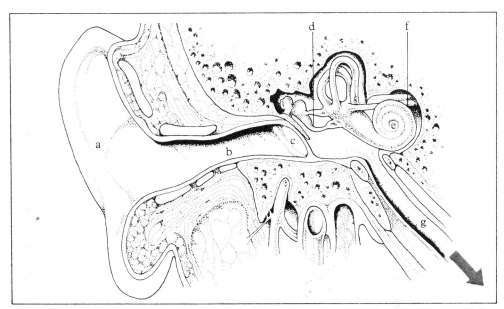

The structure of the ear. a. pinna, b. auditory canal, c. eardrum, d. small bones of inner ear, e. cochlea, f. auditory nerve, g. eustachian tube, leading to throat.

up the tiniest sound yet is able to cope with very loud noises. The ear is like a microphone: it collects sound waves, converts them to electrical impulses and transmits the sound messages to the brain. Here the noise is interpreted and this is perhaps the cleverest part of hearing because, unlike a microphone (which hears everything you point it at), the ear, or more accurately the brain to which it feeds its input, can pick out a single noise in a crowded room and shut off all the other noises so as to concentrate on that one sound.

The external or outer ear is called the pinna. This collects sound to some extent (though not nearly so specifically as it does in certain animals which can angle their ears towards sounds they want to hear) and channels it down the next part, the external auditory canal. When sound gets to the end of the short canal it reaches the eardrum – a delicate membrane of skin – and causes it to vibrate. These vibrations are transmitted to the innermost part of the ear via a chain of three tiny bones called ossicles in the middle ear. The middle ear is normally filled with air and is connected to the throat by a fine tube, the eustachian tube.

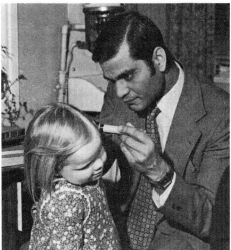

A routine ear examination at a nursery school. Hearing loss, especially in young children, must be detected early, if it is not to hinder their progress at school.

The inner ear consists of the cochlea or hearing organ and the labyrinth or balance organ. The cochlea is a snail-shaped organ full of fluid, membranes and sound receptors that have the ability to transform mechanical movement (produced by the vibrating eardrum) into electrical, nervous impulses. If the anatomical structure of the ear is impressive, the

91

power of the brain to analyse all the incoming information is even more so.

Just imagine developing a machine that could tell so many different sounds apart and identify different voices, musical instruments, bird calls and so on. Fortunately, apart from infections of the middle ear in childhood, this wonderful organ is subject to very few diseases and goes on working hour after hour, year in year out for most of our lives.

See DEAFNESS; EARACHE; GLUE EAR; OTITIS EXTERNA; OTITIS MEDIA; WAX

Eczema DERMATITIS of allergic origin which tends to run in families. The skin reaction is basically similar to that in other sorts of dermatitis, with reddening, itching, swelling, the formation of tiny blisters in the superficial layers of the skin and, later, weeping and crusting as the tiny blisters are broken by scratching. As eczema passes its acute phase the skin heals by becoming dry, scaly and thick.

Dermatitis in children may be caused by an ALLERGY to a skin irritant (allergic contact dermatitis) or to something inhaled or swallowed such as a food. In babies, it may be difficult to distinguish between eczema and seborrhoeic dermatitis. The most common type of dermatitis in children, and the most distressing, is atopic eczema, which tends to appear in children with a family history of eczema, asthma or hay fever and many affected children develop asthma in later life.

It is now firmly established that eczema is more common in infants if they have been given cows' milk instead of breast milk in the first few months of life. One large study that followed twenty thousand children for five years showed that there was seven times as much eczema in those children who had been bottle-fed as in those completely breast-fed. Babies given complementary feeds of cows' milk as well as breast milk are twice as likely to get eczema in childhood as those completely breast-fed. This survey also found that one in 20 bottle-fed babies developed eczema.

Unfortunately, just one feed of cows' milk (and all popular brands of baby milk are based on cows' milk) can sensitize a susceptible baby to cows' milk protein and cause eczema later when the baby has milk or milk products.

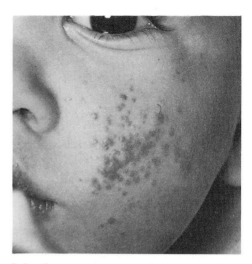

Infantile eczema.

In children from atopic families, half develop eczema if they are bottle-fed, whereas only eight per cent get it if they are breast-fed. It is thought that a baby's gut may 'leak' foreign proteins from foods other than breast milk into the bloodstream and so sensitize the baby to that protein, leading to the development of allergy. Breast milk protects against this leaking by lining the gut wall with antibodies. By the age of four to six months, most babies are producing enough of their own 'lining' antibody (immunoglobulin A) to protect themselves, and can therefore cope with foreign proteins in the form of cows' milk and other foods.

Other proteins such as eggs and wheat can also cause eczema if given in the first six months of life in particular. Some babies show a very quick reaction to the offending food, with urticaria, colic and a flushing of the skin, followed by scratching and the development of eczema, while in others the response is less clear cut and the diagnosis of eczema due to food allergy has to be made by excluding the suspected food from the child's diet and watching to see if there is any improvement over the course of a few weeks. The advice of a dietician is helpful when excluding any food from the diet.

Atopic eczema usually develops in the first two or three months of life and children tend to improve between the ages of three and five, though in some the skin lesions persist until middle age. Eczema usually appears first on the face and nappy area and spreads to the neck, wrists, hands and fronts of the legs and arms. In later childhood, eczema is more often confined to the creases of the elbows, behind the knees, the neck, face and behind the ears. Children with severe eczema often have whitish faces with thickened, dry skin.

The treatment of eczema is not yet satisfactory. A warm, moderately humid climate is the optimum and sun and salt water help in many cases. Sweating tends to aggravate the condition, so synthetic clothes should be avoided next to the skin. As wool also makes the itching worse, cotton underclothes and even top clothes are probably the best and affected babies should not crawl on woollen carpets.

The dryness of the skin can be minimized in several ways. Soaps and detergents should be avoided; oil should be added to the bath after the child has soaked in the water for some time, to rehydrate the skin: the oil then acts as a sealant, keeping the water in the skin; similarly creams and lotions are best put on to the skin after a soak in a bath. Cleansing lotions can be used in the bath instead of soap. Emulsifying ointment can be used either in the bath or applied directly to the skin.

Wet lotions applied under dressings can help in the acute stages of severe eczema but the most important thing is to prevent the child from scratching, as this aggravates the condition by leading to a vicious circle of scratch, itch, scratch. Fingernails should be kept short and drugs containing antihistamines may help control the itching.

In recent years the development of corticosteroid creams and ointments has helped the treatment of eczema enormously. The problem here is that these powerful drugs are absorbed through the skin to some extent and, if used in large enough amounts, can lead to side effects such as an abnormal thinning of the skin. Even more serious side effects can occur so these strong drugs should be used with caution.

Finally, it is worth removing items of food from the diet if it seems that any particular food leads to a worsening of the itching but the food needs to be excluded for several weeks for any real effect to be noticed.

Children with atopic eczema are at risk from developing 'eczema vaccinatum' if the virus of vaccinia infects their skin lesions. Vaccinia virus is used to vaccinate people against smallpox, so members of the family should not be vaccinated against this disease, nor should the child himself. A child with eczema can safely be immunized against diphtheria, tetanus, whooping cough, polio and (for a girl) German measles. If there is a specific history of allergy to egg protein, measles, 'flu and yellow fever vaccines should not be given.

Atopic eczema can be a very distressing condition both for the child and the family and may disrupt family life for a long time. If the child has difficulty in sleeping at night, mild sedatives (usually antihistamines) are helpful. The scratching child may be ostracized at school and needs sympathy and support both from parents and teachers. It's perhaps worth mentioning that a child with eczema is not infectious, as many people seem to think.

Educational subnormality A purely arbitrary expression used to describe children who are unable to cope with the education provided in ordinary schools in this country. Children classified as educationally subnormal do not fall into an easily recognizable group, and the decision as to whether or not to place a child in a school for the educationally subnormal is often a difficult one, requiring the advice of several experts in different fields.

Schools for these children are basically of two types, those for the mildly educationally subnormal ESN (M), and those for the severely educationally subnormal, ESN(S). The ESN(M) schools cater for those children who are able to benefit from normal educational techniques but need a higher staff ratio and more time to learn than average children, while the ESN(S) schools teach children unable to benefit from normal teaching techniques. These latter were formerly known as training centres.

There are many children who will obviously benefit from special education from the beginning of their school days. These include most children with DOWN'S SYNDROME and those definitely known to be mentally retarded, from whatever cause. These children can be assessed by doctors and psychologists with special training before starting school, so that the right sort of school is chosen. Large numbers of children are assessed to see if they need special education. Many are borderline in their performance and are sent to an ordinary school to see how they progress there. If a child gets on badly, the head teacher can arrange for special tests to be carried out by a doctor and a psychologist. Then, after discussion between the three of them and the parents, a transfer to a special school can be arranged if it is thought best for the child. Similarly, if a child does very well at an ESN school, a transfer can be made either from an ESN(M) school to an ordinary school or from an ESN(S) school to an ESN(M) school.

When a child is assessed before a school is chosen, several tests are done, including an intelligence test, vision and hearing tests and a general physical examination. The child is referred to specialists if there is any problem which may be contributing to his educational difficulties. Psychologists are well aware of the dangers of relying too heavily on the results of intelligence tests and it is unlikely that a child would be wrongly sent to a special school.

See INTELLIGENCE; MENTAL RETARDATION

Encephalitis An inflammation of the brain which can be caused by viruses and bacteria, by a special type of allergy or, rarely, by immunizing injections. Several infections can spread to the brain but the commonest in children are WHOOPING COUGH, MEASLES, MUMPS and POLIOMYELITIS. Fortunately, inflammation of the brain with these infections is rare but when it does occur the effects can be very serious. Between 5 and 20 per cent of all encephalitis cases die and a further 20 per cent are left with mental disorder, memory loss, paralysis or personality change which make a normal life difficult. However, probably fewer than one in a thousand children who get measles, for example, will suffer from encephalitis.

There has been a lot of discussion about the dangers of encephalitis following the immunization of children for whooping cough and measles but it is now widely felt that the danger of getting encephalitis as a part of the disease (should the child catch it) is more serious than that of the immunization itself. Certain children should not be immunized against whooping cough or measles because they are more likely to get encephalitis – ask your doctor if your child is one of these.

Because many children with encephalitis also have inflammation of the meninges (*see* MENINGITIS) and the spinal cord, the symptoms vary. Usually, the child is irritable, drowsy and may develop convulsions and lapse into coma. Paralysis, especially of the facial muscles, may occur. There may be a fever, headache and, in babies, screaming, vomiting and abdominal pain.

A lumbar puncture is necessary to make the diagnosis. There is no special treatment for encephalitis and the severity depends very much on the causative agent.

Encopresis The involuntary passage of bowel motions. This is normal in a baby but can present considerable problems after a child is potty trained. In an older child it is usually caused by chronic CONSTIPATION with an overflow of liquid bowel motions around a craggy mass of solid bowel motion in the rectum. The child has frequent SOILING of his pants which looks like diarrhoea and the true cause of the problem may not be discovered for some time.

Very occasionally, the passage of normal bowel motions may occur by accident and this may simply represent the child's failure to hold his motions in until he can get to a lavatory.

Some children hold in their motions on purpose, perhaps because of a conscious or unconscious desire to upset their mothers. This sometimes happens if parents are over-zealous about potty training. The desire to open the bowels may be so great, however, that the child cannot hold the motions in any longer, and so will involuntarily soil his pants.

Children who soil their pants involuntarily may have emotional problems, learning disabilities such as dyslexia or may be hyperactive. Boys are more likely to do it than girls.

Careful medical and psychiatric treatment are necessary for some children with encopresis, especially as it can cause a schoolchild to be rejected by his peers because of the smell.

Endocrine glands *See* ADRENALS; GLANDS; OVARIES; PANCREAS; PITUITARY; TESTES; THYROID

Enuresis Incontinence of urine, normal in young children. Enuresis during the day in a child beyond the age of four years, when bladder control should have been achieved, is uncommon, especially in those who no longer wet the bed. However, it can occur in perfectly normal children, for instance if the bladder is very full and the child is too shy to ask if he can go to the lavatory when he is new at school. Many young children become engrossed in what they are doing from time to time and pass water in a puddle on the floor because they can't get to the lavatory quickly enough. Dampness of the pants because of an urgent desire to pass water is also commonplace.

If a child's pants are never dry for more than half an hour, he may have an abnormality of the opening of the ureter (the tube taking urine from the kidney to the bladder), causing constant dribbling incontinence.

One in ten children with nocturnal enuresis (*see* BED WETTING) also has daytime incontinence. If the child is ever dry for a night, it is unlikely that he has any abnormality of his urinary or nervous system.

Urinary tract infection, diabetes, epilepsy, mental retardation and a defect of the spinal cord (as in spina bifida) are all possible physical causes of enuresis.

Incontinence may be precipitated by laughing, coughing or crying.

See POTTY TRAINING

Epilepsy A disorder, often with CONVULSIONS (fits), that may also cause repeated, sudden, transient losses of consciousness. There are more than a hundred causes for such attacks, so epilepsy isn't strictly a disease in itself but more a collection of signs and symptoms. The vast majority of people with epilepsy suffer from fits not known to be associated with an underlying cause. It's important to remember that not every fit is epileptic.

Epilepsy may start at any age but frequently starts in infancy. The trouble occurs because the brain produces outbursts of abnormal electrical impulses which can occur from once in a lifetime to several times an hour. Most epileptic children are normal mentally and physically when the attacks start, and most are capable of leading a happy, fruitful life, especially with the help of drugs to control the fits.

There are two common types of epileptic fit. Petit mal is the mild type in which the child loses consciousness for a fleeting moment or two (perhaps looking vacant, staring into the distance or even wetting himself) but not for long enough to make him fall down. The child comes to very quickly and carries on as though nothing had happened. These attacks can occur many times a day.

In the more serious form of epilepsy, called grand mal, the child has a 'real' fit: he loses consciousness, wets himself, shakes, clenches his teeth and falls to the ground. Such attacks may come on suddenly and for no apparent reason, may be related to a feverish illness or may be precipitated by certain trigger situations such as flashing lights or television pictures. Children with epilepsy used to be shut away in colonies but today they can be cared for at home unless they are one of the tiny minority that has grand mal fits several times an hour. Children with epilepsy need to be treated as normally as possible by their parents and indeed by all those around them. This is especially important since we now know that children with epilepsy become strange or odd as much as the result of other people's reactions as because of their own anxiety at losing control of themselves.

There's no need to feel guilty or ashamed of your child if he has epileptic fits as there's nothing you could have done to prevent them.

As for treatment, in an acute attack it's simply a matter of protecting the child from damage. Don't force anything between a child's teeth as this can be difficult and you may break a tooth. Bitten tongues heal, broken teeth don't. Don't restrain the child who is fitting or you may damage his muscles because the contraction power is so great. Make sure he can breathe. Pull him away from furniture and other objects he might hurt himself against and watch him until the fit has ended. Many children want to sleep after a fit, so make him comfortable and let him sleep. Don't call a doctor if you know your child is an epileptic unless he has very long fits or repeated fits over a short period.

The basis of treating epilepsy is to prevent the spontaneous electrical outbursts in the brain that give rise to the attacks and this can now be done successfully in most cases with drugs. In the right doses these drugs shouldn't cause drowsiness or any lack of alertness. The tendency today is to try to find the right dose of one drug to suit the patient rather than giving him many drugs in combination.

Most epileptic children go to normal schools and play all the usual games. Even swimming and climbing are to be encouraged under supervision but these children should not be too closely watched or made to feel odd.

Career guidance is essential for older children with epilepsy, but there are few jobs closed to a person with well-controlled fits.

Erection   *See* MASTURBATION

Eustachian tube   *See* EARS

Eyes   Each eye is a near perfect sphere embedded for protection in the bone of the face. A baby's eyes are relatively large (two-thirds of adult size at birth) compared with the rest of his head. Each eye has three coats which have specific functions. The outermost is the tough, fibrous one which forms the sclera behind and the cornea in front. The middle coat is made of blood vessels and forms the iris in front, and the innermost coat, the retina, is made of specialized nervous tissue.

Light enters the eye through the pupil and the amount of light allowed in is regulated by the dark iris which acts like a diaphragm on a camera lens. This diaphragm closes down in bright light and opens up in dim light. The light travels through the jelly-like fluid which fills the eyeball to the lens which focuses it on the retina. There the images of the outside world are transformed into electrical (nervous) impulses which would then go to the brain for interpretation.

The structures of the eye can be examined by a doctor with a simple hand instrument

*The eye in cross-section. a. conjunctiva,
b. cornea, c. aqueous humour, d. pupil, e. iris,
f. lens, g. vitreous humour, h. retina, i. choroid,
j. sclera, k. retinal vessels, l. optic nerve,
m. ocular muscle.*

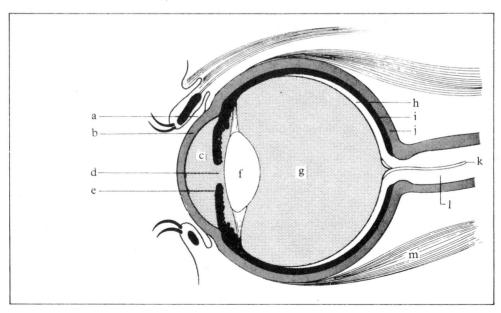

called an ophthalmoscope. He can learn much about the general working of the body by looking at the various parts of the eye because many diseases show themselves here and it is the only place in the body where he can easily look at working arteries and veins.

The eyes are moved by the action of several small muscles attached to the bones of the face. These enable us to move our eyes finely – much more finely and quickly than we could move our heads. The complexity of the co-ordination of the six muscles per eye contracting and relaxing all the time we're doing even the simplest thing is readily apparent. Any derangement of these tiny muscles means that the eyes don't move in parallel. This gives rise to a SQUINT and can also cause double vision.

The eye is protected by the eyelids, two folds of skin covered on the inside with a lubricated layer of conjunctiva which also covers the exposed surface of the eye. The lubrication is important so that small dust and grit particles don't score the surface of the cornea when the eyelids blink. The fluid for this constant 'washing' comes from the tear glands situated in the bony eye socket above the eyeball itself. Tears wash the front of the eye and pass out into the nose through the tear duct at the nasal end of the eye.

Newborn babies can see but their eyes have a fixed focus of 20cm. Many will follow a moving face if it is held 20cm away. As a baby grows older, he becomes able to focus easily on objects at varying distances.

Perhaps the greatest single advantage we have over many animals is our binocular vision. Most animals and birds have two eyes which work separately. Ours are cleverly interlinked so that we can see over a very wide area with the vision of each eye overlapping. This produces vision in depth. Try closing one eye and going about a few simple tasks. You'll see how you lose a whole dimension of vision. This also means that if there is a deficit in the vision of one eye, the other can make up for it to some extent. Binocular vision gives us the ability to judge size, shape and perspective with amazing accuracy.

See BLEPHARITIS; BLINDNESS; STYE; VISION TESTING; VISUAL PROBLEMS

Failure to thrive A term used for children who fail to gain or who even lose weight without any obvious cause. It is most often seen in babies. A thriving child is one who has a good appetite, whose weight gain is in the normal range and who is happy.

Most babies who fail to thrive do so because of environmental circumstances. They may have been emotionally deprived (for instance, in the case of LOW BIRTH WEIGHT babies reared in incubators without enough attention from their mothers); they may even have been battered or physically neglected – some perhaps not even being given enough to eat. It's important to remember that babies can become depressed and this can make them fail to thrive because they have lost their appetites and just don't seem to want feeds. Our western methods of child rearing are partly to blame for this sort of failure to thrive: mothers are taught that a baby's place is in his own cot in his own room for much of the day and all of the night. Many babies separated so much from their mothers are lonely and unhappy. Mothers are also taught that BREAST FEEDING should fit into a routine – feeds every three to five hours for a maximum of 10 minutes a side is a commonly advised schedule. It's scarcely surprising that so many babies breast-fed in this way become so hungry that their mothers have to give them complements of cows' milk, not realizing that the milk supply can be increased easily by feeding more often and for longer at each feed.

Not all babies fail to thrive because of environmental or feeding problems, however. Some have recognizable physical abnormalities, such as kidney disease, cystic fibrosis, an endocrine gland disorder, a chromosome disorder, a chronic infection or inflammation, or even a cancer. MALABSORPTION of food from the gut can also cause failure to thrive.

A child who is not growing as fast as he should may be admitted to hospital for a period of observation and routine tests. If the cause of his failure to thrive isn't readily apparent, more thorough tests are carried out.

Many families today are living in poor social circumstances, with little support for the parents from other adults. It's small wonder that their stress is often reflected in the children, who may not grow as well as they should.

See CHILD ABUSE; GROWTH; SMALL CHILDREN

Fainting A temporary loss of consciousness caused by a reduction of the blood flow to the brain. It is most common in older girls, especially in crowded, stuffy situations, when standing for long periods, and if a long time has elapsed since the last meal, causing a low blood sugar. School assembly provides an ideal environment for fainting, especially if a child has had no breakfast.

The lowered blood supply to the brain is caused by a relaxation of the walls of the veins in the legs, leading to pooling of the blood there. A hot bath makes the veins dilate and fainting is common when standing up after getting out of the bath. Anxiety makes a faint more likely, as do shock and severe pain. Some children are simply more liable to faint than others in the same situation.

A child about to faint feels 'light-headed', sweats, yawns and feels sick. He looks extremely pale. Most children know when they are going to faint and can prevent it by sitting with their heads between their knees or by lying down flat. To avoid fainting, some food for breakfast is a sensible start to the day. Many schools allow children to sit during assembly. Fresh air makes fainting less likely.

If a child faints, lay him down flat, loosen any tight clothing and let him rest quietly for a while. The loss of consciousness is only momentary – consciousness returns as soon as the blood flow to the brain is restored by the child falling into a horizontal position. Fainting is not dangerous, as long as the child does not hurt himself as he falls, and it does not endanger the brain.

Contrary to popular belief, fainting is not a sign of anaemia and is very rarely due to heart disease. Unlike loss of consciousness due to an epileptic fit, a faint does not make the child wet himself.

Schoolchildren may faint from OVERBREATHING. Young children may faint from BREATH HOLDING.

Feet Your child's feet need looking after from the very first days. Babies have pads of fat on the soles of their feet which make them appear flat. (*See* FLAT FEET.) Keep your baby out of shoes for as long as you can because a child's feet are healthier without shoes. Ensure that sleep suits, tights, socks and other clothes with built-in feet are big enough not to restrict movement of the child's toes: check this each time you wash things in case they have shrunk in the wash.

Always keep toenails clean and cut short. Cut them straight across or, in very little babies, bite them off. Check your child's shoe size regularly at a good shop that specializes in children's shoes and has the right equipment for measuring their feet. Try not to use discarded shoes from other children in the family because although they may be long enough, the width may be wrong and the second child's feet could be damaged. Many mothers put their children in plimsolls which are too small, so keep a check on all your child's footwear.

If your child wears wellingtons to school he should take a change of shoes with him because they encourage sweaty feet. Children should wear woollen or cotton socks in preference to nylon or other man-made fibres because most children's shoes have composition soles which make the feet very sweaty. Keep an eye on your child's feet for verrucae (warts on the soles – see WART) and ATHLETE'S FOOT (between the toes). If you are worried about your child's feet – see your doctor or a chiropodist. Don't attempt to cut corns, verrucae or indeed anything else off your child's feet. Leave it to the experts.

Crooked or webbed toes are fairly commonly seen congenital abnormalities. Surgical correction of crooked toes is rarely necessary unless it is impossible to buy well-fitting shoes.

See CLUB FOOT; INTOEING

Fever A rise in body TEMPERATURE can be due to many causes and often a fever occurs for no apparent reason. The body's temperature stays remarkably constant at an average of 98.4°F (37°C) but this level fluctuates in response to injury or insult to the body.

Heat is generated by the body as its cells metabolize nutrients and oxygen. The amount of blood flowing through the skin and the activity of the sweat glands normally control the loss of heat so as to keep production and loss in balance. The body's temperature varies a little during the day: it is lowest in the morning, reaches a maximum at about 10 p.m. and sinks again in the early morning.

In general, the temperature regulating mechanism of children is not as efficient as that of adults, so children get hotter in hot weather and colder in the cold. They also have higher temperatures with infections. Some children are more prone than others to running a high temperature.

Taking the temperature must be done carefully. Infants have to have their temperatures taken rectally because they might break the end off a thermometer in their mouths and

Tepid sponging to reduce a high temperature.

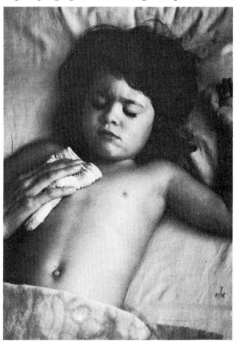

they wriggle too much to have it under their armpits. Older children will usually keep a thermometer under the tongue, where it should be left for the recommended time. It's important to ensure that the child breathes through his nose while the temperature is being taken, otherwise the reading will be inaccurate. If your child is ill, take his temperature in the morning and evening. Remember not to take the temperature soon after hot or cold drinks or food.

In children, fevers are almost always caused by infections. The child usually has a fever of abrupt onset and the temperature may rise to 105°F (40.5°C). He feels ill, loses his appetite, may have a headache, backache and pain behind the eyes and may even have a convulsion. (*See* CONVULSIONS.)

A fever is not a very good way of telling how ill your child is. A baby can be very ill yet have a temperature below normal. If your child seems ill to you, call the doctor and don't be a slave to the thermometer.

As for treatment, the child should be in bed only if he feels like it – many children with high temperatures are happier up and about. Let the child be the guide unless the doctor has told you to keep him in bed.

If the doctor thinks the child needs antibiotics, make sure you give them as instructed and complete the course. Don't stop giving the antibiotics simply because the fever has subsided, as this can produce a resistant, half-treated infection which can be very difficult to cure.

There is no need to treat a slight fever but if the temperature is very high – 103°F (39.4°C) or more – sponge your child with tepid water to reduce the temperature as this may help prevent convulsions. This is done as follows. Undress the child completely and lie him on a waterproof sheet on a bed. Cool his face, trunk and limbs with tepid water on a flannel or sponge. Cold water is not good because it makes the surface blood vessels contract and so conserve, rather than lose, heat. Wrap tepid, wet cloths around his groins and neck and check his temperature every ten minutes until it is normal. Aspirin also reduces body temperature and if given in the right dose will make the child feel better even though it doesn't actually cure the underlying cause of the fever. Aspirin probably shouldn't be used for fevers in young children unless the temperature is very high – over 103°F (39.4°C) – or unless the child has had a febrile convulsion. If your child has a fever he'll lose lots of water as sweat, so give him plenty to drink. Plain water or unsweetened fruit juice are ideal. Don't cover him with too many clothes or bedding or he'll overheat. The dangers of overheating a feverish child are far greater than those of cooling him down, so simply cover him with a light sheet or leave him naked when his fever is at its height.

Fits   *See* CONVULSIONS; EPILEPSY

Flat feet   All babies have FEET that look flat because of pads of fat on the inner sides of the soles. Even when these pads of fat disappear, many children's feet are quite normally flat. By the time a child reaches adulthood, he will almost certainly have developed feet with arches that are normal and serviceable for him as an individual. The shape of the arches in his foot depends on the shape of the bones, and provided that a child's feet arch when he rises on tiptoe and that they are fully mobile, there is never any need to worry that they will cause any problem.

If no arch develops on tiptoeing or if the foot is not mobile, your doctor may suggest referring your child to an orthopaedic consultant.

Children's shoes normally show wear to the outer side of the middle of the back of the heels. If the shoes show wear on the inner side, they encourage the child to walk with his heels slightly turned out and your doctor may advise that the shoes be fitted with some sort of

The footprints of a normal (left) *and flat foot.*

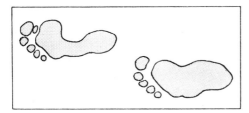

inside raise, wedge or heel. These children almost always stop wearing their shoes down on the inside of the heel by the age of six or seven years. If the shoe doesn't support the foot adequately along the inside of the arch, and especially if the child is heavy, the inner side of the upper of the shoe may be distorted and a stronger shoe or some stiffening to the shoe may be needed.

Children can wear sandals or slippers whether or not they are flat-footed, though if the feet ache or become tired, stronger shoes should be worn.

Foot exercises for flat-footed children are of no proven value, but many doctors think they are worth doing.

Fleas   Wingless insects with piercing or sucking mouth parts that bite humans. Fleas are very common on all animals and man is no exception. In this country, the human flea, cat flea and dog flea are the commonest types that bite humans.

Fleas bite through the skin, suck up blood on which they live and leave an itchy red spot. (*See* ITCHING.) The irritation is caused by the injection of the flea's saliva, which can give rise to unpleasant side effects in sensitive individuals.

More seriously, fleas can spread plague, typhus and a more uncommon disease called tularaemia.

Fleas are best controlled with insecticides, which should be applied not only to household items such as furniture, carpets and beds, but

The human flea (left) *and the dog flea, which also bites humans.*

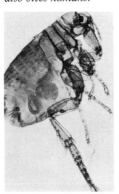 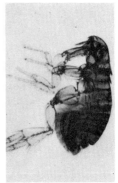

also to pets. Beware of using any insecticides with children about and keep the containers well out of their reach. Powdered insecticides are often completely effective against animal fleas if used on carpets alone and then removed with the vacuum cleaner. If you have any trouble talk to your local environmental health department who will come and de-flea the house for you for a modest fee. Cats and dogs should be disinfested regularly.

The bites themselves need little treatment other than a soothing lotion such as calamine. Antihistamine creams can help, though they can cause a sensitivity reaction on the skin. Antihistamine tablets can be useful if there are lots of bites or if the itching prevents sleep.

See BITES AND STINGS; PETS

Fluoride A naturally-occurring mineral present in drinking water in many areas. It is now artificially added to drinking water in some parts of the world in order to prevent DENTAL CARIES (dental decay).

Dental caries is an almost universal disease in the western world where only three in a thousand people are unaffected by it. Today in the United Kingdom 37 per cent of all people over the age of 16 have no teeth of their own, and dental decay and gum disease are to blame.

In 1916 it was noticed in a certain area in the USA that children had mottled teeth, but it wasn't until 1931 that dentists associated mottled teeth with the water supply, which was found to contain fluoride. As well as being mottled these children's teeth were almost free from caries. It was soon realized that fluoride in as tiny a concentration as one part per million in drinking water could cut down dental decay yet cause no mottling.

Carefully controlled studies have shown that dental decay can be reduced by at least half in fluoridated areas. Thirty per cent of the children aged 12 to 14 in these areas were free from caries altogether in one study. This protection also continues into adult life.

Seventy million people in the USA and a quarter of the population of Holland drink fluoridated water. In Britain the Department of Health and Social Security has left it up to area health authorities to decide whether or not they want to add fluoride to their drinking water.

The greatest single objection to fluoridation is over personal liberty. People fear mass medication and wonder where it will all end. If very large amounts of water are drunk (in tea, for example), teeth can become mottled by the fluoride but this slight chance seems an inadequate reason for opposing fluoridation.

Babies living in areas with low levels of fluoride in drinking water should have fluoride drops or tablets from the age of six months until they are 12 years old. This is because the teeth are developing their enamel during this period and the fluoride acts by strengthening enamel against tooth decay. Fluoride toothpaste has been shown to help get fluoride into the tooth enamel and fluoride can also be applied as a jelly by your dentist. Fluoride paste should not, however, be used by children who swallow toothpaste because it has been shown that repeated ingestion of such paste can cause fluoride toxicity.

As the enamel in the teeth doesn't start forming until after birth, a mother cannot help protect her child's teeth by taking fluoride tablets during pregnancy.

Fontanelle (soft spot) At birth a baby's skull bones are not joined rigidly together but are loosely jointed so that they can override each other as the baby's head is forced down the birth canal, and grow as the brain inside grows.

Where the bones meet there are six small spaces called fontanelles. The most obvious are the anterior and posterior ones which are both in the centre line on top of the baby's head. All the fontanelles close over with bone as the baby grows but the last one to go is the anterior (front) one. This can be felt as a soft spot until about 15 months. It is usually completely closed over by 18 months. The posterior (back) fontanelle usually closes by three months.

Sometimes you'll see the fontanelle pulsating and this is normal. It's important to treat the area over the soft spot exactly like the rest of the baby's head. If you don't wash over the soft spot because you're afraid of damaging it (which you won't) your baby will be more likely to get CRADLE CAP.

The fontanelle can sometimes help doctors in diagnosis. If a baby becomes severely dehydrated (after diarrhoea and vomiting for example) the fontanelle appears sunken. If a child has a raised pressure inside the skull, the fontanelle bulges outwards. If you are worried about your baby's fontanelle, ask your doctor's advice.

See HYDROCEPHALUS

Food allergy *See* ALLERGY; ASTHMA; ECZEMA; HYPERACTIVITY; MILK; SUGAR INTOLERANCE

Foetal distress The term used when a foetus is short of oxygen. Insufficient oxygen may be caused by many factors, including a poorly functioning placenta and obstruction of the umbilical cord by a knot or a loop around the baby's neck.

Signs of foetal distress are staining of the amniotic fluid with meconium (the thick, green substance in the rectum, normally passed after delivery), an irregularity and slowing of the heart rate, and excessive movements by the baby.

Some maternity units take samples of blood from the baby's scalp during labour, if foetal distress is suspected, and measure the amount of oxygen in this blood. If the foetus is shown to be short of oxygen by this method or by clinical judgment alone, the delivery may be speeded up.

See ASPHYXIA; BRAIN DAMAGE; CEREBRAL PALSY; CHILDBIRTH

Food The source of the essential nutrients for life. Food can be solid or liquid but in whatever form it's taken it has to provide energy for body movement and heat and 'building blocks' for growth and repair. The latter is especially important in children because growth during childhood is so rapid.

Food is composed of many types of nutrient but the main ones are carbohydrates, fats, proteins, minerals, vitamins, water, and dietary fibre.

Carbohydrates occur in foods as starches, sugars and cellulose (or similar substances). They are all either simple glucose or multiple units of it. Sugars and starches are man's main source of energy all over the world. Most carbohydrates are eventually converted to simple sugars during digestion, and glucose is the main energy source for the body.

Carbohydrates are found in abundant supply in our modern diet because we add so much sugar to our foods. Lactose in milk and fructose in fruit and honey are just about the only naturally-occurring sugars and we don't eat much of those compared with foods laden with added sucrose. The starch in flour products and potatoes has been our main source of carbohydrate for centuries and continues to be so today.

Although all sugars and starches provide the same amount of energy per unit weight eaten, they have different effects on the body. Too much sugar causes tooth decay and too much carbohydrate almost certainly causes OBESITY, with all its associated diseases.

Fats include not only the 'obvious' fats such as fat on meat, cooking oils, butter and margarine but other less obvious fats in milk, nuts, beans, lean meat, fish (especially herring and mackerel) and several other animal and plant foods. They provide twice the amount of energy (calories) per unit weight as do carbohydrates and so are very fattening. Fats play an important role in making our food palatable and, because they are digested slowly, make food satisfying to eat.

Proteins are the body's building and repair materials and are made up of units called amino acids. About twenty amino acids are combined in a large number of ways to produce the many proteins that make up our bodies. 'Essential' amino acids cannot be made by our bodies and therefore have to be eaten but 'nonessential' ones are made by the body.

Most animal protein foods (meat, fish, eggs, milk, cheese, poultry) are high quantity protein foods. Most people eat too much animal protein in the western world although there is no need to eat meat, fish or cheese every day. Many plant foods also contain valuable protein. Excess protein (after body building and repair have been satisfied) is broken down into glucose in the body and used as energy. Also, if there is too little energy-producing food (fat and carbohydrate) available to the body, protein is broken down to produce energy. This is why we need a balanced diet of all the three main nutrients, fats, carbohydrates and proteins.

Water makes up about two thirds of the body's weight and is used to distribute most of our nutrients through the body in solution. Man can't live long without water (probably only a few days) but can live for weeks without food. Water is obtained from solids as well as drinks and the body's water balance is controlled by the kidneys. Water intake has to be varied according to the body's needs and we have a thirst mechanism that tells us whether we need more fluid or not. If we drink when we are thirsty, the body's systems will look after the rest (unless there is a disorder of any of the vital systems).

Dietary fibre. Roughage in food used to be thought of as useless or even possibly harmful to our bowels. We now know that foods high in dietary fibre (roughage) are essential to the normal working of our bowels and indeed to many other body systems. Wholemeal flour (and its products), fruit and vegetables and bran-containing breakfast cereals are the best sources of fibre and are readily available to us all. The child who eats a diet rich in fibre will never be constipated and may even be protected from certain diseases in later life.

Minerals have three main functions. They are essential for the building of bones and teeth (calcium, phosphorus and magnesium); are essential in solution to control the composition of the body's fluids (especially sodium, chlorine, potassium, magnesium and phosphorus) and lastly are essential to many enzymes and other vital metabolic systems in the body. Iron, for example, is vital to the formation of blood. There is usually no need to concern yourself with the mineral content of your child's food. Provided he is getting a well balanced diet, containing all the main food groups, he'll be unlikely to go short of minerals.

Vitamins. We all need vitamins to maintain our health and children are no exception. A balanced, normal diet probably contains all the vitamins we need but it has been suggested that some children need additional vitamins. For details of when and how to give vitamin supplements *see* BABY FEEDING; BOTTLE FEEDING; BREAST FEEDING; WEANING.

Vitamin A is mainly found in dairy products (milk, cheese and butter) eggs, fish liver oils and green vegetables. It is added to margarine. Vitamin A is necessary to keep the body's linings healthy and is also essential for perfect vision. Poor vision in dim light is often the first sign of a deficiency of this vitamin.

Vitamin B is in fact a group of vitamins widely distributed in many foods but especially in pork, dairy produce, liver, potatoes, yeast and wholemeal flour and its products.

Vitamin C (Ascorbic acid) is found in fruit and vegetables. This vitamin is easily destroyed by heat so cooking fruit and vegetables destroys most of it as does adding hot water to vitamin C-containing drinks. A lack of vitamin C causes SCURVY but this is rarely seen in Britain. One of the main functions of vitamin C is to help the body resist infections and a school of medical thought believes that it is protective against the common cold. This has yet to be proven.

Vitamin D. A vitamin found in similar foods to those containing vitamin A. Humans also produce their own vitamin D in the skin (*see* RICKETS) on exposure to sunlight. Vitamin D is necessary to enable the body to absorb calcium and phosphorus from the diet and so is vital for the growth of healthy bones and teeth. A lack of this vitamin causes rickets.

Infants and young children need good, balanced diets in order to grow healthily. Babies rely on milk for their total food intake and obviously breast milk is ideal (*see* BREAST FEEDING). Cows' milk is a reasonable substitute but breast milk is greatly superior, not simply as a food but in many other ways. A mother should breast feed her baby for at least four to six months (and longer if possible). Solids should not be introduced before the age of four to six months (*see* WEANING).

Schoolchildren grow very fast and are very active and they need lots of food in comparison to their size. For example, the food requirements of a nine- to twelve-year-old girl are greater than for most grown women.

For most children in Britain there is very little chance that they'll go without food so MALNUTRITION in the classic sense won't occur. However, overnutrition is just as dangerous to their health and a close watch should be kept on children's weight to see that they aren't becoming obese. Moderation and balance are the keywords in child nutrition – don't let your child over-indulge in any one food (except for short periods when it is probably a food fad) and ensure that his diet contains a balanced mixture of all the main food groups.

Food poisoning An infection of the bowel caused by consuming contaminated food or drink. It's usually characterized by DIARRHOEA and abdominal pain and sometimes there is vomiting and a fever.

Food poisoning is caused by certain bacteria – salmonella, staphylococci, clostridia or E. coli. Some of these bacteria cause GASTROENTERITIS by their presence in the bowel while others produce poisonous toxins which act on the body in the absence of the bacteria themselves. One of the most serious types of food poisoning, typhoid, is caused by a strain of salmonella. However, other strains of salmonella are much more common in this country and produce milder diseases.

Salmonella food poisoning produces fever, colicky abdominal pain, nausea and vomiting, aching limbs and diarrhoea, all of which come on between 8 and 24 hours after consuming infected food. The illness usually lasts less than a week. Most people are completely better by this time but some 'carriers' continue to harbour the bacteria and so endanger others around them. In young babies salmonella infection can be fatal if the child becomes grossly dehydrated with untreated diarrhoea and vomiting.

Salmonella food poisoning is probably the commonest of all and is the type that goes round schools and other institutions. These infections occur most in the summer months when the bacteria breed very quickly in unrefrigerated food.

The way to prevent salmonella food poisoning is to be hygienic in the preparation of food and scrupulously careful in its cooking. Hands should always be washed before and after handling meat and poultry especially. Food poisoning can also be transmitted by infected utensils and cloths, so these should be washed regularly in hot, soapy water. If you have diarrhoea or your child has food poisoning and your work brings you into contact with other people's food, you should stay at home until the infection is past. Anyone with diarrhoea should be scrupulous over washing his hands after opening his bowels, to avoid passing the infection on.

It's important too to look after meat and poultry at home. Make sure that joints are small enough to eat within a day or two. Never reheat food half-heartedly – either recook it properly or eat it cold. Remember that high temperatures kill salmonella but rewarming encourages them to breed. Always keep meat and poultry in a refrigerator both before it is cooked and afterwards before you use up the rest the next day.

Staphylococci produce toxins which cause staphylococcal food poisoning. The onset is usually a lot quicker than salmonella poisoning (two to six hours is common). The whole course of the illness is shorter and recovery is usually within a few hours. Processed peas and various canned meats have been known to contain staphylococcal toxins – the bacteria being drawn in through faulty seams of the can.

When travelling abroad, unless the water is known to be safe, it's wise to boil it before it is used for drinking, washing the mouth or cleaning the teeth. Ice cubes and even commercially bottled soft drinks may also be contaminated with certain organisms. Raw vegetables, salads, shellfish, ice-cream and cream may be contaminated, and meat should be well-cooked.

Treatment of food poisoning is usually simple. The child should rest in bed if he's ill or weak enough but will usually want to be up. The prime danger lies in losing large amounts of body water through vomiting and diarrhoea. This must be replaced. Should the child become seriously ill and unable to take fluids by mouth he'll have to go to hospital and have fluids intravenously, so call your doctor.

Antibiotics are not usually necessary and will not hasten recovery. Call your doctor if your child vomits for more than six hours or his condition deteriorates. A vomiting baby will need medical attention sooner.

Thirty to fifty people die every year from food poisoning in Britain – they are mostly very old or very young.

As with so many other infections in babyhood, a breast-fed baby is protected to a large extent by anti-infective factors in his mother's milk.

Food fads *See* APPETITE

Foreign body Children are especially prone to getting foreign bodies stuck somewhere in themselves. They stick beads, pencils, beans and small toys, for example, into their ears, noses and vaginas and also get splinters in their hands and knees and grit in their eyes.

Splinters are probably the commonest foreign bodies. They should be gently dislodged with the point of a sterilized needle and removed with fine tweezers. To sterilize a needle, pass it through a flame until it becomes red hot and then let it cool. Don't let it touch anything else before using it. Finally, a small adhesive dressing may be necessary. If you think your child has a deep puncture wound, or splinters in or near a joint you should tell your doctor or go to an accident and emergency department at a hospital. A very deep splinter, nail, or wire injury may also need medical advice. Splinters of glass can be especially nasty. They are very sharp, can enter the skin almost painlessly and are difficult to locate even with X-rays. If you're ever in doubt as to whether your child might have a glass splinter, see your doctor. Don't poke around in a wound yourself.

After a fall, particles of wood, grit, or earth can remain in a wound however well you clean it. It's important that these are removed or the wound may become infected and very difficult to treat. Severe grazes with gravel or other dirt should be cleaned thoroughly by a doctor who will then apply proper dressings. Remember that unless a wound heals quickly and effectively it may leave an unsightly scar.

Grit in the eye is a common complaint. If your child comes to you with a red, watering eye, the chances are that he has a piece of grit in it. Ask him if he can feel anything sharp there. Encourage him to blink so that this, together with the watering of the eye, will flush it out. Try to stop him rubbing his eyes as this might rub the foreign body into the delicate cornea and scratch it. If the foreign body doesn't come out of its own accord, pull down the lower lid and remove the grit with the corner of a handkerchief. If you can't see the speck of grit, get him to tell you if it seems to be under the upper lid. If it is, put a matchstick on the upper lid and pull the lid upwards over the matchstick so that you can see the underside. Then, when you can see the grit, remove it with the end of a wisp of cotton wool.

Children often stick things in their noses and ears. If you see something right at the outside of the ear canal, remove it gently but, if it's deep inside, get a doctor to remove it with

If a small piece of grit gets stuck in a child's eye, and the child cannot remove it by blinking, pull down the lower lid in case you can see it there (a). If not, you may find it under the upper lid by pulling the lid upwards over a matchstick (b).

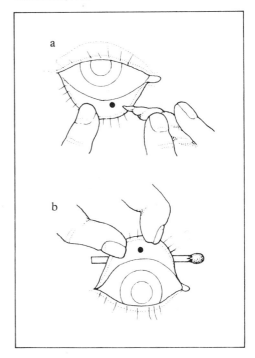

a

b

proper instruments. Poking about in your child's ear can be dangerous because you may break the eardrum. Similarly, with the nose, leave it to a doctor to remove beads, beans and so on. Remember that a nosebleed or a pussy discharge from one nostril may be caused by a foreign body in the nose.

Children swallow all kinds of foreign bodies. The vast majority pass through the bowel uneventfully and come out the other end within a day or two. Occasionally though the swallowed object lodges in the gullet (the oesophagus). Open safety-pins are quite often found in babies of 7 to 15 months of age and coins, hair-grips, buttons, marbles and small toys may be found in older children. The child gags or chokes, and swelling of the local tissues can even obstruct the windpipe. A foreign body stuck in the gullet needs urgent medical attention. Either call an ambulance or take the child to hospital by car if you can be sure to get there quickly.

Children may also inhale foreign bodies. These can get stuck either high up in the larynx or right down in the lungs themselves. If the latter happens, the doctor will need to pass a tube down the airway and look directly into the lungs. He can then remove the object with long tweezers.

Some small girls poke things up their vaginas. The parents first become concerned because their daughter has a discharge for no apparent reason. Here again, the child should be seen by a doctor, who will remove the foreign body.

Prevention must be foremost in a parent's mind. Keep small objects out of young children's reach. Never leave safety-pins around – they're extremely dangerous and very difficult to remove from inside a child. Don't set a bad example by holding pins and other objects in your mouth because children always imitate. Don't encourage your children to play with food – especially peanuts, which if tossed into the mouth as a game can do a lot of harm if they end up in the lungs.

Fracture A break in a bone. Children get fractures relatively often because they play rough games and are learning to do new things such as ride bicycles. Sometimes fractures occur after the slightest injury and at other times you may be surprised that your child hasn't broken something after a serious fall. Young bones are more supple and heal more quickly than those of adults.

The main problem facing a parent is to distinguish between a bad sprain and a fracture

Four common types of fracture. a. greenstick, common in children, who have more supple bones than adults, b. simple (closed), c. compound (open) when the bone pierces the flesh, d. comminuted (shattered).

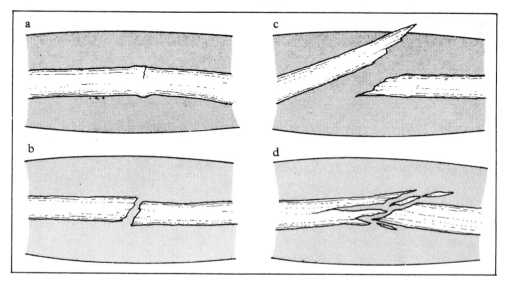

because both are painful and cause swelling. (*See* SPRAINS.)

If the fracture is large and the bones are clearly out of alignment, the fracture is obvious. Such serious fractures have to be reduced (put back into place) by a doctor and this will need an anaesthetic. If you think your child may have fractured a bone, do not give him any food or drink until he has been seen by a doctor because an anaesthetic should not be given on a full stomach.

More often a fracture isn't this obvious. A child with a sprain will be able to put some weight on the damaged limb and will be able to use it to some extent, unlike a child with a fracture. Interference with the use of the affected part is a good indication that it might be fractured.

The final diagnosis of a fracture relies on X-rays. Often the bone doesn't actually break right across but simply bends. This type is called a greenstick fracture because it's rather like bending a green stick. The next most common fracture is a simple (closed) fracture. In this, the bone breaks cleanly in one place. This can usually be set easily and soon heals. A compound (open) fracture is one in which the bone pierces the skin. This is a dangerous fracture because there's usually damage to the tissues, and nerves and arteries can be severed. Such a fracture needs surgical treatment in hospital. A comminuted fracture is one in which the bones have shattered and an impacted fracture is one in which the bone ends are rammed into each other. Any but the simplest of fractures can cause SHOCK.

The treatment of fractures involving long bones is remarkably straightforward – at least in principle. The first thing is to kill the pain and immobilize the broken part. Splinting (immobilization) prevents the broken ends of the bones doing further internal damage and helps reduce pain. In an emergency a broken leg can be bound firmly to the other leg which then acts as a splint, and an arm can be bandaged to the body. If in any doubt, do nothing and call an ambulance.

Once in hospital the bone will be set and fixed in place so that healing can begin. Bones take a long time to knit and six to ten weeks is not uncommon. A plaster of Paris cast supports a fractured bone as it heals.

There is one potentially dangerous fracture in children that needs immediate medical attention – the skull fracture. If ever your child hits his head and loses consciousness, even for a short time, it's wise to take him to the accident and emergency unit of your local hospital. A child's skull can be fractured without there being a head wound and, conversely, even quite serious head wounds need not be accompanied by a fracture. If ever your child becomes drowsy, vomits, or loses pale or blood-stained fluid from his nose or ears after a fall, get medical help at once.

G

Galactosaemia A condition in which the sugar galactose is present in the blood in abnormally large amounts. Galactose is formed in the body by the action of lactase on the lactose in milk, which in this condition acts as a poison to affected babies. The most usual type of the disease is due to a deficiency of an enzyme which normally metabolizes galactose. Without treatment, the baby may die. Those who survive develop a mental defect, cataracts and liver damage.

Affected babies appear normal when they are born but within a few days become listless, lose their appetite, vomit and lose weight. Treatment involves the withdrawal of milk from the baby's diet and its replacement with a specially prepared and commercially available lactose- and galactose-free milk. Early treatment results in the disappearance of symptoms, though cataracts may later need to be removed by operation. As the child is weaned on to solid foods, care must be taken to avoid milk-containing foods (other than those made with the special milk). Some medicines and tablets contain lactose. A pharmacist can tell you which to avoid.

Galactosaemia is thought to be inherited via recessive genes from both parents. In a baby born into a family with a history of the condition, blood can be tested at birth so that treatment with the special milk can be started straight away to avoid problems.

Gastroenteritis Inflammation of the stomach and bowels causing DIARRHOEA, with or without VOMITING and other symptoms. It may be due to non-infective dietary factors such as a reaction to fruit juice or an allergy to cows' milk, but the term gastroenteritis is commonly used to apply only to those cases of diarrhoea which are secondary to infection. The infection can be anywhere in the body, though most often it's in the urinary tract or ears (OTITIS MEDIA). It may also, of course, be a specific infection of the stomach and bowels themselves. It is now thought that when diarrhoea is caused by an infection elsewhere in the body, the organisms reach the stomach and bowels via the bloodstream.

Gastroenteritis caused by direct infection of the stomach and bowels may be caused by infection with bacteria, (salmonellae and shigellae, E. coli, staphylococci or TB bacilli); viruses; parasites (amoebae, causing amoebic dysentery, especially in tropical countries); or small organisms called protozoa (Giardia lamblia, again seen mainly in the tropics). Gastroenteritis caused by salmonella or shigella infection is commonly known as FOOD POISONING.

E. coli gastroenteritis is spread by person-to-person contact, infected objects, possibly by droplet infection, and also by infected food and drink thus making E. coli infection another cause of FOOD POISONING. This sort of gastroenteritis may be difficult to distinguish from that caused by salmonellae and viruses without a bacterial culture of the motions. Tonsillitis, urinary tract infection, otitis media or, in babies, intussusception, may all mimic this condition.

The illness is caused both by toxins produced by the bacteria and by the bacteria themselves. They can be carried in the bowel or respiratory tract of people who have no symptoms and the illness tends to occur more in the summer. Though children of any age can suffer from E. coli gastroenteritis, those under the age of 18 months are most prone to it. In fact, up to 80 per cent of all cases are aged under six months.

E. coli gastroenteritis has an incubation period of two days, followed by watery diarrhoea containing mucus. Bowel motions are passed between five and ten times a day. In older children there are few other symptoms or signs and the illness is over in three to seven days. However, in babies the illness is not only worse but also more dangerous and up to five per cent (more in certain outbreaks) may die as a result of dehydration and the subsequent disturbances of body salts caused by the diarrhoea and vomiting. It's very important not to wait until a baby has signs of dehydration before getting medical help. Prompt treatment can be life-saving and involves restoring the lost body fluids.

If a baby has diarrhoea only and is being breast-fed, his mother should carry on breast feeding only but should breast feed more often to provide more fluid. If he is bottle-fed and has severe diarrhoea your doctor may advise stopping the cows' milk formula and replacing it with a special solution made up with the correct concentrations of glucose and salt. If a breast-fed baby is vomiting as well, he may tolerate a glucose-salt solution better than breast milk. The breast milk supply should be kept up in the meantime by regular expression or pumping of the breasts. If a baby cannot keep enough fluid down by mouth, he'll need to be given fluid intravenously and this means that he'll have to be in hospital.

Some strains of E. coli cause dysentery similar to 'proper' Shigella dysentery. The incubation period of this severe form of gastroenteritis is 18 to 24 hours and there is a sudden onset with watery and often bloody diarrhoea, nausea, vomiting, crampy abdominal pains, a persistent desire to open the bowels, muscle aches, shivering and headache. Medical attention is needed.

Antibiotics are not given routinely for E. coli gastroenteritis because they are of no proven value. However, they may be given to very ill children or to those whose symptoms are prolonged.

E. coli gastroenteritis is prevented by breast feeding babies completely for the first four to six months, because such babies have organisms (lactobacilli) normally present in their bowels which make it difficult for E. coli bacteria to get a hold there. Breast milk also contains various anti-infective factors, including specific antibodies to E. coli in some mothers. Very few cases of E. coli gastroenteritis are seen in exclusively breast-fed babies. People dealing with babies or young children, especially if they prepare food for them, should be extremely careful that they wash their hands before touching food, after

going to the lavatory and after blowing their nose.

Viral gastroenteritis due to the rotavirus is now increasingly recognized and has helped solve the puzzle of why stool culture used to reveal no infecting organisms in half of all cases of gastroenteritis. This infection is seen mainly in the winter and is highly contagious. After an incubation period of 6 to 24 hours, the child has a fever and vomits, then has diarrhoea, abdominal pain and distension. Sometimes there is also an upper repiratory tract infection. The symptoms last for three to ten days and treatment simply involves replacing lost fluids. Antibiotics don't help in this case.

Genes *See* CHROMOSOMES

Genetic counselling The advice given to parents who run the risk of producing a child with an inherited illness or malformation.

Counselling by experts is offered at several centres throughout the country but for many conditions the general practitioner or paediatrician can give adequate advice without recourse to a specialist genetic counsellor.

A genetic counsellor needs to know exactly what the condition is that is being discussed and this may involve special diagnostic tests on parents, children or relatives. Once he knows exactly what he is dealing with, he can explain how the condition is inherited so the parents have a clear understanding themselves.

Second, he can give estimates of the risk of the parents having a child with the condition and then discuss how they should come to a decision as to whether or not to take the risk. If the risk of having a child affected with a serious condition is high, then he might explain that in their place he would think twice about running that risk. Conversely, if the risk is low he may advise them to discount it for all practical purposes.

A genetic counsellor meets many different sorts of problem, from the parent with a port wine stain birthmark who wants to know if his child will be affected, to the mother of a child with spina bifida who wants to know her chances of having a second affected child.

Sometimes he has the unpleasant task of informing relatives of his patients that they may also be at risk of producing affected children.

Several inherited conditions can now be detected early in pregnancy by tests of the baby's blood or of the amniotic fluid. Where this is so, a genetic counsellor can explain how early in pregnancy the parents would need to approach the obstetrician for the relevant test to be carried out. If the unborn child were affected, abortion would be offered.

See AMNIOCENTESIS; CHROMOSOMES; CONGENITAL ABNORMALITIES; INHERITED DISEASES.

Genius *See* GIFTED CHILD

German measles (rubella) A mild, infectious, viral disease.

After an incubation of two to three weeks there may be mild catarrhal symptoms, followed by swelling and tenderness of the lymph nodes at the back of the neck and behind the ears, which is the characteristic feature of

The distribution of the German measles rash.

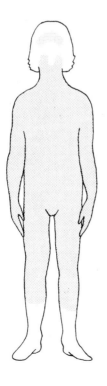

German measles. Twenty-four hours or more later, the rash starts behind the ears and on the forehead and spreads over the body. The flat pink spots may converge so that the skin simply looks red and flushed all over. There may be some itching and the temperature is usually normal. Inflammation of the eardrum may cause earache. Older girls in particular may develop swelling and tenderness in several joints, and this usually disappears within two weeks. There is no specific treatment for German measles but isolation is recommended until the child is better and for at least four days after the rash has first appeared.

Always ask for your doctor's advice if you think your child has German measles because, if he has, you must keep him away from any woman who might be pregnant. The trouble is that a woman may be pregnant but not know it in the earliest weeks, yet it is then that her foetus is most vulnerable to German measles if she is not already immune. This means that a child with German measles should not be taken to public places and that you should warn anyone visiting you in case they get the infection and pass it on to a pregnant woman. A person with German measles is infectious seven days before the rash appears.

If a woman is infected during the first three months of pregnancy, she may have a spontaneous abortion (miscarriage) but if her pregnancy continues without treatment, the baby could be born with one or more of various disorders, including some degree of deafness, a cataract or a congenital heart deformity. Even in late pregnancy, there is still some danger. If a pregnant woman knows she has been exposed to German measles, antibody tests should be done as soon as possible to determine whether or not she was already immune. If she is not, an injection of gamma globulin may help abate the infection.

One attack of German measles usually provides life-long protection, so it's useful to remember if your daughters have definitely had it because it means you can reassure them should they become pregnant and come into contact with the disease.

A baby is protected for the first five to six months of life by antibodies acquired from his mother across the placenta (if she herself is immune to German measles). Rubella vaccination is now offered to all schoolgirls (even if they are thought to have had German measles) in an attempt to protect more women of child bearing age than would be protected by the immunity developed through natural infection. It is important that a woman should not become pregnant within two months of being vaccinated or, indeed, of having the disease itself.

Gifted child A child with superior intellectual ability, as opposed to one who has exceptional skill in bodily co-ordination or aesthetic sensibility, in mathematics, music, art, dance, or athletics for example. A gifted child, however, may also be unusually creative or talented in one or more areas.

Research shows that gifted children tend to have fewer neurotic tendencies, to be more self-sufficient, less submissive, and to compare favourably with other children as regards physical characteristics. However, they have their own special problems. Some are easily bored by their parents or by the school curriculum geared to the average child. Others deliberately under-achieve so that they are accepted by the less bright children in their peer group and, as a result, their teachers and parents do not suspect the brilliance of their INTELLIGENCE (they usually have an IQ of 150 or more). The first time that many gifted children are recognized for what they are is when their parents or teachers can't cope with their 'difficult' behaviour. Others can't find intelligent enough company among children of their own age and may become unmanageable. The problems for the parents of these children may be considerable and it helps them to be in touch with other parents of similarly bright children.

Although it is not easy to predict future intelligence in a baby, a baby that is especially alert and a toddler who talks early and fluently may be showing the first signs of intellectual brightness. Gifted children often need less sleep than their fellows and a gifted pre-school child is likely to have a tremendous interest in everything and to want to read and write and find out about unusual subjects. Long after other children have gone out to play or have become fed up with what they've been doing, the gifted child will still be at it because of his exceptional powers of concentration and tenacity. The typical gifted child has insatiable curiosity, unflagging energy and may be a considerable strain for his parents to amuse.

While it is commonly accepted that talent and creativity can be initiated and encouraged by training, and that creative potential can be stifled by social, emotional and intellectual deprivation, we in the West do not provide special educational opportunities for gifted children as does the USSR, for example. It's left up to parents and individual teachers to provide stimulating opportunities for gifted children, both at home and at school, in such a way as to help them fulfil their potential and avoid frustration. If gifted children can work and play together sometimes, this helps minimize their feelings of apartness. Perhaps the most important task for *any* parent is to help his child fit into society and get on with as many different people as possible. This is as true for a gifted child as it is for a child of normal intelligence.

Gingivitis Inflammation of the gums. The gums are normally pink, firm and finely stippled. With gingivitis they become swollen, reddish-blue and may bleed. If your child's gums bleed (for example during toothbrushing) you should see your doctor or dentist because healthy gums should never bleed.

Gingivitis is usually caused by plaque – the slimy coating that forms on teeth and causes decay. This same substance destroys the fine fibres that tether the teeth in the jaws, so that the teeth become loose and may even fall out. Gum care is important because gum disease is responsible for the loss of more teeth than tooth decay itself. Most gum disease occurs in adults but bad oral hygiene habits start during childhood. Daily brushing with a good nylon brush is the best prevention against gum disease at any age.

After or during a serious illness, a child's resistance to infection may be so lowered that bacteria that would never normally do so can get a hold in the mouth. Children on antibiotics sometimes get a white covering over

111

reddened areas in the mouth and gums – this is THRUSH and can be quite easily treated by a doctor. Some children on phenytoin (Epanutin) – an anti-epileptic drug, get swollen gums. These should be reported to the doctor and will not improve with better brushing and oral hygiene.

See DENTAL CARIES

Glands Groups of cells that make a secre-

The location of the endocrine glands. Each produces hormones which control different processes in the body. a. pituitary (growth and functions of all other glands), b. thyroid (rate of metabolism), c. parathyroids (use in the body of calcium and phosphorus), d. thymus (in children, development of immunity system), e. adrenals (metabolic response to stress and physical effort), f. pancreas (levels of blood sugar), g. testes (production of sperm and male sex hormones) or ovaries (eggs and female sex hormones).

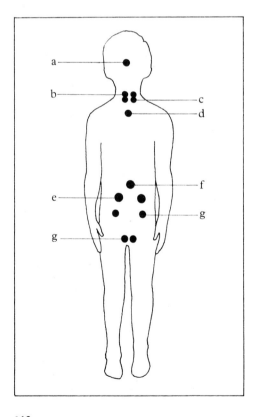

tion. The body has numerous glands of two basic kinds. The first type (exocrine) produces secretions that go directly to where they are needed. Examples of these are the sweat, milk, salivary and digestive glands. The second (endocrine) produces HORMONES which then pass into the bloodstream to be circulated all over the body. The word is also used for the lymph nodes. (*See* LYMPHATIC SYSTEM.)

If your child is overweight, it's very unlikely he has anything wrong with his 'glands'. The chances are that he's simply eating too many refined foods. Fewer than one per cent of all fat people have anything wrong with their hormones.

See ADRENALS; OVARIES; PANCREAS; PITUITARY; TESTES; THYROID

Glandular fever A disease thought to be caused by viruses that causes swelling of the lymph nodes and the spleen. It is uncommon in children but common in late teenagers and young adults. It usually begins with a sore throat which may also be ulcerated. The nodes or 'glands' in the neck may be large, and the child feverish. Many children are wrongly labelled as having the disease. The diagnosis can only be confirmed with special blood tests and there is no specific treatment.

A child who has had glandular fever may feel ill or depressed for weeks or even months.

Many parents are worried that this condition is highly infectious but this seems not to be the case. Spread within families is rare and it seems that very intimate contact is necessary to spread infection – hence it has been called the 'kissing disease' in America.

Glomerulonephritis *See* NEPHRITIS

Glue ear Almost ten per cent of schoolchildren have some sort of hearing loss. The commonest reason for this is glue ear – the presence of fluid in the middle ear which is sticky and glue-like. Fluid is a poorer conductor of sound than the air normally present in the middle ear and so causes some degree of DEAFNESS.

The basic cause of glue ear is poorly functioning eustachian tubes. This may be associated with enlarged ADENOIDS (which

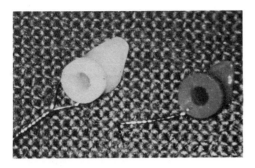

Two grommets (magnified 5 times) which are inserted in the eardrum after an operation to remove fluid from the middle ear, to allow any remaining fluid to drain away. They usually fall out by themselves once the ear has healed.

block the openings of the tubes into the throat and so don't allow fluid in the middle ear to escape) viral infections, chronic sinusitis, or allergy, and is aggravated by repeated upper respiratory tract infections. Large adenoids are by no means always the culprit – in two-thirds of children with glue ear, the adenoids are small or have already been removed. Children with CLEFT PALATE are also prone to glue ear. Initially, the fluid in an ear with a poorly functioning eustachian tube is runny but in some children it eventually becomes thick and glue-like. Usually both ears are affected.

Glue ear can cause recurrent EARACHE, hearing loss and even occasionally speech problems. The child may have a feeling of fullness in his ear and the ear may click when he swallows or moves his jaw. Ear, nose and throat experts disagree about the outlook and the need for treatment. Many believe that glue ear eventually leads on to permanent damage to the middle ear with hearing loss, so if initial treatment with antibiotics (for any underlying bacterial infection) and decongestant medicines and nose drops, and treatment of any allergy makes no difference to the symptoms of glue ear within about six weeks, an operation may be performed. This is done to prevent glue ear and so reduce the educational and social disadvantages suffered by a child with hearing loss. Other specialists believe that there is no conclusive evidence that glue ear results in permanent deafness or that an operation necessarily influences the

long-term outcome, except for recurrent or chronic glue ear.

If an operation is decided upon, the ENT surgeon removes the fluid from the middle ear by suction via a hole he makes in the eardrum and he may also insert a little plastic drain (a grommet) through the eardrum which allows the remaining fluid to drain down the external ear canal and lets the ear heal. This is not permanent and usually falls out between two months and two years later. If the adenoids are enlarged, they are removed at the same time so that they cannot block the openings of the eustachian tubes into the throat and cause fluid to build up inside the middle ear.

Some children show a temporary improvement after adenoidectomy and the insertion of grommets, only to become deaf again later. Yet others regain their hearing months after the operation, while some improve spontaneously while waiting for the operation.

Six months after an operation there is no difference in the hearing whether a grommet has been put in or whether the fluid was simply sucked out, though the hearing is better for the six months after an operation if a grommet has been inserted, and this is a long time for a child to have improved hearing. There is, however, a long-term side effect of having a grommet inserted through an eardrum: the drum can become thickened, which may theoretically lead to hearing loss in later life.

Children with grommets in their ears should only be allowed to swim if they wear a properly fitting earplug, as the middle ear can become inflamed following the entry of chlorine-containing water via the grommet.

It has been suggested that some cases of glue ear are caused by incompletely resolved bacterial infections of the middle ear due to treatment with antibiotics to which the bacteria were partially resistant or due to too short a course of the antibiotic. There is no proof of this idea, but it is sensible always to give your child a full course of any antibiotic prescribed by your doctor for a middle ear infection.

See EARS.

Gluten sensitivity   *See* COELIAC DISEASE

Goitre   An enlargement of the THYROID

gland. Enlargement may occur for several reasons and usually represents an attempt by the thyroid gland to make more thyroid hormones. If too few hormones are produced, a hypothyroid condition results, whereas over-production causes symptoms of hyperthyroidism. Frequently, however, the enlargement produces just the right amount of thyroid hormones so there are no symptoms of hormone lack or excess.

A baby may be born with a goitre and this can cause problems not only from lack of thyroid hormones but also with breathing (the enlarged gland pushes on the windpipe). A congenital goitre like this can be caused by the mother having taken antithyroid drugs or medicines containing iodides (certain cough medicines and asthma remedies) during her pregnancy, and it disappears spontaneously. Treatment may hasten the process. A rare cause of congenital goitre is an overactive thyroid, frequently associated with Graves' disease (a form of hyperthyroidism) in the mother. This type is transitory, though it may need treatment in the first three months. Another cause is a defect in thyroid hormone synthesis which is hereditary and may produce hypothyroidism needing treatment with thyroxine. Finally, iodine deficiency in the pregnant mother can cause goitre in the baby but this is scarcely seen today in the West.

One of the most common causes of goitre in childhood, increasingly widely recognized, is lymphocytic thyroiditis (a type of inflammation of the thyroid gland) thought by some experts to affect one per cent of all school children. The underlying cause of this disorder of immunity is unknown. Girls are affected between four and seven times as often as boys, the disorder tends to cluster in families and it is seen most commonly after the age of six, reaching a peak at adolescence. A few children have symptoms of hypothyroidism and these and a few others may need treatment with thyroxine.

Some adolescent girls develop a goitre thought by some to represent the increased need for thyroxine at this time. Occasionally, treatment with thyroxine is suggested.

Rarely, treatment with medicines containing iodides can produce goitre in children,

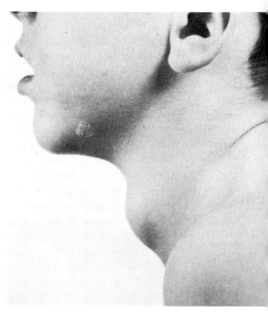

A goitre in the neck caused by enlargement of the thyroid gland.

though there is usually an underlying abnormality of the thyroid in the first place. Certain other drugs, for instance, lithium, can cause goitre.

Iodine deficiency goitre is rarely seen today because of the addition of iodine to table salt and a better all-round diet. This used to be a very common condition in certain areas of Britain and was called Derbyshire neck since it was commonest in Derbyshire (where the people ate few foods rich in iodine).

Other causes of goitre in childhood are infection (rare) and hyperthyroidism (also rare) usually due to Graves' disease – the commonest cause of thyrotoxicosis. Children with Graves' disease usually develop symptoms during adolescence. Girls are more often affected than boys and the tell-tale signs are emotional disturbance, sweating, tremor, prominent eyes and weight loss. They are often tall for their age. Treatment may be with antithyroid drugs or by the partial removal of the thyroid gland by surgery.

Gonorrhoea A type of venereal disease seen more commonly than ever before in children and adolescents, and caused by oval-shaped bacteria called gonococci. If a newborn baby is infected as it comes down the mother's infected birth canal, the eyes and eyelids may be affected. (*See* STICKY EYE.)

Young children can contract the disease by contact with infected parents but older children and adolescents usually catch the infection by sexual activity. After an incubation period of three to five days, the infection produces a discharge (from vagina or penis), painful urination, itching of the genitals and possibly vaginitis (inflammation of the vagina) in girls. (*See* VAGINAL DISCHARGE.) Unfortunately, gonorrhoea can be present without symptoms, and this means that someone can infect another person (or his or her own child) without knowing. Fifteen to thirty per cent of women with gonorrhoea have no symptoms.

Apart from the local genital signs and symptoms, gonorrhoea can cause skin lesions and arthritis. Gonococcal arthritis is now the commonest cause of painful joints in the adolescent age group and occurs more frequently in girls. The diagnosis in a person with symptoms is often easy. A sample of the discharge shows the organism responsible but the emergence of drug-resistant organisms is making gonorrhoea more difficult to treat. Prevention can be achieved to some extent by the use of a sheath during intercourse. A physical barrier like this reduces infection rates, whereas girls on the Pill can harbour the organism and infect their sex partners easily.

Gonorrhoea is now the fastest growing epidemic of infectious disease known to man and much of the growth in numbers has occurred among the young. Unfortunately, the long-term effects in girls and women are serious. The infection can permanently block the fallopian tubes and may make the woman unable to conceive. In certain areas of the world it is the commonest cause of infertility.

With the explosion in teenage sexual activity parents today must be doubly careful to advise their children about the dangers of gonorrhoea. Certainly it's treatable, but by the time a girl realizes she has it (and many have no symptoms) her reproductive capacity may be finished for ever and she may have spread the disease to others.

Graves' disease *See* GOITRE

Growing pains Children often complain of vague aches and pains in their legs – usually in their thighs and calf muscles – and because a cause is rarely found such pains have come to be known as growing pains. Growth is, of course, quite painless, so this is a misleading term.

The aching usually starts in the evening though occasionally it may wake a child at night. It always disappears by the morning. There are no other signs of illness and the pain is often made better by massaging the affected muscles. Parents are frequently concerned about the possibility of RHEUMATIC FEVER but the two conditions are quite distinct. A child with rheumatic fever has a fever and other signs suggestive of heart involvement, and the typical pains are felt not in the muscles but in the joints themselves.

Growing pains may be caused by the exercise that a child has had during the day – in other words, simple muscle fatigue. There is no need to limit exercise and parents should be careful not to show undue concern over a condition which is harmless and self-limiting.

Growth One of the outstanding features of the human race is the length of time children take to grow to adult size. Growth in all other species of animals is completed far more quickly. Physical growth of the body is usually measured in terms of HEIGHT and WEIGHT, though each part of the body grows at a different speed and some parts finish growing sooner than others. The brain, for instance, grows more quickly than the rest of the body in the first ten years, then slows down. The sexual organs hardly change at all during early childhood but rapidly increase in size at PUBERTY. The thymus gland grows rapidly for the first five years but actually becomes

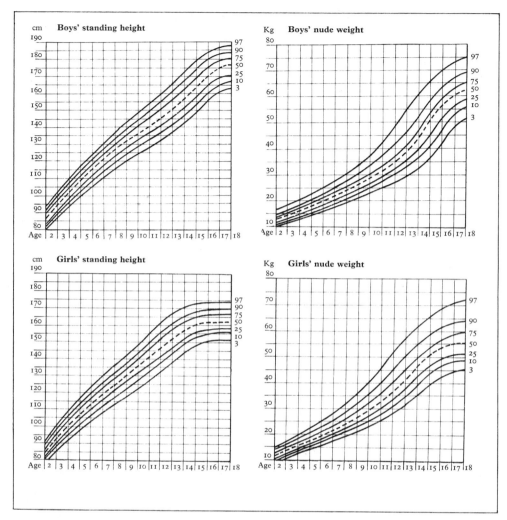

Average height and weight from 2 to 18 years. The figures at the end of each curve show the percentage of children smaller than the values plotted.

smaller from puberty onwards.

Measurements of the height and weight of large numbers of healthy boys and girls of different ages have led to the construction of height and weight charts. Measurements of an individual child can be plotted to indicate whether they fall within the average range of whether the child is abnormally tall or short, heavy or light for his age. When physical growth and DEVELOPMENT are complete, the body may be said to have reached physical maturity.

Growth is at its maximum in the foetus but continues at a high level during the first few weeks after birth and throughout the first year. From the age of two or three, the rate of growth slows down, becoming slowest of all just before the onset of puberty. Puberty, which occurs earlier in girls than in boys, brings with it an adolescent spurt of growth which continues until adult size is reached.

Other parameters of growth include the development of the mind, the emotions and the spirit.

See LOW BIRTH WEIGHT; SMALL CHILDREN

H

Habits Habit spasms or tics are irritating nervous habits often affecting the head and shoulders. Some children sniff, blink or make silly movements with their nostrils or shoulders and others rub their faces repeatedly.

Many tics start as being useful: for example, a child will toss her hair back to get it out of her eyes but may continue to do so even after it's been cut.

Tics are not the child's fault but can be infuriating to those around him. Try to ignore them as much as possible and find out if there's anything that might be worrying him. Being tough with a child with a tic usually does more harm than good.

Other children have repetitive habits which may start in infancy. Some babies rock interminably and noisily: this usually starts around nine months. Other children bang their heads against hard objects and even rock back and forth at the same time.

None of these tics does any harm to the child, even head banging, so there is no need to be anxious on this account.

Most of these repetitive habits stem from a lack of security in the child (often the result of anxiety or boredom at being separated from his mother) and represents the child's attempt to comfort or console himself. Try not to leave your child alone if he is awake and try to involve him in whatever you are doing, even if only as an observer. Your doctor or health visitor will help you sort out the problem if necessary.

See BED WETTING; BREATH HOLDING; DIRT EATING; HEAD BANGING; NAIL BITING; THUMB SUCKING

Haemolytic disease of the newborn *See* BLOOD GROUPS

Haemophilia An inherited blood disorder caused by a deficiency of one of the blood clotting factors.

Haemophilia is a rare disease, affecting only one or two children in every 100,000. Almost all cases are passed on by a sex-linked recessive gene which means that females are unaffected and simply carry the disease, whilst males are affected. New tests can detect female carriers of haemophilia fairly accurately, allowing GENETIC COUNSELLING if necessary for daughters of families with a history of haemophilia.

Children with haemophilia are liable to bleed at the slightest provocation, and often the first sign is an abnormal amount of bruising following minor falls while learning to walk. Small cuts bleed for hours or even days instead of only for a few minutes. Perhaps the most uncomfortable part of the disease is the haemorrhages that occur into joints, which cause pain, swelling and limitation of movement and, if repeated into the same joint, eventual permanent damage. The degree of the deficiency of the clotting factor involved determines the severity of the disease.

Treatment of haemophilia is primarily by prevention of injury, though it's sensible not to protect your child so much that he becomes fearful, loses much of the fun of life and doesn't learn to be independent. A baby's cot can be padded and he should be watched carefully as he learns to walk. A protective helmet may help guard the head and face, while knee pads can be sewn inside trousers. Later, thick or special protective clothing can be worn to prevent superficial skin grazing, but the only way of preventing joint haemorrhages is by avoiding rough play and games. Because bleeding can occur if teeth are removed by the dentist, even more care than usual should be taken to make sure the child's teeth don't decay. (*See* DENTAL CARIES.) The natural shedding of the teeth does not cause bleeding.

An acute bleeding injury needs to be treated with a transfusion of plasma, a plasma concentrate, or pure clotting factor from a normal person to replace the missing clotting factor and minimize the amount of blood loss. Initial first aid measures include the application of ice packs and pressure over the bleeding or damaged part.

Your doctor will probably arrange for your child to be linked with a special haemophilia centre if there is one in the neighbourhood.

See BLEEDING

Halitosis (bad breath)   There is one major cause of bad breath in children: severe dental decay (*see* DENTAL CARIES).

Certain diseases such as tonsillitis and appendicitis can cause bad breath but you'll know your child has something wrong with him in other ways than by his bad breath.

Constipation is not a cause of bad breath, as is commonly supposed. A very few children have bad breath for no apparent reason.

Hallucinations   False perceptions (visions, sounds, smells and other sensations) that have no basis in the real world. An illusion (such as performed by a magician) is 'real' but fools the senses. Hallucinations are very different and much more serious because, unlike the magician's trick, there is no basis in reality for them. The person who suffers from hallucinations believes they are real and often they alter his life considerably. Someone who persistently has hallucinations needs medical attention because the vast majority of such people are schizophrenic.

Schizophrenia is rare in children but is often first seen in the late teens. It fills about one fifth of all hospital beds in the UK and one person in a hundred is likely to suffer from the condition at some time.

Children can experience hallucinations when they have a very high fever or just as they are going off to sleep but if your child has one at any other time, he should have medical attention.

If your older child has hallucinations, bear in mind that he might have taken a hallucinatory drug. Get medical help.

Hare lip   *See* CLEFT LIP AND PALATE

Hay fever (allergic rhinitis)   An allergic condition of the nose and eyes usually caused by an ALLERGY to the proteins in plant pollens. Other foreign proteins may also be responsible. The body's reaction is for the mucous membranes of the nose, and perhaps also of the

sinuses, to produce CATARRH and for the conjunctivae of the eyes to become inflamed. Attacks of hay fever are commonest in the summer months, the worst months being from May to July. Hay fever (along with asthma and eczema) often runs in families.

The trouble starts with itching of the eyes, nose, palate, throat and ears which is soon followed by sneezing, swelling and redness of the membranes of the nose and also a discharge from the nose (which may be watery or profuse). Because of this, the nose becomes blocked. The eyes are red and water profusely. There is sometimes a headache. Attacks can last for hours or even weeks and depend upon the pollen count in the air, weather conditions and many other factors.

Some children have all these signs and symptoms from an allergy to a food, house dust, cat fur or moulds, for example, and so have symptoms outside the pollen season as well as during it.

A child who suffers a lot from hay fever may have a horizontal crease across his nose near the tip caused by the repeated upward rub he does when his nose irritates. This movement may persist as a habit even when he isn't actually suffering from hay fever.

Once the offending allergen has been isolated, prevention can do much to help. Clearly you can't remove your child from pollen but house dust and moulds can be controlled by keeping the house scrupulously clean and cats, for example, can be given away. The child may improve with a course of desensitizing injections (*see* DESENSITIZATION).

If these injections don't work, then the child will need treatment during attacks. Antihistamines are useful but can make him sleepy. Decongestant nose drops should only be used in the short term, but decongestant drugs given by mouth can be helpful. Steroids are rarely used because though they are very effective they are too dangerous a group of drugs to be taken repeatedly except for serious medical conditions. Sodium cromoglycate has proved a very useful drug in the prevention and treatment of hay fever.

Head banging   Rhythmical head banging is seen in children usually between six months and a year old and rapidly becomes a habit. While the child probably enjoys the repetitive movements, banging against hard or sharp surfaces such as unprotected cot sides can cause bruising or callus formation of the skin over the head, or a bald patch, though any more serious injury is highly unlikely. Rubbing the head can also cause a bald patch.

Head banging sometimes begins if a child is bored and left unamused for long periods in a cot. Some mentally retarded children bang their heads but head banging certainly doesn't cause retardation, as many parents fear. By far the largest group of head bangers do it purely out of habit.

It's a good idea to make sure that your child is not left awake in his cot for long periods alone and that he is not bored during the day but given plenty of love and stimulation. Make sure that whatever he usually bangs his head against is soft and unlikely to hurt him. Cot bumpers can be bought or you can make your own with little effort.

Headache Young children rarely complain of headaches so, if they do, they should be taken seriously. Older children and adolescents may get recurrent head pains but they are usually quite harmless. Most parents fear the worst when their children get headaches but there are dozens of causes for headaches in all but the youngest of children.

Headaches can arise from the meninges (the delicate coverings of the brain itself); the blood vessels inside and outside the skull; the nerves inside the skull, and even the nerves in the upper part of the neck.

MIGRAINE is caused by a temporary narrowing of the arteries inside the skull with a widening of those outside it but is an uncommon cause of headache in children. A much more common cause is the onset of an infectious fever. Fevers produce dehydration and it's probably this that causes the headache along with the direct effects of the infecting agent on the brain and its coverings. The classic infection of the meninges (MENINGITIS), can produce a headache in children, but the chances that a child with a headache has meningitis are very small indeed. If he has a sudden change of mood, becomes irritable,

vomits, has a stiff neck or fever – then these things may point to meningitis. Any child who develops these symptoms out of the blue or as a result of another childhood infection should be seen by a doctor urgently.

A headache can be part of the aura that precedes an epileptic fit and can also occur after the attack. Tension headaches due to constant contraction of the neck and shoulder muscles are sometimes seen in children. These headaches are dull and steady, get worse as the day goes on and go with sleep. They are rarely seen before adolescence.

Depressed and anxious children commonly suffer from headaches. They have them continuously, in contrast with other headaches which come and go. The child may look sad, speak only in a whisper, have a poor appetite and sleep badly. The problem with these headaches is that they seem so serious that the child is often subjected to unpleasant and extensive investigations to try to find a cause for them. Of course, all the tests are negative.

Lastly, the headache every parent fears – that caused by a BRAIN TUMOUR. Because of the growth of a tumour inside the rigid skull, the pressure rises, causing a headache. Brain tumour headache is often worst after a change in head position and first thing in the morning. Any child with a headache on awakening must see a doctor.

Headaches are not caused by bad teeth or constipation. Eye strain is a rare cause.

Head injury Children quite often fall and bang their heads. The problem for a parent is to decide whether that particular bang on the head is serious or not.

Babies and toddlers, especially when they're learning to walk, fall and bang their heads time and again yet seem to come to no harm. As they get older and more adventurous they fall from heights, which can be dangerous. If a child loses consciousness for even a short time after a fall, call the doctor.

When children fall, they often cut their heads. If there is any sort of wound you should take a child to hospital, because any bang hard enough to break the skin may have fractured the skull or done deeper damage. You must also get medical help if he vomits after a head injury, loses blood from his nose, ears or mouth or watery fluid from his nose or ears, or if he stays pale or behaves strangely after a fall. The doctor will need to know how far the child fell and on to what surface.

If your child falls asleep after an accident, watch him carefully. If his breathing becomes abnormal, call the doctor. If he won't wake easily, get medical help.

When the doctor sees your child he'll stitch up any obvious wounds and X-ray the skull to look for fractures. There's nothing easy about assessing head injuries, especially in children, and the child may need to be kept in hospital for 24 hours' observation. This is usually just a precaution but hospital is the place to be if anything should go wrong.

Even if the skull isn't actually fractured, there may be a large swelling after a head injury. This is usually caused by blood leaking from blood vessels under the scalp but is only a big bruise.

When the scalp is cut, it bleeds a lot because it is so well supplied with blood vessels. If your child has a head injury, don't panic because there seems to be so much blood. Stop the bleeding if you can and wipe away the mess. The trouble often turns out to be much less serious than it at first seems. All it needs as a first aid procedure is for you to press hard on the area through a handkerchief until the bleeding stops or slows. These cuts almost always need stitches because you can't bandage the scalp easily.

If ever you are in doubt about a head injury – get medical help at once.

Hearing *See* DEAFNESS; EARS; HEARING TEST-ING

Hearing testing Perfect hearing is vitally important so that a child can both learn to use language and communicate with other people. Any degree of hearing loss can interfere with these processes, but the sooner that DEAFNESS is recognized, the sooner appropriate treatment can be started. While not all deaf children can be cured, most deaf children can be helped (perhaps with special training by their parents, special schooling, or the use of a deaf aid) to make the best possible use of

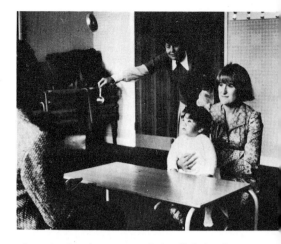

A routine hearing test at a baby clinic involves distracting the baby, who sits on his mother's lap, shaking a rattle at his side (so that he cannot see it) and seeing if he turns towards the sound.

whatever hearing they have and, if necessary, to learn other ways of communicating.

In order to detect any hearing loss as soon as possible, all parents in this country are offered routine hearing tests for their children. The newborn baby is first tested for his response to sound when he has his examination by the doctor soon after birth. The doctor may ring a bell near his ear while he is crying to see if he quietens, for example. The health visitor or doctor carrying out routine developmental checks will ask from time to time about the baby's response to sound and whether he is making baby sounds in the normal way. If there is any reason to be concerned, extra tests can be done. Round about $7\frac{1}{2}$ months, a hearing test is carried out with the baby sitting on the mother's lap (ideally being distracted by a helper in front of him) and with the doctor or health visitor behind him and his mother. Various sounds are then made to either side of the baby, a certain distance away from his ear and on a level with his ear. These sounds include the ringing of a bell, the rustling of tissue paper, the sound of a spoon being stirred in an empty cup, a rattle, and various vocal sounds. Though many things may interfere, it is useful as a screening test, and any baby who doesn't seem to respond normally is either tested again or is referred to an ear, nose and throat specialist.

Several tests are available for older preschool children and most are based on games which require the child to hear. Various types of audiometer can be used to test hearing (*see.* AUDIOMETRY) and are especially useful for school-age children.

In children whose hearing is difficult to assess, it is possible to measure electrical changes in the brain in response to different sounds by doing an EEG (electroencephalograph). This test is also used if there is a strong likelihood of a baby being born deaf, as a result of the mother having had German measles in early pregnancy, for example.

Other tests of hearing can help the specialist determine first, the type of deafness; second, the extent to which it hinders the child in normal everyday life; and, last, how best it can be treated.

See EARS; GLUE EAR; OTITIS MEDIA

Heart A four-chambered muscular pump situated in the left side of the chest. The heart is divided into two halves, left and right, handling oxygenated and deoxygenated blood respectively. Each side of the heart has an upper collection chamber or atrium, a set of valves through which the blood passes to the lower pump chamber or ventricle and an outflow vessel. Blood can flow only from the upper chamber to the lower when the mitral and tricuspid valves are open. These valves also prevent reverse flow.

Blood which has performed its oxygen- and nutrition-giving tasks to the body is collected by veins which open into the big collecting veins known as the inferior and superior venae cavae. Thus all the venous blood from the body ends up in the right atrium. This chamber contracts and pumps the blood through the tricuspid valve into the right ventricle below. The valve then closes and the blood is pumped up into the vessel which takes it to the lungs to be re-oxygenated.

Once its oxygen has been replenished, the blood returns to the heart, entering the left atrium. This contracts and forces the blood into the biggest and most muscular chamber of all – the left ventricle. The blood is then

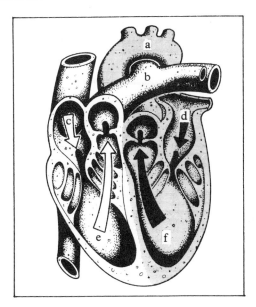

A cross-section through the heart. a. aorta, b. pulmonary artery, c. right atrium, d. left atrium, e. right ventricle, f. left ventricle.

passed out into the aorta under pressure high enough to push it round the body.

The heart is about the size of a fist and is made of a very special type of muscle that beats spontaneously even when outside the body. The beating is controlled by a sophisticated set of nervous pathways in the heart itself. The heart is a remarkable organ. It contracts about 70 times a minute in adults all our lives: that's over a 100,000 beats a day for 70 years or 2,575 million beats in a lifetime. At birth the pulse rate is about 140 and falls to around 100 at three years. It goes on falling in rate until middle age when it is about 70 beats a minute.

Every single beat is controlled by the heart's pacemaker, which disciplines the natural tendency of each part of the heart to contract at its own rate into a concerted effort. So it is that all the four chambers and the four sets of valves (two in the chambers and two in the outflow vessels) work with split-second accuracy to ensure that the body gets the blood it needs every minute of our lives. The pacemaker's activity is modified by sympathetic and parasympathetic nerves. (*See* AUTONOMIC NERVOUS SYSTEM.)

The heart is the most demanding muscle in

121

our bodies and uses a great deal of the oxygen supplied by the lungs. The blood needed to provide the oxygen and nutrients for the heart reaches the heart muscle via the coronary arteries. These come off the aorta and give the heart a high pressure supply of blood even before the rest of the body gets its supply.

See HEART CONDITIONS; HEART MURMURS

Heart conditions A careful examination of the HEART forms part of the doctor's routine examination of the newborn baby.

Similarly, during early childhood, it's well worth having your child's heart listened to routinely by your clinic or family doctor, as a heart condition may otherwise go unrecognized. Though some congenital heart conditions improve spontaneously, others get worse as the child grows older and may sometimes prove fatal without medical or surgical intervention.

Many newborn babies have HEART MURMURS but the vast majority of these murmurs are innocent – they don't represent an abnormality and often disappear in a short time. Others point to an underlying congenital heart abnormality which will usually need investigation and perhaps even treatment. Some congenital abnormalities of the heart are apparent at birth but others are not diagnosed until the child is older.

The abnormalities which may be present in the heart at birth include narrowing of the heart valves, a hole between the upper or lower chambers of the heart, the persistence of foetal blood vessels which normally close around the time of birth, and more complicated conditions such as Fallot's tetralogy, the classical blue baby condition, in which there are several defects. Some children are born with a normal heart on the right side of the chest instead of the left.

A blue baby is one with a heart abnormality which causes a mixing of the blood from the two sides of the heart, so that the arteries of the body are supplied with blood which is poor in oxygen. This should not be confused with blueness affecting some newborn babies after a difficult labour. (*See* BLUE BABIES.) A severe heart abnormality may lead to signs of heart failure, including poor colour, very quick

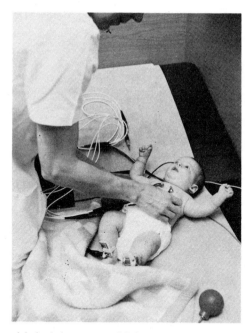

A baby being prepared for an electrocardiogram (ECG), which demonstrates abnormalities by recording electrical changes produced by the heart muscle.

breathing, and swelling of the limbs and face.

A child with congenital heart disease needs an antibiotic if he is going to have a tooth extracted, to prevent dislodged bacteria from the tooth socket reaching the abnormal heart tissue via the bloodstream and setting up infection in the heart.

Children with bad congenital conditions can often do a surprising amount. Most can be trusted to rest when they have tired themselves and they sometimes get into a squatting position to help the blood circulation. The child grows up to be more independent if he is not constantly told to stop and rest. However, tiredness should always be taken seriously and treated by rest.

Heart massage A procedure performed to save life when there is no heartbeat. How can you tell if a child's heart has stopped beating?
1) He'll be unconscious.
2) He'll look pale or blue-grey.
3) The pupils of the eyes will be large.
4) There'll be no pulse at the wrist or in the

neck (felt at the side of the Adam's apple).

If ever a child is in this state, you'll need to take emergency action. Lie the child on a hard surface on his back. If he's in bed, pull him on to the floor. Give one sharp, hard blow with the side of your hand over the lower left side of the breastbone. This may 'shock' the heart into re-starting. If the heart still does not beat, send someone for an ambulance while you do the following.

Kneel on the child's right side and put the heel of one hand over the lower half of the breastbone (not over the upper stomach). The rest of your hand shouldn't press on the chest at all. Place the heel of your other hand over the back of the first and rock your body backwards and forwards without flexing your arms. Keep your hands in position all the time and, in a big or older child, depress the breastbone about two inches, 80 times per minute.

In small children, use one hand only at 100 beats per minute and in babies, use two fingers at 110 beats per minute. In babies, press higher up the breastbone so as not to damage the delicate and large liver.

Whatever the child's age, continue until:
1) The child looks better.
2) His pupils return to their normal size.
3) The neck pulse returns.

Once a pulse has returned *do not apply further heart massage.*

Whenever the heart stops, breathing will stop too so you'll also need to do the KISS OF LIFE. To do both if you are alone, inflate the lungs quickly, then do 15 heart compressions and repeat this until help arrives. If you have help, get one person to do mouth-to-mouth resuscitation (the kiss of life) while you do the heart massage. He breathes one breath and you do 5 heart compressions. Get a rhythm going and keep it up until recovery occurs or professional help arrives.

Heart murmurs When a doctor listens to a child's HEART with a stethoscope, he is listening to the rate of the heart beat, its rhythm, its character and for any extra noises such as murmurs. Besides putting the stethoscope over the lower left ribcage in front, he will also listen in several other places on the front of the chest wall, over the back and also over the great blood vessels in the neck.

The heart beats are associated with the closing of the two main sets of heart valves, whereas murmurs are associated with normal or abnormal currents of blood flowing through the heart. They may be short or long, may be heard in one of several places, may be high or low-pitched and may disappear altogether if the position of the child is altered.

Many murmurs of childhood are innocent, associated with normal eddy currents of blood flowing in the heart. Your doctor may suspect that your child's murmur is innocent and yet want to see him every six months or so – this is good practice and there are large numbers of children throughout the country who are being observed in this way. Innocent murmurs almost all disappear completely and are present in up to half of all newborn babies. Other murmurs may be due, for instance, to a hole between either the upper or lower pair of heart chambers or to a narrowing of one of the outflow vessels. Treatment depends on the heart abnormality present.

Some children are noticed to have a murmur during the course of a minor infection and this kind disappears as the illness gets better.

See BLUE BABIES; HEART CONDITIONS

Heat rash A rash caused by profuse sweating and overheating of the skin. It is usually due to wearing too many clothes in too hot an atmosphere. The baby or young child sweats and gets a faint red rash in the sweaty, overheated area. The rash is usually seen in the skin creases, and on the face, neck and shoulders, where there are most sweat glands. Sometimes the mother thinks the baby is crying because he's cold and so puts on even more clothes. Babies can get overheated very easily and in conditions that may surprise an adult. The baby may be fine one night and too hot the next, and mothers find it difficult to judge how much clothing to put on their babies at night.

Rather than dressing your child for the season, dress him for each day. The climate may be so unpredictable that you can't make assumptions about what clothes will be best. Don't put wool directly next to the skin but use a cotton vest first. Keep man-made fibres away from the skin as they can be especially bad for trapping sweat.

Cooling the baby cures the rash and calamine lotion helps the itching.

It's worth remembering that if you go on holiday to a hot place you should keep the baby somewhere cool and shaded from the sun. Babies can't tolerate direct sun like adults and can get heat rashes, become dehydrated and be very unhappy.

See HEATSTROKE; SUNBURN

Heatstroke A condition that occurs with prolonged exposure to heat. The body is usually kept at its TEMPERATURE of 98.4°F (37°C) by a clever balance of heat production and loss. The balance is controlled by the temperature-regulating centre in the brain and normally doesn't allow a shift of more than a few fractions of a degree in either direction.

When a person (especially a small child or baby) is exposed to heat (usually the sun) for a long period or even for a short, intense period, the sweat glands seem to switch off temporarily and the body cannot cool itself down. The heat-regulating mechanism fails and the body begins to heat up. The child feels and looks red and very hot, may be confused, has a rapid pulse, inco-ordinated movements and eventually becomes delirious and ends up in a coma. The conclusion is death if treatment isn't instituted quickly. Recent reports suggest that this condition can occur – albeit rarely – in babies who are wrapped up too warmly by their mothers, especially during minor illnesses.

Body temperature in this condition can go up to 108°F (42.2°C) and beyond, but anything over 106°F (41°C) produces permanent damage. The brain cells are literally cooked like the white of a boiled egg and so cannot function properly afterwards. Convulsions may occur with these high temperatures too. (*See* FEVER.)

Treatment involves cooling the child slowly by removing clothes, tepid sponging and fanning. If your child has heatstroke, call a doctor and don't start cooling him yourself except for removing his clothes and directing a fan on to him. Too rapid cooling can be dangerous.

To prevent heatstroke, you must look after your really young children who cannot look after themselves. Older children may go into the shade when they get too hot but babies and little ones won't. Get children used to heat slowly and don't let them go out in the sun for hours on end on the first day of your holiday. Make sure they all drink plenty of fluids and put suntan creams on to protect their skins. Every year thousands of families suffer from problems with overheated children on holiday or in closed cars standing in the sun but with a few basic precautions it need never be you.

See SUNBURN

Height A baby's height (or more accurately length) is measured preferably with the help of two people and a flat board with head and foot rests. It is impossible to predict the adult height of a child until he is at least two. With the improvement in nutrition and general living standards in this century, there has been an increase in the height of our children. Children of different families and races show inborn differences in height.

A child's height can be compared with that of the 'average' child by plotting it on a special chart. As children grow at different rates according to the time of year, whether or not they have been ill, and whether or not they have reached puberty, a single height reading is of little predictive value and serial readings taken every six months or so are of more value.

The typical height charts used in schools and clinics throughout the country are based on measurements taken from large numbers of normal children. If a child's height is said to be on the 50th percentile, this means that he is average in height – 50 children out of every 100 would be taller than he and 50 would be shorter. Similarly, for example, a child whose height was on the 10th percentile would be relatively short, though still within normal limits. If a child's height is thought to be especially great or small (usually if it falls outside the 3rd or the 97th percentile) an expert opinion can be sought from a paediatrician, though it is usually sensible to repeat the measurement after six months or so before taking this step.

An important point for parents to remember is that the adolescent growth spurt begins and ends on average two years earlier in girls than in boys, so for much of their teenage life girls tend to be taller than boys of the same age.

Obviously a major cause of small or great stature is having short or tall parents, though other factors, including some diseases and emotional deprivation also influence height. Parents frequently worry that their sons will be short or that their daughters will be tall. Fairly accurate height predictions can now be made by looking at bone X-rays during childhood and it is occasionally thought worthwhile to influence the eventual height with hormone treatment, albeit for purely cosmetic reasons.

See FAILURE TO THRIVE; GROWTH; SMALL CHILDREN

Henoch-Schönlein purpura (Henoch-Schönlein vasculitis; allergic purpura) A condition in which there is a skin rash, sometimes combined with abnormalities of the joints, gastro-intestinal tract and kidneys. It is more common in children than in adults, mostly affecting those from two to eight years. Twice as many boys are affected as girls. The cause is unknown, though it may be associated with an allergy or a sensitivity to a drug. Some experts suggest that a streptococcal infection may precipitate it.

Affected children develop small weals or flat or slightly raised patches which become 'purpuric' – red or purple due to tiny haemorrhages under the skin. The colour of these patches fades gradually (like a bruise) though new crops may continue to appear. The underlying abnormality is an inflammation of the small blood vessels of the skin and the rash is seen mainly on the legs, though the rest of the body may be affected. Other skin rashes may be seen, including itchy, swollen patches (angioneurotic oedema) on the scalp, eyelids, lips, backs of the hands, tops of the feet, the back and the genital area.

Two out of three affected children develop arthritis, especially of the knees and ankles. The swelling and tenderness usually disappears after a few days but may recur. Again, two out of three children have gastro-intestinal symptoms such as colicky abdominal pain, perhaps with vomiting. There may be bleeding from the gut, which may be severe enough to cause black bowel motions, and

blood may sometimes appear in the vomit.

Up to half the affected children have involvement of their kidneys, causing NEPHRITIS, but this is only severe in a very small number. The nephritis of Henoch-Schönlein purpura may develop up to one or two months after the condition was first diagnosed. It has usually disappeared within six months.

Rarely, there may be involvement of the brain, liver, spleen, heart and certain other parts of the body.

Henoch-Schönlein purpura may last for up to six weeks, though mild cases last only a few days. However, relapses may occur even when a child seems better. There is no specific treatment, except for the alleviation of symptoms such as pain in the joints. Rest does not improve the healing process. Steroid drugs may be advised for some children.

Hepatitis An inflammation of the liver commonly caused by a virus. Jaundice is usually present and the liver may be enlarged.

The foetus of a mother with hepatitis, especially serum hepatitis (see below) can be infected. If a pregnant woman contracts hepatitis, an injection of gamma globulin may protect her foetus.

A very young baby may suffer from infectious hepatitis transferred from his mother, though the risks to the baby are not as great as experts used to think they were. A mother with hepatitis who has a young baby need not be separated from her baby because he will already have become infected long before her symptoms appear because the incubation period is so long.

Hepatitis in early infancy can be caused by a variety of viruses including the Coxsackie and Herpes simplex viruses and the cytomegalovirus. Occasionally infectious hepatitis leads to cirrhosis in later childhood.

In older children hepatitis follows approximately the same pattern as that seen in adults. There are two main types – infectious (epidemic) hepatitis, usually spread by faecal contamination of drinking water or food, and serum hepatitis, transferred by the use of contaminated syringes and needles. The incubation periods of these two types are very different. That of infectious hepatitis is 14 to 40 days, whilst that of serum hepatitis is 60 to 160 days. There is no cross immunity between these two types of hepatitis.

The child infected with either type of hepatitis virus is usually unwell for four to five days before jaundice appears and a loss of appetite may be the most obvious complaint. There may be upper abdominal pain, he may seem generally unwell and his breath may smell foul. His urine becomes dark with bile and his liver may be enlarged. As the jaundice appears, the child feels better and his motions become pale. The 'yellow' phase of the disease lasts from two to four weeks. A child may have hepatitis with all the classical signs and symptoms and yet not be jaundiced. The child who has had hepatitis feels weak and tired for weeks or even months after the disease.

The diagnosis can be difficult to make if there is no jaundice and appendicitis may be suspected. Some experts maintain that the family of an affected child should receive protective gamma globulin but this is not routinely given.

Treatment is with bed rest when the symptoms are bad and the child should have a high calorie, high protein diet. Restriction of fat in the diet is unnecessary. Bed rest doesn't seem to produce a more rapid recovery and as soon as the child feels well enough (even if he is still jaundiced) he should be allowed up.

Rare cases of hepatitis include certain drugs and infection with amoebic dysentery.

Heredity *See* CHROMOSOMES

Hernia Otherwise known as a rupture, a hernia occurs when there is a defect or weakness in the muscular wall of the abdomen which allows a small part of the intestine to push itself out of the abdominal cavity to form a visible lump. There are two types of hernia in children, an UMBILICAL HERNIA near the UMBILICUS or navel and an inguinal hernia in the groin.

Umbilical hernias are very common in babies. When the umbilical cord detaches itself from the baby's body, it may leave a temporary area of weakness in the muscle wall. A small part of the bowel can then protrude through this weakness, under the skin, and it is the bulge that is called an umbilical hernia. When the child's abdominal pressure is raised (when he coughs or cries, for example) the hernia is seen to bulge even more, but there is no need to stop a child crying because of this. These hernias are especially common in babies of African origin and almost all disappear by the age of five without treatment. Doctors used to put binders around the abdomen to hold the hernia back but this has been shown to be unnecessary and even on occasions harmful. If they do not close spontaneously, a simple operation can be performed to close them.

Inguinal hernias are seen less frequently and are much more common in boys. When the TESTES are developing they start life inside the abdominal cavity. They migrate into the scrotum down a canal in the groin called the inguinal canal. This canal usually closes as soon as the testis has passed through but, if it doesn't, a little knuckle of bowel can push through it, causing a bulge in the groin which can sometimes even go into the scrotum.

This lump, like an umbilical hernia, is more easily seen when the child coughs. But, unlike an umbilical hernia, whose wide mouth always allows the contained bowel to slide in and out easily, an inguinal hernia can trap the bowel and cut off its blood supply. This is dangerous because it can damage and obstruct the bowel. The dangers of strangulation of the bowel are very great in the first six months of life, so if your child has a hernia of this type, your doctor may advise an operation. The operation is short and simple if the hernia is caught early, so do report a lump in the groin of your baby or young boy as soon as you see it.

Herpes simplex A very widespread virus that can cause several infections, including cold sores, a venereal disease, encephalitis, hepatitis, and a generalized infection of newborn babies. The latter can usually be avoided by delivering the child of an infected mother by Caesarean section.

Cold sores sometimes appear for no apparent reason, while on other occasions they follow colds or other mild illnesses. Some people come out in cold sores when exposed to the sun, some when they're under stress, and some girls have them particularly at period times.

The first infection a child has is rather different from subsequent ones. He complains of ulcers inside the mouth which may be so painful that he cannot eat or drink. There's very little that can be done but the condition subsides quickly of its own accord. Second and subsequent infections don't cause mouth ulcers but give rise to a readily recognizable rash around the lips.

This rash is itchy and composed of a mass of tiny blisters that rupture and become encrusted. Sometimes a secondary bacterial infection sets in (IMPETIGO) but if this doesn't happen, the condition cures itself within a week or so. Young babies don't seem to get cold sores and indeed they are uncommon before school age.

Herpes virus can be spread by sexual contact and can cause fever, swelling of the lymph nodes in the groin and pain on passing urine, as well as infection of the cervix in females and of the penis in males. A baby born to an infected mother acquires the infection during birth and may develop local infection of the eyes, mouth or skin or even a generalized infection which may be fatal. Older, severely malnourished babies may also suffer from a severe generalized infection.

ENCEPHALITIS can also be caused by this virus and is responsible for a high mortality rate.

Hiccups A short, sharp noise (really a short inbreathing cough) caused by the spasmodic contraction of the diaphragm. Newborn babies normally hiccup from time to time and may even hiccup in the womb before birth.

Older children may hiccup because of indigestion, an overfull stomach and even with 'flu. In children the cause is almost never serious and hiccups can be cured by many old wives' tricks such as breathing into a paper bag.

If your child has hiccups that go on for more than a day, consult your doctor.

Hives See URTICARIA

Hodgkin's disease A CANCER of the LYMPHATIC SYSTEM not commonly seen in children. The first sign of the condition is usually an enlargement of the glands at the back of the neck but occasionally those in the armpits and groins may enlarge first. The nodes are firm, separate and not painful. The diagnosis is made by examining one of the removed nodes under a microscope.

The treatment of Hodgkin's disease depends (as does the outcome) on the stage of the condition when it is diagnosed. X-ray therapy is used for the early stages and drugs later. Without treatment Hodgkin's disease is eventually fatal but 80 per cent of children can be cured in the early stage. Even children first treated in the later stage are alive and well in large numbers as long as six years after the diagnosis with modern drug treatment. Hodgkin's disease, like childhood leukaemia, was almost untreatable only a few years ago but today neither condition need fill parents with fear.

Hormones Substances produced by the endocrine GLANDS. Hormones are passed directly into the bloodstream which distributes them round the body where they control and regulate various physiological processes. If any particular endocrine gland produces too much or too little of its hormones, illness can result.

The master gland of the endocrine system, controlling the fine balance of all the hormones, lies in the skull just beneath the brain and is called the PITUITARY gland. This gland controls the action of the others (the OVARIES, TESTES, ADRENALS, and THYROID).

See PANCREAS

Hospital Among children aged 17 in 1975, one in two had been an in-patient in hospital by the age of seven! Three-quarters of a million children are admitted to hospital each year, whether as an emergency or as a planned admission, so it's obviously sensible to prepare both yourself and your child for the strong possibility of this happening.

In recent years several researchers have highlighted the fact that many children, and especially those under five, react very badly to being in hospital. They may become withdrawn or angry because they feel they have been rejected or betrayed, and may not return to normal for some time after getting back home. Detailed work has shown that this sort of emotional response is normal in under-fives left in hospitals without their mothers. Their misery or even frank DEPRESSION can be prevented completely by the admission of a parent – usually the mother – to the ward. Young children in particular need their mothers with them because they cannot understand that they have not been permanently deserted when their mothers go home, even with the best nursing attention. More and more hospitals are offering overnight accommodation to mothers of children under five (on the basis of an official recommendation) in an effort to make hospital admission a less traumatic experience.

If it is impossible for a parent to accompany the child into hospital, several measures can make the parting easier for him. Careful explanation beforehand about what will happen is helpful except for very young children. Bringing the hospital, nurses and doctors within the realms of the child's experience by pointing the hospital out, talking about the people, and using specially produced books about hospitals, making sure the child has some familiar objects with him, never leaving him without first telling him that you are going, reassuring him constantly that you will come back and that he will come home soon, and perhaps leaving something of yours or sending him a letter or postcard every day, will all help.

Children in long-stay hospitals have worse problems and the best thing in these circumstances is for one nurse on each shift to take special responsibility for the child so that he has someone in particular to relate to. One special nurse or other 'parent-figure' for each child in hospital is also arranged by some enlightened hospitals for short-stay children whose mothers can't be with them.

Unrestricted visiting has been recommended as a standard in all children's wards, with parents welcomed by the staff and often even working with them. Many hospitals, however, still restrict visiting because of old-fashioned and misguided ideas about what is best for children.

A ward in which visiting is frequently neglected or discouraged is the special care baby unit. Surprisingly, mothers often think that their newborn babies don't need them. However, there is mounting evidence that the baby separated from his mother doesn't thrive or feed as well as when she is there, sleeps badly and is more irritable. There is also evidence that mother-baby BONDING is impaired if the mother isn't with her baby as much as possible, so it seems sensible to spend as much time with the baby as you can. Some hospitals have special baby care units with rooms for mothers adjacent to the unit. The mothers co-operate with the nurses with the simpler baby care tasks and also find it very much easier to get breast feeding established.

See LOW BIRTH WEIGHT

Hydrocele A collection of fluid around the testis that makes the testicle look bigger than it should. Sometimes a hydrocele is present at birth and both sides of the scrotum may be affected.

The fluid almost always goes of its own accord and does no permanent damage. Should it not disappear by the age of four or five years, it may have to be drained by a small operation, but this is rarely necessary.

Hydrocephalus (water on the brain) A condition seen in three in a thousand children in Britain in which the head is enlarged because of excessive cerebro-spinal fluid in the brain. The fluid is produced by a special part of the brain's blood system and normally circulates between the coverings of the brain and spinal cord and inside the brain and cord as well. This fluid normally carries nutrients to the brain and spinal cord and acts as a hydraulic buffer to them so that they don't get damaged as we move about. In hydrocephalus there is too much fluid so that pressure builds up in the cavities of the brain and the bony skull enlarges.

Hydrocephalus may be seen alone or together with SPINA BIFIDA.

Hydrocephalus can be caused by several things but the commonest cause in a baby is a blockage in the flow of cerebro-spinal fluid due to a malformation of the brain. When it develops later in babyhood it is usually

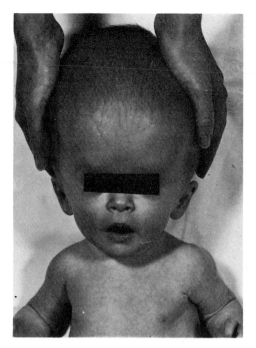

A baby suffering from hydrocephalus –
excessive cerebro-spinal fluid in the brain.
Regular measurements of a baby's head are
taken to detect this condition in its early stages.

due to meningitis or a tumour. In an older child, the skull sutures and fontanelles are closed, so hydrocephalus causing enlargement of the skull can't develop. This leads to a rise in pressure inside the skull.

Although some cases are diagnosed before birth, the majority don't even show up until after the first few weeks or even months of life. Routine regular measurements of the circumference of the baby's head and feeling the anterior FONTANELLE of the skull to see if it is bulging are a great help in the early detection of hydrocephalus and this is one reason why you'll see doctors measuring around your baby's head and feeling the soft spot.

If untreated, the skull sometimes enlarges at the rate of an inch a month and the child's appearance can become very distressing. The forehead bulges, the whites of the eyes are clearly visible as a rim above the iris, the scalp thins and the skin becomes shiny with easily visible veins. Eventually the brain can be so severely damaged by the pressure of the fluid

that permanent mental retardation is caused.

Surgery can offer a lot to these children today. If there is an obstruction to the flow of the fluid, it can be bypassed with plastic tubes that take the fluid into the heart. This has revolutionized the outlook for many babies because whereas two-thirds of them used to have a very short life span, today after operation about two-thirds of them live.

Hyperactivity (overactivity) A disturbing condition in young children which is ill understood and may not always be recognized. Nine times as many boys as girls are affected.

Hyperactive children are often prone to cot rocking and head banging as babies and go on to be disruptive at school and at home. They may be of above average intelligence but this is not always so and many have learning difficulties. They are very excitable, cannot sit still for long, sometimes have difficulties with co-ordination, and may need little sleep. There may be a history of headaches, asthma, catarrh, hay fever and other respiratory problems.

Medical opinions as to the cause of hyperactivity vary and the diagnosis is made very much more frequently in the USA than in the UK. Many parents feel instinctively that it is a behavioural problem which can be overcome by proper handling of the child but there is good evidence that many such children are adversely affected by certain food colourings and flavourings. Good results have been achieved by keeping such children off all foods containing these chemicals but this is difficult to carry out in practice.

Environmental changes may play a part in the production of hyperactivity. It has been known for some time that children with high levels of lead in their bodies tend to be hyperactive (*see* LEAD POISONING). Other heavy metals can cause hyperactivity in certain animals and research is under way to see if these substances may also be implicated in children.

Hypermetropia *See* VISUAL PROBLEMS

Hyperventilation *See* OVERBREATHING

Hypospadias *See* PENIS

129

Hypothermia A lower than normal body temperature which can be dangerous, especially in premature babies. For details of the body's temperature control mechanisms, *see* TEMPERATURE.

A premature baby loses heat easily because its heat-regulating centre is immature and because there is less insulating fat than in a full term baby. Babies suffering from oxygen lack may also have a lowered body temperature. Because of the dangers of excessive cooling, the environment of these babies should be kept between 70–80°F (21–26°C), which is most easily achieved in an INCUBATOR. Newborn babies don't respond to cold by shivering, as do adults. It appears that in order to raise their body temperature in cold surroundings they mobilize energy from specialized fat stores – a mechanism seen in many animals.

An unexplained fall in body temperature in a baby may be due to an infection or a metabolic disorder.

Many mothers worry a great deal about their babies getting cold and may keep their rooms too hot. Unless a baby is premature (and assuming that he is sensibly dressed for the type of weather), a room temperature of about 60°F (15.5°C) is quite warm enough. The baby who sleeps next to his mother at night is naturally kept warm by the heat of her body.

Hysteria A medical term for a condition in which there is a loss of body function without any obvious disease. Almost any part of the nervous system can be affected but the loss of function that occurs happens at a subconscious level. Hysterical children don't deliberately produce their symptoms, although malingering can be a form of hysteria.

Hysteria has been recognized as an epidemic condition for years, and young women and girls seem most prone to it. Over the centuries there have been many such examples. In recent years an epidemic of a mysterious 'virus illness' caused fainting among schoolgirls in Derbyshire: this turned out to be a type of hysteria.

In everyday speech the term is used rather loosely to describe any seemingly exaggerated behaviour. The peculiar physical and mental changes that occur among young girls at pop concerts, for example, are usually hysterical and soon disappear.

Hysterical fits in children can resemble epileptic fits very closely but are easily distinguished once the features of each are known. First, there's usually a neurotic background and, second, these children rarely hurt themselves, bite their tongues or wet themselves during a seizure, unlike a child having an epileptic fit. Also an epileptic child will often sleep after a grand mal fit and awake with a headache. This almost never occurs in a hysterical fit.

I

Immunity Although the body has good mechanical barriers (the skin and mucous membranes) to keep it free from external contamination, some potentially harmful bacteria and viruses still get through and are coped with by the body's immunity system. When, for example, the body is invaded by bacteria for the first time, local protective mechanisms (inflammation) come into play, together with a general reaction including fever. However, at the same time there is a specific immune response: the bacteria are 'recognized' as foreign or antigenic, engulfed by white cells (phagocytes) in the liver and spleen if they invade the bloodstream, and otherwise engulfed by local white cells and swept along in the lymph to the local lymph nodes or spleen. Here other white cells (lymphocytes) respond by producing specific antibodies and by developing a memory for that particular foreign protein so that the next time an infection occurs, the body's reaction can be faster.

These 'memory cells' explain why the body's immune response to a first infection takes longer than its response to further infections: with a second infection the antibody production system is ready to go immediately and reaches much higher antibody levels. IMMUNIZATION against infectious disease is commonly (though not always) carried out in several stages in order to prime the immunity system, so that if natural infection occurs, the system has the best possible chance of overcoming it.

Unfortunately, not all antibody responses are advantageous to our bodies – sometimes the system goes wrong and the body produces antibodies against its own cells which are treated as foreign for some unknown reason, as in certain sorts of thyroid, arterial and skin diseases, called auto-immune diseases.

Immunological factors are also involved in the body's reaction to cancer of some of its cells and to the transplant of organs from another person.

Several rare diseases in children (including agammaglobulinaemia), are due to a deficiency of the immunological tissue.

ALLERGY occurs if the body's immunity system over-reacts to a foreign substance, such as grass pollen, cat fur or food.

Immunology, the study of immune systems and the way diseases affect them, is a relatively new and fast-growing science and has revolutionized our understanding and treatment of many diseases.

Immunization Immunity to disease can be acquired by getting the disease itself or by active or passive immunization. If a child has actually suffered from an infection, he will have developed his own antibodies to that disease and so is unlikely to contract it again. However, rather than wait for children to get certain infections it's wiser to ensure that their antibody levels are built up artificially by immunization.

With passive immunization, the antibodies are produced by another person or animal and injected into the child. With active immunization, a child is given a weakened form of the organisms, which then produce a mild form of the disease and in so doing stimulate the production of protective antibodies.

Some immunizations provide lifetime protection (such as DIPHTHERIA) while others last a very short time (such as influenza).

A child is born with immunity to some diseases because antibodies may pass across the placenta from the mother if she herself has had or has been immunized against these diseases. After birth, a breast-fed baby continues to get valuable antibodies in breast milk and especially in the colostrum produced in the first few days after birth. Breast milk contains other anti-infective factors besides antibodies and bottle-fed babies miss out on these completely.

As the baby matures he becomes able to manufacture his own antibodies and so can cope with the challenge of illness himself.

Today's children are immunized in infancy against diphtheria, WHOOPING COUGH, TETANUS, POLIO and MEASLES. Routine VACCINATION against SMALLPOX is no longer considered advisable as the disease has been eradicated worldwide.

Immunization schedules vary, but one method is to have the first injection of triple vaccine (diphtheria, tetanus and whooping cough), together with oral polio vaccine, at about three months; the second dose follows six to eight weeks later; and the third dose six months after that. Measles vaccine is often given in the second year.

Having your baby immunized is very important because it means that he'll probably never get the diseases in question or, if he does, they will be in a very mild form.

Immunization against GERMAN MEASLES (rubella) is now offered to girls of about twelve years. This is to prevent them contracting the disease when they are pregnant, when it could harm their unborn baby.

BCG vaccine against TUBERCULOSIS is given to adolescent children if necessary – a skin test is done first to ascertain whether they need it. In certain circumstances younger children are given the vaccine.

It's a good idea to keep a record of all your child's immunizations and to take it with you when you go to your clinic or doctor. This is useful especially if your child has an accident as the timing of his last tetanus immunization will determine whether or not he will need a BOOSTER.

Should your baby be unwell on the day he's meant to be immunized, ask for your doctor's advice because immunizing babies who are ill can be dangerous. However, the common cold or 'snuffles' without a fever should not put you off having your child immunized. Vaccines are also available when necessary for cholera, typhoid and paratyphoid, influenza, anthrax, yellow fever and rabies.

Impetigo A contagious skin condition usually of the face, scalp or hands, seen mostly in schoolchildren and caused by staphylococci or streptococci. Outbreaks occur in schools and other places where children mix closely. Sometimes it is seen as a complication of ECZEMA, cold sores, SCABIES or URTICARIA that has been scratched.

Affected skin is covered with yellowish-brown crusts. Healing tends to occur from the centre, leaving rings of reddened skin.

If your child has impetigo, don't feel guilty because you think it's due to poor hygiene. Infections such as this can be contracted by the cleanest children.

Treatment is with an antibiotic ointment (usually containing tetracycline) but tetracycline tablets may also be necessary. Any really thick crusts can be gently removed with warm water and cotton wool, but be very careful to wash your own hands thoroughly after touching the infected skin as impetigo can spread through a family like wildfire.

Your child can go to school if his impetigo is loosely covered to prevent him scratching it and spreading the germs with his hands.

Incest Sexual relations between two people in the same family prohibited by law from having intercourse. It is practised worldwide. Incest is officially rare (fewer than three hundred cases a year are reported) but is known to be very much more common than the statistics suggest. In certain countries incest is accepted in ceremonial circumstances.

Many brothers and sisters play with each other sexually, but then they also play in this way with other children and anyway it is very rare for either type of relationship to culminate in intercourse. No harm comes from this play unless there is guilt either at the time or later.

The commonest form of incest occurs between father and daughter. Mother-son relationships are far less common. Such relationships may or may not harm the child but often the guilt associated with this, the last social taboo, is too much for the child to bear and she ends up being psychologically or even physically affected by the relationship. In one survey of 36 girls who had paternal intercourse, 11 developed certain promiscuous character disorders (some of them became prostitutes); five later became frigid (with marriage problems); five became psychotic, though it was impossible definitely to link the two; and in 15 there were no detectable psychological effects at all.

Perhaps surprisingly, the mother usually tolerates the incestuous relationship between her husband and daughter and some mothers even connive at it. They probably do this for a number of reasons. First they fear they might lose their husband if they create a fuss so in the interests of keeping the family together they don't; second, they fear that their husband will be jailed; and third, subconsciously they may feel that as they are now menopausal and often less interested in sex than they were, they would prefer their husband to have sexual relationships with someone inside the family rather than outside it. Why fathers have these relationships is not known and there are many theories, but many of the offending fathers are not mentally stable and large numbers are alcoholic or have aggressive and disordered personalities. No social class is exempt from having incestuous relationships.

Treatment has until recently been very poor. The damage has been done before the incest is revealed. Jailing the father may break up the family, and, if not, the facts show that once out of prison he starts all over again. Separating father and daughter does not work because the man turns to his next daughter. Some success has been achieved with psychotherapy but supportive care such as is being offered at incest centres in the USA is probably the only way of coping with this difficult problem.

Incubator A specially constructed chamber in which to keep babies too small, immature or ill to be nursed in a cot. The commonest reason for babies to be nursed in incubators is prematurity. Many babies born too early or light-for-dates need to be protected in a controlled environment.

Most incubators are box-shaped containers on legs or wheels that stand at waist height. The baby's bed is covered with a perspex dome. A thermostatically controlled heater keeps the air warm and the air is circulated in such a way as to prevent the build-up of carbon dioxide from the baby's lungs. An incubator is virtually closed off from outside but the baby can be seen through the dome. Portholes at the sides allow doctors, nurses and mothers to handle the baby, if necessary using gloves which are fitted as part of the incubator.

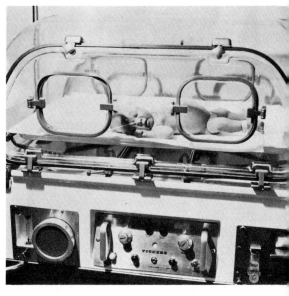

An incubator may be vital to protect a very small or ill baby from extremes of temperature, and can be filled with oxygen-enriched air if the baby is having difficulty breathing.

There are several different kinds of incubator but they all provide certain essential things. First, a pre-term baby cannot control his body temperature properly: the incubator is thus kept at a steady temperature to protect him from the cold. Second, the incubator keeps the baby relatively free from infection. Because premature babies are so small and immature, they cope very badly with infections, so this function of the incubator can be life-saving. Third, an incubator is a closed chamber and so can be filled with air rich in oxygen if the baby's breathing is poor.

Really small babies – less than 3lb (1360g) in weight – start off with many odds stacked against them. An incubator allows the environment to be regulated, so the baby has the best chance of survival. The modern incubator helps the caring staff that man the premature baby units in our hospitals to save thousands of babies' lives every year.

We now know that the separation of a baby from its mother in these early weeks can have long-term adverse effects. Because of this it is highly desirable for every baby who has to be cared for in an incubator to have as much contact with his mother as possible. You can breast feed (if necessary by expressing or pumping milk to be given to the baby via a tube or dropper) and touching and caressing him will still be as valuable as if your baby was quite healthy. Remember, the baby is still yours, so keep in close contact with him for both his sake and yours.

Infectious diseases *See under name of disease*

Influenza An infection of the upper respiratory tract, usually starting with a cold and perhaps a sore throat, that is caused by viruses. It generally lasts only a few days. 'Flu usually occurs in epidemics during which the very young in particular are at risk from dying of secondary bacterial infections.

In 1918-19, twenty million people died in 'flu pandemics, and since then there have been other big epidemics which have killed large numbers of people. The last two big 'flu epidemics were in 1957 and 1968 and were known as 'Hong Kong 'flu' and 'Asian 'flu'. Three kinds of influenza virus are recognized – A, B and C. Type A is especially liable to change and this is one of the great problems in creating an effective vaccine against 'flu. However, routine immunization against 'flu is not recommended for normal children.

As with some other infectious diseases, the immunity conferred by one infection lasts a very short time. This is why people get 'flu many times.

Unfortunately, we can pick up our influenza viruses from animals as well as from other humans. Pigs were, only a few years ago, responsible for a particularly potent type of 'flu that caused many deaths among young, healthy people in the USA. This led to a massive immunization programme against the so-called swine 'flu but the programme was halted because some deaths resulted from the vaccine itself. A great deal of research is under way to find a really effective way of making a suitable vaccine fast enough to keep up with each change in the 'flu virus.

There is no effective drug treatment for the viral infection which is the basis of 'flu because drugs powerful enough to kill viruses also damage the body cells in which the viruses live. The incubation period is usually 36 to 48 hours. The onset is sudden, with a high fever, sweating, aches in the limbs and back, a cough, sore throat and painful eyes. In young children there may be diarrhoea and vomiting, croup or nosebleed.

Bed is the best cure for 'flu in the older child. Give him plenty to drink and treat his FEVER if necessary. Don't be surprised if your child doesn't want to eat – he'll come to no harm for a day or two. Keep other children away and don't allow dirty handkerchiefs to collect in the house. Either wash them at once with the washing machine set at its hottest; boil them if you have no machine; or use paper hankies and burn them or flush them down the lavatory.

Treatment with antibiotics is only effective if there is a secondary bacterial infection such as PNEUMONIA, OTITIS MEDIA, SINUSITIS or MASTOIDITIS.

Though there is no specific treatment for 'flu, don't hesitate to ask for your doctor's advice if you are worried about your child. The worst symptoms usually go within three or four days but the child may feel weak or depressed for weeks afterwards.

Inherited diseases Those diseases which run in families. It's always distressing when a child develops an unpleasant disease or is born with a deformity, but it's doubly so for the parents if they feel it might in some way have been their fault.

One of the most difficult things about deciding whether a condition is in fact inherited from one or both parents is the ruling out of environmental factors that could have caused the problem. For example, children born to mothers who took thalidomide were severely deformed yet this was clearly due to the drug and not to the parents being abnormal in any way. It may well be that many more diseases and deformities than we realize are tied to environmental factors such as the mother's diet, drugs or infections during pregnancy, but only time and more research will tell. We discuss the congenital malformations elsewhere (*see* CONGENITAL ABNOR-

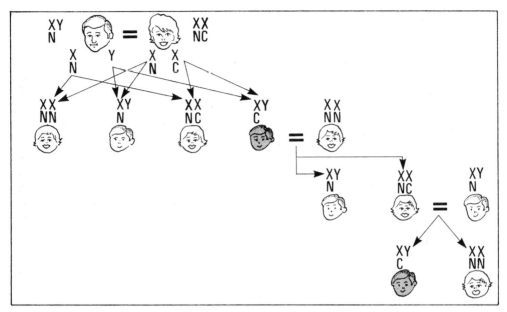

MALITIES) so here we'll deal with other inherited diseases.

One of the commonest to run in families is DIABETES in which the child inherits the potential for the disease rather than the disease itself. Other diseases such as TB and some types of cancer also run in families: that is to say it's the potential to develop the disease that's inherited, and not the disease itself. Under certain environmental conditions the child may develop these diseases if he has the underlying potential. Asthma, eczema and hay fever similarly run in families but not every child in the family necessarily suffers from any of these complaints.

The genes are the parts of the CHROMOSOMES that carry the details of inheritance and more is being learnt about genetic structure and function every year. It has been estimated that each of us has about ten potentially harmful genes in our sex cells which may be transmitted to future generations.

Nature rejects many of her worst mistakes by aborting abnormal foetuses spontaneously – sometimes even before the woman realizes she's pregnant (she simply thinks she's had a

The family tree shows how colour blindness, usually due to a sex-linked recessive disorder, may be transmitted. N, the gene for normal vision, is dominant, and when present overrules the action of C, the gene for colour blindness (which is present only in the female X chromosome).

heavy period). Probably as many as one in five of all conceptions fail to reach a stage in which they can survive outside the womb, and some of these have genetic defects.

Some inherited diseases are caused by the presence of an abnormal genetic structure in one parent only (dominant or 'sex-linked recessive' conditions). Others are caused by the inheritance of abnormal genes from both parents (recessive conditions) and yet others by a spontaneous change (mutation) that may occur in the genes of normal parents.

Many inherited diseases are caused by inborn errors of metabolism due to the faulty action or even a complete absence of particular enzymes in the body. These result in a build-up of certain body chemicals or a lack of others and it's these that produce the symptoms of the disease. PHENYLKETONURIA is relatively common. Albinism (*see* ALBINO) is another such inherited condition, as is GALACTOSAEMIA, a condition in which the child cannot change lactose (milk sugar) into glucose.

The study of genetics is now well advanced and today's parents can be advised by a genetic counsellor as to the likelihood of their having a baby with an inherited disorder. There should be a unit with a genetic counsellor attached to one of the hospitals in your region. (*See* GENETIC COUNSELLING.)

Most of the inborn errors of metabolism are carried from generation to generation by recessive genes in normal people who nevertheless have the potential to produce children with one of these diseases. Such parents are called carriers. If two carriers of the same abnormal gene have children, they have a one in four chance of producing a baby with this particular error of metabolism; three out of four of their children will either be completely normal or carriers themselves. This sort of knowledge is of value when people who are known to be carriers want to marry. It's also important to be careful of marriages involving relatives. Only a half to one per cent of all marriages involve first cousins but a third of all the cases of one particular inherited disease are produced by these marriages.

In families with a history of a sex-linked recessive disorder such as HAEMOPHILIA, a pregnant woman may be offered an AMNIO-CENTESIS to see if her unborn child is a boy or a girl. If it is a boy, and thus has a one in two chance of being affected by the disease, she may wish to have an abortion.

In certain inborn errors of metabolism the effects of the enzyme deficiencies can be overcome (e.g. galactosaemia and phenylketonuria). One day we may even be able to cure these diseases by genetic engineering. However, advances in genetics must be slow and well controlled because once we have the knowledge and ability to alter genetic structure, we have the potential to alter it for the worse, which worries many people.

Insect stings *See* BITES AND STINGS

Insomnia *See* SLEEP

Intelligence Definitions of intelligence are always unsatisfactory as so many abstract factors are involved. In practical terms, a useful way of assessing intelligence is by observing how a child or adult copes with a new situation: the more able he is to handle the problem, the more intelligent he is likely to be, though this also depends on his personality. An intelligent person not only deals with new situations more capably but also usually learns from experience better than a less intelligent person would. He is therefore more able to manipulate his environment to suit himself.

We have become accustomed to equating intelligence with ability to pass intelligence tests. Unfortunately, these tests are limited in what they can measure and simply demonstrate to the examiner how able the examinee is to answer the questions and perform the tasks set in the test. These IQ or intelligence quotient tests, as they are called, do however have a useful function in assessing how well a child will be able to cope with formal schooling. But two children with the same intelligence quotient will not necessarily be equally intelligent in the wider sense of the word. They may have an equal ability at vocabulary scores, 'draw-a-man' tests, arithmetical tests and so on, but they will probably have widely differing abilities in such day-to-day activities as dressing, catching the bus, settling down to work alone, getting on with other people and learning from experience. This latter group of abilities is much more important overall in adult life, especially for those of low formal intelligence, as success in these spheres determines whether or not they will be able to live normal lives or will always need supervisory care.

In Britain there are special schools for those of low intelligence, as assessed both by intelligence tests and a more general assessment of the child's abilities. (*See* EDUCATIONAL SUBNORMALITY.)

Some countries have special schools for GIFTED CHILDREN – children with unusually high intellectual ability. The reasoning behind this is that they can nurture their most capable children in the hope that these children will do great things for the good of their country. In others, the cleverest children go to the same schools as the rest, even though many of them have problems such as difficulty in getting on with others and boredom in class when the teacher goes too slowly for them.

Though many people prize intelligence in their children, it certainly is not the be-all and end-all of human virtues. Many intelligent people do not know how to get the best out of their lives or how to be happy, whereas many less intelligent people live far happier and more fulfilled lives. Striving for academic, or any other sort of success for one's children is understandable but not necessarily a good thing. Instead, the child should be given opportunities, in this case the right environment for learning, and allowed to go as far as he wants to in the academic field. Though the intelligent child can nearly always have academic success, it will not necessarily make him happy.

See BEHAVIOUR; MENTAL RETARDATION

Intoeing   *See* PIGEON TOE

Intussusception   A condition in which a piece of the bowel telescopes into the part in front of it, rather like a sock being turned inside out. Intussusception is seen in previously well babies, usually between the ages of 3 and 12 months. It is a dangerous condition because the blood supply of the affected part of the bowel becomes obstructed, leading to gangrene and death if it is not treated.

A baby with an intussusception has sudden attacks of severe pain together with screaming and straining. Attacks sometimes recur at very short intervals and the child may at first be apparently quite well between them. He looks very pale during an attack and may also vomit and have a slight fever. Eventually he goes into a state of shock. During the first few hours of being ill he passes normal bowel motions but later the typical 'red currant jelly' stools of intussusception may be passed. These consist mostly of blood and mucus.

Treatment is by an emergency operation, carried out as soon as possible. Occasionally the bowel may right itself while the child is waiting for the operation.

IQ   *See* INTELLIGENCE

Iron deficiency anaemia   *See* ANAEMIA

Itching   Irritation in the skin relieved by a painful stimulus such as scratching.

One of the commonest causes of itching is a dry skin, caused by too much washing, the excessive use of soap or detergents, or sunburn. Drugs can also cause itching as part of a hyper-sensitivity reaction. Chemicals, hair dyes, cosmetics, plants and scores of other everyday things can produce itching, and often it's not easy to track down the cause. Flea bites, scabies and other skin conditions may cause itching and it may also be caused by allergy, such as eczema, urticaria or dermatitis, or even by getting too hot (prickly heat).

Athlete's foot and other fungal infections of the skin are itchy, as are several generalised diseases such as Hodgkin's disease, jaundice, uraemia, diabetes, and some infections such as chickenpox.

Itching around the anus is known as pruritus ani, and around the vulva, pruritus vulvae. Threadworm infection can cause itching in these areas as can scabies and lice. Older girls may get itching of the vulva caused by a vaginal discharge.

Neurodermatitis is an uncommon condition that results from scratching irritating skin. The sites most commonly affected are the elbows, knees and ankles. There is no underlying disease of the skin. This type of itching is probably of neurotic origin and can eventually lead to almost continuous scratching.

The treatment of itching is, if possible, to remove the cause. If this can't be done, antihistamine tablets are of use but can make the sufferer sleepy and so must be used with caution. If necessary, sleeping medicines at night will ensure that the child gets some sleep in severe cases of itching.

If your child has itching that goes on for more than a day or two, consult your doctor.

J

Jaundice A yellow staining of the skin and whites of the eyes (as well as other body tissues) by bilirubin formed by the pigment from broken down red blood cells.

Jaundice occurs for one of three reasons:
1) The liver enzymes are unable to metabolize bilirubin adequately.
2) Too many red blood cells are being broken down.
3) There is an obstruction to the flow of bile from the liver to the intestine.

So-called physiological jaundice occurs in many newborn babies because the liver enzymes can't cope adequately with the excretion of bilirubin produced by the breakdown of red blood cells. Excess bilirubin in the foetus passes across the placenta to be metabolized and excreted by the mother, so as long as the baby is in the uterus it is protected from the accumulation of bilirubin. As the liver is more likely to be immature in premature babies, these are more likely to have physiological jaundice. This type of jaundice appears on the second or third day after birth and disappears spontaneously within a week in full term babies, and a bit later in premature ones.

Jaundice caused by Rhesus incompatibility is less of a problem than it used to be (*see* BLOOD GROUPS). This sort of jaundice is either present at birth or develops in the first 24 hours. Incompatibility between the blood groups of the mother and baby other than Rhesus incompatibility can also cause jaundice.

Among the many other causes of jaundice in the newborn are internal bleeding; certain drugs; thyroid deficiency; and congenital abnormalities of the bile ducts. Jaundice persisting in a newborn baby after leaving hospital should be reported to your doctor. Some breast-fed babies develop jaundice on the third day that lasts for several weeks, but this 'breast milk jaundice' rarely reaches dangerous levels and it is only necessary to stop breast feeding temporarily if the bilirubin level is very high. Recovery from jaundice may be delayed by an insufficient milk intake associated with restricted and scheduled feeds.

If the blood level of bilirubin that has not been metabolized by the liver is very high, it can cause brain damage, so the level is carefully watched by the doctors looking after the baby. A high level can be treated with phototherapy, by putting the baby under the light from a fluorescent tube. More severe or persistent jaundice may need to be treated by an exchange transfusion.

Babies with any sort of infection can become jaundiced (though this is unusual) because infection may prevent the liver from functioning properly. Such babies are usually obviously ill from the underlying infection which needs suitable treatment. HEPATITIS, a viral infection of the liver itself, causes jaundice in children of any age.

In older children and adolescents there are other causes of jaundice, and gallstones (a common cause of jaundice in adults) are now being seen in adolescents with increasing frequency.

Since jaundice is not a disease but only a symptom of an underlying disease, the cause must always be sought and treated. If ever your baby or child looks yellow, he must be seen by a doctor.

Jealousy Jealousy between brothers and sisters is so common as to be considered absolutely normal. Many psychiatrists think that if there is no sibling rivalry in a family, something must be wrong and that this normal emotion must be buried in the subconscious minds of the children, ready to cause trouble later.

Many parents notice signs of jealousy in their children for the first time when a new baby arrives. Although all the children in the family may feel some degree of jealousy because of the amount of time their mother has to give up to the new arrival, the former youngest child is usually most affected. Many people have tried to work out the ideal age gap between children to minimize jealousy, but this is difficult as so much depends on the way the situation is handled by the parents and on the personalities of the individual children. One of the commonest age gaps these days is two years but this can prove to be awkward because of the very nature of two-year-olds – demanding and egocentric. A smaller age gap can mean that the mother doesn't have enough time to devote to the one-year-old who is developing so fast in language and other skills, and a bigger gap means that the children can easily feel so different in age that they don't play well together.

Jealousy can reveal itself in many ways. The child can be obviously aggressive towards the baby or even to the mother. He may withdraw affection from his mother and become quiet and sad. He may forget the skills he has learned and start wetting or messing his pants, feeding himself with his hands and demanding a bottle or a cuddle at awkward times.

The best way to cope with all this is to make sure that the other child or children are given plenty of love and attention so that they feel secure again in their mother's affection, as jealousy is basically caused by a feeling of insecurity. Make sure that each child gets his fair share of your time each day, though there is no need to pretend that the baby is not getting his fair share as well. Seeing you look after and take a joy in your new baby should be an enriching experience for each child in the family, as long as they are not left out in the cold.

Feed times can be difficult with a toddler around, so try to make sure that you have everything that the toddler might want, such as a potty, a drink, books and so on, before you start feeding the baby. It's quite easy to make feeding time a special time for the toddler as well.

Jealousy also crops up between older members of the family and you will have to work out the solution each time according to the individuals involved. Great patience is often necessary because jealousy between children often lasts a long time and can be very demoralizing to the parents who have to listen to the constant squabbling. Here again, remember that reassurance and extra demonstrations of your love will help a lot towards recovering the self-confidence that has often been lost in such a situation.

See AGGRESSION

Joint pains *See* ARTHRITIS; GROWING PAINS; RHEUMATIC FEVER

K

Kidneys The kidneys are a pair of abdominal organs, situated one each side high up in the small of the back, that extract water and waste products from the blood and convert them into urine. Each kidney is protected by fat and lies under the lower back part of the rib cage. Each is about 11cm long and 6cm wide in an adult and correspondingly smaller in children.

A kidney is divided into two main parts: the outer part or cortex surrounds the paler, inner medulla. A kidney has about one million subunits which produce urine as a kind of filtrate from blood. About one fifth of the total output of blood from the heart goes to the kidneys.

The kidneys produce urine which is passed

Diagrammatic cross-section of a kidney.
a. cortex, b. medulla, c. artery, d. vein,
e. ureter.

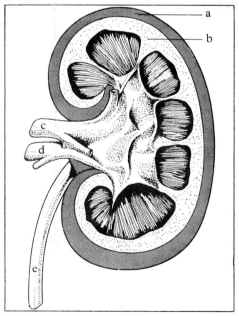

into the ureters. These are the paired, thin tubes that convey urine from the kidneys down to the bladder which lies in the pelvis behind the pubic bone. Very little goes wrong with the ureters but a kidney stone can sometimes get stuck in the tiny tube as it passes down to the bladder. This can produce extremely severe pain. The bladder holds the urine until the child is ready to pass it. The only common bladder problem is CYSTITIS, in which the urine becomes infected, usually as part of a generalized urine infection (*see* NEPHRITIS).

Although tumours are rare in very young children, the kidney is the site of one of the most common, a Wilms' tumour, which usually first shows as a lump in the abdomen. Treatment is by removal of the kidney.

Not only do the kidneys excrete various waste substances from the body in the urine but they also conserve useful substances that would otherwise pass out in the urine. This reabsorption is a critical part of the function of the kidneys. They also produce a substance known as erythropoetin which stimulates the bone marrow to produce red blood cells. Two other substances, renin and angiotensin, are produced in the kidneys and these help to control blood pressure.

But one of the most important functions of the kidneys is to regulate the pH (acidity and alkalinity) of the body. When we eat certain foods they tend to produce an excess of acidic substances in the blood. This is quite normal. The kidneys help to maintain the acidity of the whole body and its fluids at the correct level by several processes of secretion and reabsorption of chemicals as the urine is produced.

Rather like the heart, the kidneys go on functioning constantly throughout our lives, producing thousands of gallons of urine and keeping our body fluids in perfect balance.

Should the kidneys go wrong or fail completely sophisticated tests can be done to find the cause. Kidney machines can take over the work of the failing kidneys but in the long term a transplant is the ideal solution.

Kiss of life (mouth-to-mouth resuscitation) You may be able to tell if your child has stopped breathing by putting your cheek against his mouth to feel for breaths. You may

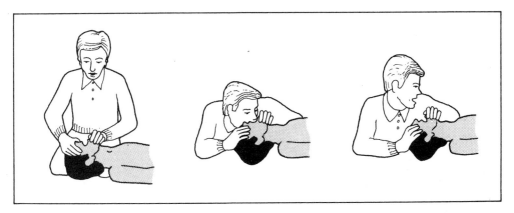

How to do the kiss of life. Make sure the child's head is tilted well back so that his tongue does not obstruct his windpipe.

notice that there are no chest movements but this is sometimes difficult if he is wearing lots of clothes. If you have a mirror handy, place it in front of his mouth and see if it steams up.

Once you've decided he's stopped breathing, you must act quickly.

Lie him on the ground on his back (unless he's vomiting) and see if there's anything in his mouth that's obviously obstructing his breathing. If there is, remove it. If not, tilt his head backwards as far as possible so that the nostrils point directly up at you. Cup one hand under his chin and, with the heel of the other hand on his forehead, ensure that his head is tilted right back. In an older child squeeze the nostrils closed with the fingers of the hand that is on the forehead and, after ensuring that his mouth is open, breathe firmly, but not hard, into his mouth. As you turn your head away to take another breath, watch for the chest to fall. Repeat this procedure either until professional help arrives or until the child starts to breathe spontaneously. Try to blow a breath into the child every five seconds or so. You can give the first few breaths much more quickly but then settle down to a rhythm.

Don't blow too hard or you may blow air into the stomach down the gullet. You'll be able to tell if you're doing this because the abdomen will swell. This may make the child vomit which is unpleasant for you and hazardous for him because he may inhale it.

In young children, put your mouth over both nose and mouth when blowing air in and use much less force than in an older child. In babies, only use the amount of air you can hold in your cheeks – *don't blow from your lungs*.

If there is no heart beat, *see* HEART MASSAGE.

See ASPHYXIA; COMA

Knock knees Many three-year-old children have knock knees: in fact some splaying out of the lower legs is seen in three-quarters of

Knock knees.

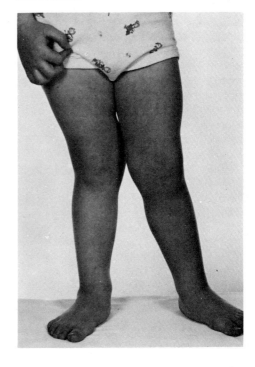

normal children between three and three and a half years.

Obese children are more likely to be affected, simply because their excess weight puts a strain on the mechanical structure of the knee joint. With time alone these children lose their knock-kneed appearance and by the age of seven years their legs look quite straight in almost every case. The overweight child should be helped by his parents to lose weight, when his legs should straighten faster than if he were allowed to go on carrying excess weight around.

The child who, when examined by the doctor, with his knees together and his legs straight, has a distance of more than two inches (about five centimetres) between his ankles, should be seen at regular intervals by the doctor for observation of his knees. He may be wearing his shoes down on their inner sides and an inside raise may be recommended for the sole and heel.

While the cause of knock knees proper is usually obesity, some rarer diseases such as RICKETS can be the culprit. A one-sided deformity is nearly always pathological. The child with true knock knees which aren't getting better, with one-sided knock knee, or with severe knock knee at any age needs medical supervision.

Very occasionally, an adolescent child can develop knock knees which, if severe, may need surgical treatment. Obesity is nearly always a factor in these children, so there is always a chance that alert parents may be able to prevent the condition from worsening by helping the child with his diet.

L

Lactose intolerance *See* SUGAR INTOLERANCE

Language A child develops speech as the result of the many complex processes involved in language development. Although we tend to concentrate on how many words a child can say and on how well he says them, speech or verbal expression is less important to a child's language development than his 'unspoken language' ability – the ability to listen to what is said, to understand its meaning, and mentally to pick out the words he needs in order to express himself. Once the child knows what he wants to say, provided he has had experience of the words necessary to say it and has remembered these words, then speech is just a question of practice and the correct action of the muscles and nerves involved in speech production. The intellectual processes involved in language are all-important.

Until a child realizes that a word is a symbol for something, he cannot be said to be using language as such, although he may say words and occasionally by chance use them in the right context. This symbolic understanding of words develops along with the understanding of other symbols, such as the fact that a toy car represents a real car and, later, that a picture of a car also represents a real car. When a young child starts playing with toys in a meaningful way, perhaps using a toy tea set to make a cup of tea, or loading a toy lorry and putting the driver in place, then we know that he is using these toys as symbols of the real things and it is likely that he is also at the stage of understanding words as meaningful symbols and of picking out words to express what he wants to say. True language has started to develop.

Symbolic understanding develops at different times in different children, depending partly on the amount of language experience they have had, but it is usually seen when a child is about 15 to 18 months old. From this age, the child rapidly develops the ability to relate ideas and concepts to one another. For instance, at two years old, a child can usually relate two words and will correctly respond to the suggestion that he should, for example, 'put the spoon in the cup'. He may do this before if the objects are pointed out, but this is not the same as doing it simply after listening to a spoken instruction, when the verbal symbols are all-important. At this age too, another form of symbolic understanding can be seen, corresponding with the use of words as symbols: the child matches pictures of objects to toys – both symbols of real things.

The months before symbolic understanding is reached are vital for language development. A baby makes various cooing and gurgling noises and learns to experiment with sound production. He learns to recognize certain sounds, for example his mother's voice. He learns to listen to sounds and eventually, at about eight months, he'll realize that some sounds have meaning – perhaps he'll recognize that the words 'time for milk' mean that milk is going to appear, because the words are always followed by milk. He doesn't of course, know what the actual words mean, but they are a signal. At the same time he begins to realize that certain objects have meaning, that his cup, for instance, means a drink. It isn't until he is nine months to a year old, however, that he realizes that other cups are also used for drinking. When this happens, he is at the stage of recognizing groups of objects that have a common use. This is obviously necessary before he can use words as symbols.

The babbling of the six-month-old baby gradually develops into double syllables without meaning, such as 'mama'. By the time he is ready to use words properly, his ability to produce sounds is good because he has been experimenting for so long. None the less, his progress with speech still depends first and foremost on the continued development of language – a highly complex business.

See BEHAVIOUR; LANGUAGE PROBLEMS

Language problems A child whose speech development is slow in the early years may need specialist help and advice if he is not to be at a disadvantage when he starts school. Of course, many children are simply slower than average at learning to speak and in time become as skilled as the quicker ones. However, others may have more complex reasons for their delay: for example, they may not be able to hear or interpret the speech of others, and accurate diagnosis is helpful in sorting out their problems.

If your child's speech does not seem to be developing normally, ask your clinic or family doctor or your health visitor for advice. If necessary, your child will be referred to an assessment clinic to be seen by a speech therapist and a doctor experienced in the full examination necessary to assess the cause of the delay. In some areas, parents can contact the speech therapy clinic direct for advice.

Some of the more serious causes of slowness in starting to use speech are mental retardation, deafness, emotional disorders, autism and parental neglect in the form of emotional deprivation. Many more children, though, are simply under-stimulated at home and don't have enough opportunity to experience and acquire language. Others have all the opportunity they need and yet are slow to start. A child exposed to several languages at home may be slower than average in starting to speak.

If your child is a slow starter, you will probably be advised to use simple language with a small vocabulary, repeat words often, and to have as much one-to-one time with your child as you can. It's a good idea not to bombard your child with too many words, as he may 'turn off' if you do, in the same way that many people do who have the radio on all day without actually listening to anything. Although you pay particular attention to what you say to your child, don't expect him to talk back. That will only happen when he is ready.

A speech therapist is *not* a person who teaches children to speak with beautifully clear diction – her time is spent with more serious problems than poorly pronounced vowels. Much of her time may be devoted to assessing and treating the cause of language delay in pre-school children. Special tests are used to ascertain the child's ability both to express himself verbally and to understand spoken language. The parents may be instructed on how to help the child at home. However, many speech therapists see children with language delay at regular intervals, either individually or in groups, to expose them to a wide range of linguistic experience and to help them overcome their difficulties before they go to school.

Therapy can help the cerebral palsied child with difficulty in speaking and again the parents will probably be taught the rudiments of treatment by the therapist. Children with cleft palate may need prolonged help from the speech therapist, as may children with certain other conditions affecting speech.

Perhaps the most common request for speech therapy comes from the parents of children of two to five years who are not speaking clearly, substituting some consonants for each other and leaving others out. While time alone improves their speech, the speech therapist can offer parents guidance on how to help the child and may herself treat some children.

See AUTISM; DEAFNESS; LANGUAGE; STAMMER

Laryngitis An inflammation of the vocal cords of especial significance in younger children, because any narrowing of the young child's relatively smaller airway by inflammation is likely to cause breathing problems. Laryngitis is more common in the winter months and there is often a family history of the condition.

Acute laryngitis is usually due to a viral infection and can occur with a cold, pharyngitis, 'flu, measles, or other childhood infections. The main symptoms are hoarseness of the voice, a sore throat, a cough and CROUP.

Infection in children is rarely of the larynx alone but is combined either with infection of the upper respiratory tract or as part of acute laryngo-tracheo-bronchitis. This latter condition is usually seen in children under five years and can cause severe difficulty in breathing due to obstruction of the flow of air through the larynx by its swollen walls. Pneumonia or otitis media may complicate laryngitis.

Treatment includes humidification of the air the child is breathing (preferably with cool vapour) and antibiotics if there is thought to be an underlying bacterial infection. An emergency tracheotomy may (rarely) be necessary if there is acute airway obstruction causing severe difficulty in breathing.

Acute laryngitis together with spasm of the larynx can cause the characteristic crowing sound of croup.

Laxatives Substances that encourage the emptying of the bowel. Laxatives are also known as aperients, purgatives and cathartics.

Laxatives have been used extensively for centuries but they should not be necessary in a breast-fed baby or in a child eating a diet high in all forms of dietary fibre.

Many parents worry if their children don't have their bowels open every day at the same time and are tempted to give them laxatives regularly. This is bad because the long-term use of certain laxatives can permanently harm the bowel and render it incapable of passing motions along in the usual way. Gradually, higher doses of laxatives are necessary. Certainly it's convenient if a child gets used to going to the lavatory each morning, but this is mainly for practical reasons rather than medical ones. A child that puts off going to the lavatory because of the morning rush or because he's embarrassed will almost certainly become constipated.

If your child is constipated, encourage him to eat more fruit and vegetables and bran-containing breakfast cereals. Make sure he is drinking enough as well.

If he ever complains of extreme pain or bleeding when he opens his bowels, he may have an ANAL FISSURE accompanied by CONSTIPATION and needs to be seen by a doctor. Some children may need temporary treatment with laxatives by the doctor if they have severe constipation accompanied by SOILING.

There should really never be any need to give your child laxatives. You should not give laxatives to a child if there is any chance that he has an inflamed appendix (*see* APPENDICITIS).

Lazy eye *See* SQUINT

Lead poisoning An excessive accumulation of lead in the body from the swallowing or inhalation of lead-laden material. Children who suck things painted with lead-containing paint or who eat flakes of this paint can suffer seriously from lead toxicity. Older houses which have lead water pipes can also be a source of lead poisoning. If you live in a house with lead pipes, always run the water for a few minutes before drinking it. Other sources of lead include red lead in putty, lead-containing cosmetics such as surma, and an Asian baby tonic which is imported into Britain.

There have been suggestions that lead from petrol fumes can cause lead poisoning in children living in areas with a lot of traffic. The lead from the fumes ends up in household dust, soil and even home-grown vegetables. However, experts are not agreed that lead in petrol fumes has a major effect on the intellectual or behaviour development of children in these areas.

In young children, stomach pains, sporadic vomiting, loss of appetite and constipation are common signs and the nervous system is also affected. This shows itself as a loss of recently acquired developmental skills, irritability and lethargy. Severe, long-term lead poisoning can cause hyperactivity, aggressive behaviour and even encephalopathy – involvement of the brain with vomiting, fits, unsteadiness, impairment of consciousness or even coma.

Diagnosis of lead poisoning involves tests of the child's blood, urine and tissue levels of lead, and tests to measure the amount of lead in the child's environment.

Treatment includes removing the child from the source of lead, treating the underlying anaemia and using drugs to bind the lead in the body.

See DIRT EATING

Left-handedness If children are allowed to choose which hand to use for any given task from babyhood onwards, about 11 per cent of boys and seven per cent of girls are found to be left-handed at the age of seven years. About 25 per cent are ambidextrous, using the left hand for some tasks and the right for others, though few are perfectly ambidextrous – content to use either hand for any task. The remainder are right-handed.

Being left-handed is not so much of a handicap nowadays, because children are allowed to write with their left hand and adults are allowed to use their left hand in sports, for example. In industry, special tools are sometimes provided. Because of this there's no excuse for a parent to try to influence his obviously left-handed child to use his right hand. This will only cause the child anxiety when he finds he can't live up to his parents' expectations without considerable difficulty. If, however, your young child uses both hands and seems to show no preference during his second year, by all means encourage him to use his right hand by passing him things to hold in that hand whenever possible.

There have been many theories as to the cause of left-handedness but we still don't know the whole answer. There may be a genetic basis but it's rare for identical twins both to be left-handed, so the answer obviously isn't that straightforward. Left-handed children may show a preference for using their left foot, but this is not always true. The use of the left eye in preference to the right when one eye only is needed is not connected with left-handedness.

Much has been written about left-handedness and reading difficulties but the consensus is that there is no connection between the hand used and the child's progress in learning to read or spell. Confusion has arisen over this subject in the past because more boys are backward readers than girls, and more boys are left-handed than girls, so the incidence of left-handedness in backward readers is higher than the overall average.

Another bogey that haunts the parents of left-handed children is that their children may stammer. This is another old wives' tale. There are no more left-handed people or people who have changed the hand they prefer to use among stammerers than among normal people. Perhaps earlier this century when educationalists thought it wise to put pressure on left-handed children to make them write with their right hands, children with an inborn tendency to stammer started to do so because of the anxiety caused by the teachers and parents. Certainly there is no other link. (*See* STAMMERING.)

So, if your young child seems to like using

his left hand more than his right, let him. Being left-handed is quite normal and shouldn't hinder him unduly at school, at home or at work later. However, we live in a world dominated by right-handed people and using even common household gadgets can be very difficult for the left-handed. If you're right-handed, try opening a can with your left hand using a normal can opener and you'll see what left-handed people go through when using right-handed things. There are shops today that sell implements and goods for left-handed people, including left-handed playing cards!

Leukaemia A CANCER of the white BLOOD cells.

Like most cancers, leukaemia is a killing disease but it is especially emotive when it affects children. Leukaemia usually first shows itself as extreme paleness, often combined with an increased tendency to bleed or bruise. All children look pale from time to time and most children bruise when they knock themselves; but of all the pale children with bruises, only a tiny fraction are suffering from leukaemia, so don't worry unnecessarily. The commonest sites for bleeding are the gums and other mucous membranes, but the bruises can be found anywhere. A child may also have pains in his limbs or an unexplained fever.

Although there has been a lot of public interest and a great deal of research into a cure for leukaemia, no sure cure has been found. However, today's leukaemic child will almost certainly live longer than he would have done even ten years ago. In 1968 a survey of leukaemic patients showed that those who survived for more than five years represented less than one per cent of the leukaemic patients from which they were drawn. Today the chances of a complete 'cure' are very much greater. One survey showed that 70 per cent of those surviving for four years had a life span within normal limits.

Great advances have been made in treating leukaemia and five-year survival figures are now up to 50 per cent in some studies. Perhaps as many as one third of children with leukaemia can actually be cured. Treatment includes chemotherapy (drug treatment), radiotherapy and blood transfusions. Long-term

follow-up of a child once diagnosed as having leukaemia avoids confusing a remission of the symptoms with a cure.

Many mothers are worried if they have to have an X-ray in pregnancy because they have heard that leukaemia can be caused by X-raying the foetus. It's true that large doses of X-rays have caused leukaemia but today's doctors are very careful about ordering X-rays for women who are (or might be) pregnant, and the risks from the occasional X-ray are almost nil. Dental X-rays taken with modern, safe equipment do not harm the unborn baby either but for safety it is best to wear a lead apron when you have dental X-rays done or if you hold your child while he has an X-ray examination.

If you think your child has leukaemia, see your doctor. He won't think you're worrying unnecessarily and a simple blood test will settle the matter.

Lice *See* NITS

Limp The commonest cause of a limp is an injury which would cause pain if the full weight of the body were to be taken by the leg. The injured leg thus takes only a fraction of the weight while the good leg is quickly swung forward and the child walks with a characteristic dip towards the side of the injury. Damage to any weight-bearing part of the leg – the foot, bones, or joints – can cause such a limp.

An injured, limping child can usually point to the injury easily, so that the correct treatment can quickly be started.

Other causes of limping can be more difficult to sort out. They range from simple things such as badly fitting shoes and verrucae on the sole of the foot, to infection of the hip joint, slipped epiphysis in the hip, PERTHES' DISEASE and undiagnosed or inadequately treated CONGENITAL DISLOCATION OF THE HIP.

A limp should never be ignored, so get medical advice unless there is an obvious and trivial cause which you can put right.

See FRACTURE

Lips Very few conditions affect the lips but those that do can be unpleasant for the child. Cleft lip is discussed elsewhere (*see* CLEFT LIP AND PALATE).

Dryness of the lips with subsequent scaling and cracking is common in children. It may be caused by a sensitivity to substances in toys and foods or by the child simply licking his lips with his tongue. This wetness dries in the wind and causes chapping and further irritation. The best treatment is to use a bland ointment to break the cycle.

Softening and cracking of the angles of the mouth can also be caused by THRUSH or it may be an early sign of riboflavin deficiency.

Cold sores (caused by HERPES SIMPLEX) occur around the lips as a collection of tiny transparent blisters on a red base. They itch and burn and usually disappear in a week or so.

Lisping A substitution of spoken sounds caused by a defect in speech. The most usual type involves the pronunciation of 'S' and 'Z' as 'Th'. Children may lisp as a normal part of their development, because they have lost their front teeth, or temporarily during an emotional upset. Dental deformities can be corrected and a lisp can also be helped by speech therapy.

There are more serious causes of lisping, of which partial deafness and cleft palate are two. You'll probably know if your child has either of these and will already be under the care of a doctor who will also reassure you about your child's lisp.

Liver The body's largest organ, the liver is situated just below the diaphragm on the right. It is so large that it stretches across the top of the abdominal cavity almost to the left side and 'sits' on top of the right kidney and the stomach.

The liver is probably the most complex organ of the body but basically it has two functions – it produces bile and plays a vital role in metabolism. Blood from the large vein that drains the gut empties into the liver. From this blood, the liver extracts glucose and turns it into a storage substance called glycogen. Amino acids from food are also changed by the liver and the resultant ammonia formed is converted to urea which is passed out in the urine.

Bile pigments (which give stools their brown appearance) are also produced by the liver and passed to the gall bladder in bile. The gall bladder stores bile until it is needed, when it contracts and squeezes the bile into the first part of the small intestine to aid digestion. The liver also produces blood constituents essential for blood clotting, and stores vitamins A, B, D and K. It controls to some extent the production of red blood cells elsewhere in the body, helps regulate blood volume, and is one of the main sources of body heat.

Fortunately, few diseases affect the liver in children, but JAUNDICE is a condition which is commonly seen in babies. The liver is responsible for dealing with the products of broken down red blood cells when they reach the end of their natural life (about 120 days). If, for any reason, the liver can't cope then these products build up and produce a yellow coloration of the skin and whites of the eyes known as jaundice.

Infection of the liver (HEPATITIS) is a rare cause of jaundice in the newborn and is almost always viral in origin. The baby doesn't need to be isolated from its mother. Babies with any infection can become jaundiced but the sensible use of antibiotics to cure such infections before they get too serious has helped reduce this kind of jaundice.

Long sight *See* VISUAL PROBLEMS

Low birth weight On average, babies born in the western world weigh 7lb (3200g) or more at birth. Any baby that weighs less than 5½lb (2500g) is known as a 'low birth weight baby'. Two-thirds of low birth weight babies are premature or 'pre-term' (born before 37 weeks) and one-third are 'light-for-dates' (underweight for the duration of pregnancy). About seven per cent of all babies come into the low birth weight category.

Why some mothers go into labour too early and produce a small baby is not always known, but pre-eclamptic toxaemia, twins, antepartum haemorrhage and diabetes are among the possible causes. Women who smoke tend to have light-for-dates babies and a poorly functioning placenta can also be responsible for a baby that is too light in weight relative to the length of pregnancy. It's important to say that unless a pregnant mother's diet is ex-

147

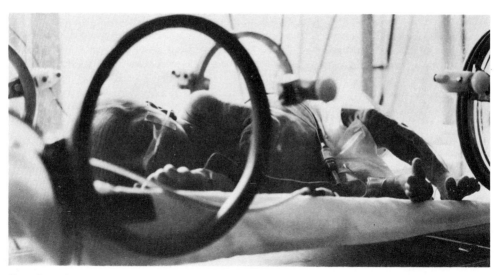

One of a pair of twins born at 31 weeks, weighing less than 5lb (2250g) at birth.

tremely poor (which is unlikely in the West) there is no danger of 'starving' the foetus and it's certainly wrong to eat for two.

A premature baby looks different from a full term one. His skin is red, wrinkled and covered with fine hair. His head is in fact small but looks big in comparison with his body. The eyes may stay closed and very premature babies cannot suck. Because specialized parts of the brain aren't properly developed he can't maintain many of the basic functions a normal baby can.

A very small baby thus presents all kinds of problems, such as trouble with breathing, feeding, JAUNDICE, temperature control, resistance to infection and poor liver function. Because of these potential hazards a very high proportion of low birth weight babies spend some time in a special care baby unit and many have to be nursed in incubators or under radiant heaters until their body systems mature sufficiently to take over. (*See* INCUBATOR.) It has been found that breast milk is nearly always best for low birth weight babies (except the very small or ill who need to be fed intravenously). Those babies too young to have an adequate sucking reflex may be given the milk by a tube through their nose into their stomach, or by a dropper. The mother should express or pump her milk frequently to stimulate the milk supply and should offer her baby the breast often as soon as he shows any signs of developing a sucking reflex.

From the point of view of the relationship between the mother and baby, it's just as important for the mother to be near her low birth weight baby in the special care unit as if he were born of normal size. Some hospitals have good facilities for mothers to sleep near their babies in these units, but even if the mother is sleeping a long way away, if she is well, she should still visit her baby frequently and spend as much time as possible nursing him (under supervision) and getting to know him. Separation from the mother may be one of the reasons why low birth weight babies cry more than full term babies for the first few months of life.

About one in ten of all low birth weight babies suffers from the RESPIRATORY DISTRESS SYNDROME. Bleeding into the brain is another potentially dangerous complication in a baby of low birth weight.

Hospital policy does not generally allow a baby to go home until he weighs more than 5lb (2250g). A better guide is his behaviour, how easy he is to manage, and how well his mother can handle him. Some of these babies sleep a great deal, may need waking for feeds, and still need special care, even after the weight reaches 5lb. A premature baby may need extra iron later because he has missed out on the last few weeks in the uterus when the mother would have passed iron across the placenta to the liver.

Once your baby is home, try to treat him normally. This won't be easy because you're bound to be more sensitive about his well-being than other mothers. Today, a small baby, although he is at a disadvantage at first, need not be a source of ongoing worry to you. By the age of a year, or even sooner, most premature babies have caught up with their full term peers. Premature or light-for-dates babies usually grow up to be perfectly normal, healthy children and adults. Continuing improvement of living standards means that there are increasingly fewer premature babies born.

A baby born prematurely should not be thought of as delicate for the rest of his infancy. This outlook would be bad for him and the rest of the family.

See BABY BATTERING

Lumbar puncture   *See* MENINGITIS

Lungs   The two organs of breathing situated one in each side of the chest. Each lung is covered on the outside by a thin membrane called the pleura and is divided by a deep fold which runs obliquely down its length. The right lung has three lobes and the left two.

Air enters the body through the windpipe (trachea) and then goes to the lungs themselves via large airways called bronchi. These branch repeatedly, rather like an upside-down tree, until the branches become extremely fine. At the ends of these branches are millions of tiny air sacs called alveoli. Air goes down this branching system and ends up in the alveoli where, because it is so close to the capillaries, it gives up its oxygen to the blood and picks up waste carbon dioxide formed in the rest of the body and carried to the lungs by the blood. Because we need so much oxygen for our bodies to function properly, the blood supply to the lungs is very great, as is the area for oxygen exchange. It's been calculated that if an adult's lungs were stretched out flat, their area would be equal to that of a full-size tennis court.

The airways of the lungs are lined with fine hair-like structures that trap dust particles and waft them out of the lungs. Larger foreign bodies such as plastic toys, peanuts and beads

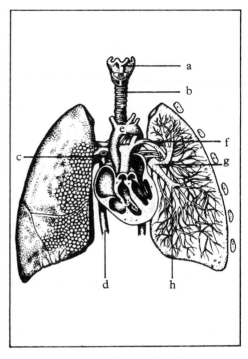

The heart and lungs. The left lung is drawn in section to show the bronchi. a. larynx, b. trachea, c. superior vena cava, d. inferior vena cava, e. aorta, f. pulmonary artery, g. left main bronchus, h. small bronchus.

can, however, find their way into the lungs of little children who play with these things in their mouths. If your child inhales a FOREIGN BODY, he must see a doctor as a matter of urgency.

The lungs and bronchi can be affected by various diseases in children. (*See* ASTHMA; BRONCHIOLITIS; BRONCHITIS; PNEUMONIA; RESPIRATORY DISTRESS SYNDROME; WHEEZING.)

Lymphatic system   Lymph is a colourless fluid formed in the tissue spaces all over the body and carried in vessels back to the bloodstream. It transports digested fat to the body's cells, keeps the tissues moist and takes special cells from the lymph nodes (or glands) all over the body. The lymph nodes are found along the major lymph channels and are roughly bean-shaped. They occur singly all along the lymphatic system and in clusters in the groins, under the arms and in the neck.

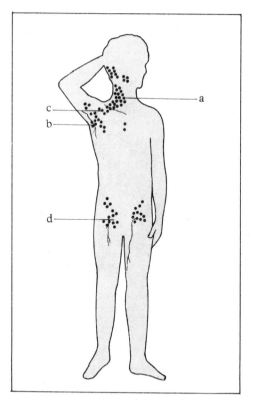

The superficial lymph channels reach every part of the body, and flow into regional groups of lymph nodes (shown). Deeper channels and nodes occur in the internal organs. a. cervical, b. axillary, c. subclavian, d. inguinal nodes.

They act as a filter for the circulating lymph and so prevent foreign matter, especially bacteria, from being transported further round the body. You'll have noticed that when your child gets a sore throat, the lymph nodes in his neck swell up and are tender. They do this because they are producing millions of tiny cells to fight infection and produce antibodies.

Lymph nodes also swell when they are trapping cancer cells, so if your child ever has swellings or lumps (especially in the three areas we've mentioned) that are not associated with infection, see your doctor.

As well as the lymph channels, there are three other parts of the body that play an important role in the lymphatic system, the SPLEEN, the LIVER and the THYMUS. The spleen has the most lymphatic tissue in the body and

lies just above the stomach under the left side of the rib cage. The thymus lies in the chest and is at its largest in childhood. It decreases in size until it almost disappears at puberty. It can't be found at all in most adults. The thymus plays a key role in a child's ability to resist infection. Children also have considerable amounts of lymphatic tissue in their TONSILS (*see* TONSILLITIS), ADENOIDS and around the small intestine. Pain in the tummy, often quite severe, can be caused by an inflammation of this lymphatic tissue due to infection – a condition called mesenteric adenitis. This inflammation subsides, like that of the nodes in the neck, once the infection is over.

If, for any reason, lymph flow is interrupted, tissue fluid accumulates in the tissues and that part of the body swells with oedema. The most dramatic example of this is seen in a tropical disease called elephantiasis in which the lymph nodes are blocked by parasites and the legs swell to an enormous size – hence the name elephant leg. This particular cause of swollen legs is not seen in the West.

If your child has an infected area of skin (a boil, for example) you may notice long, thin, red lines radiating away from it. This is called lymphangitis and is evidence of spread of the infection up the lymphatic channels. If this occurs, get medical advice at once.

M

Malabsorption A phenomenon common to a large and varied group of conditions resulting in poor absorption of one or more nutrients from food. The additional symptoms produced are not only those caused by a lack of the malabsorbed substances but also those caused by the presence of these unabsorbed substances in the gut.

Disorders causing malabsorption include SUGAR INTOLERANCE; CYSTIC FIBROSIS; COELIAC DISEASE; cows' MILK protein intolerance or 'ALLERGY'; vitamin B_{12} malabsorption; parasite infestation (uncommon in Britain); and the absence of part of the bowel (after an operation for volvulus, for instance).

Finding the underlying cause of malabsorption in a child involves taking a careful history of the food the child eats, a physical examination, tests of the stools and blood, and certain other specialized tests, for example for cystic fibrosis. Some of these tests may have to be carried out in hospital. Treatment depends upon the underlying cause.

Maladjustment A maladjusted child is one who is unable to cope adequately within the structure of the family or who is unable to fit into a group of normal children of the same age and intellectual ability, or in society as a whole. Some children have difficulties all the time, others only temporarily, and the difficulties are sometimes experienced only at home or at school. The behaviour disturbance may show itself as undue aggression, withdrawal, or an inability to form good relationships. One result may be poor educational progress. Poor vision, imperfect hearing or a physical handicap may cause the behaviour disorder, so a full assessment of the child is essential to decide on suitable help. To untangle the problems can

be very time-consuming and long-term counselling for both child and family may be necessary.

Being misunderstood because no one realizes what his problem really is puts extra stress on the child's emotional adjustment. This adds greatly to his difficulties.

Any signs of behaviour disturbance should be discussed as early as possible by the parents between themselves and, if they are unable to help their child, they should seek outside help. This help can be given initially by the GP, head and class teachers, school or clinic doctor. If necessary the family should be seen by a paediatrician or a child psychiatrist in a hospital, or referred to a child guidance clinic.

Usually the child is best kept in his own school to avoid further disruption of his life, but sometimes one of the special schools for maladjusted children is recommended.

Malnutrition Bad nutrition. The vast majority of children in the world are malnourished. Two-thirds of the world's population suffers from the effects of too little food and many of the rest suffer from the effects of too much. Both are forms of malnutrition. Malnutrition is usually taken to mean undernutrition which is sadly very common today in large areas of the world where famine and other natural disasters are a part of life.

Children need a balanced diet to remain healthy and grow and develop properly. A deficiency of any part of their diet can produce illness. It's easy to think that in a welfare state children are not malnourished but

A malnourished (in this case, undernourished) child, showing the typical wasted limbs and swollen abdomen.

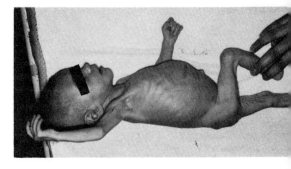

this is, unfortunately, not true. Children eating an unbalanced diet can become vitamin deficient and coloured children in particular who are not getting enough sun or foods containing vitamin D may develop RICKETS due to a deficiency of vitamin D. Babies unsuccessfully but solely breast-fed (*see* BREAST FEEDING) and babies fed on cranky diets of one sort or another (such as fruitarian or certain macrobiotic diets) may also be seriously malnourished.

Over-nutrition and OBESITY are greater dangers in western society, and overweight probably does more to hasten our deaths in the western world than any other single factor.

See FOOD

Mastoiditis   The mastoid sinus lies in the mastoid bone behind the ear and communicates with the middle ear. When a child has an infection of the middle ear (OTITIS MEDIA), the mucous membrane lining the mastoid sinuses is also affected. If the infection spreads to the bone itself, acute mastoiditis is produced, with redness, tenderness and swelling behind the ear.

Nowadays, treatment of middle ear infection with antibiotics has made mastoiditis, with its serious complications, unusual.

See SINUSITIS

Masturbation   Playing with or caressing the genitals to give pleasure or even sexual climax (orgasm). The term is generally used to mean the sexual stimulation of the genitals by the person himself.

Masturbation is common in people of all ages and in both sexes and in fact is probably universal. There is nothing perverted or peculiar about masturbation – most children simply find it pleasant. Most parents feel guilty or uneasy at the thought of their children masturbating but this is almost always because of their own sense of repressed sexuality and hangups from their own childhood when masturbation was said by some to cause blindness or insanity.

Almost all babies touch their genitals at some time, boys more than girls because there's something obvious and easy to touch. Soon they find it's pleasant and they may

get an erection (for instance if the bladder is full). Some babies rub or rock themselves rhythmically, look into the distance in a glazed sort of way, puff or go red in the face, relax and then go to sleep. Many parents whose children do this worry that they might have an over-sexed child on their hands but clearly this is complete nonsense. If your young child's masturbation in front of other people worries you or them, get round it somehow by diverting his attention or moving him somewhere else if you see him starting. Don't be cross or make him feel guilty as this could make him feel ashamed of his genitals and sexuality later in life.

If you ignore genital play and masturbation, both you and your baby will be a lot happier. Any reasonably intelligent child will soon sense your disgust or guilty feelings, so be open and reasonable and all will be well. If you keep trying to distract his attention, he'll be frustrated and will soon be secretive about masturbation. There is no magic age at which sexual pleasure becomes allowable.

If a child becomes addicted to masturbation, this is usually a sign of serious underlying problems. Family tensions and obsessive parental prevention of the child's normal handling of his genitals can cause this type of obsessive masturbation.

Masturbation may be a part of the sex games that little children play. Here again, it's a perfectly normal part of growing up and certainly isn't a sign of perversion. Cope with the situation exactly as with masturbation and you won't go far wrong.

Measles   A highly infectious disease of childhood that occurs in epidemics.

Measles is a viral illness that starts off rather like the common cold. It's also caught in the same way, by droplets from the nose and throat of an infected person. The incubation period is about 10 to 12 days but the child may become infectious to others as early as seven days after exposure to the person he caught it from. He should be isolated from the seventh day after exposure until about five days after the rash has disappeared.

The first signs and symptoms of measles are slight to moderate fever, conjunctivitis, a

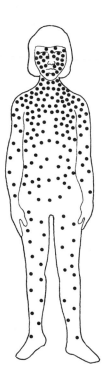

The distribution of the measles rash.

cough and a cold. There are also small white spots (Koplik's spots) on the lining of the cheeks.

The rash begins on the third or fourth day and is first seen on the neck and behind the ears. It then spreads to involve the face and the rest of the body. Small, flat, red spots join up to form irregular red patches and by this stage the child is usually on the mend. The rash of measles is not itchy. As the typical measles rash appears, the temperature rises abruptly and may reach 104 or 105°F (40 to 40.5°C). Other symptoms include loss of appetite, swollen nodes in the neck, abdominal pain, diarrhoea and vomiting and earache due to an inflamed eardrum. Within two to three days of the rash spreading to the legs and feet, the fever and other symptoms usually subside rapidly.

The only way to make the child feel better during measles is to relieve any unpleasant symptoms. Tepid sponging (*see* FEVER) will lower his temperature if it is unduly high. If the light hurts his eyes, draw the curtains. He may be completely disinterested in food: this doesn't matter at all for a few days but make sure that he has plenty to drink. He only needs to be in bed if he feels like it.

Measles is not serious in itself but its complications can cause long-lasting effects if they are not treated adequately. Pneumonia, bronchitis and middle ear infection (otitis media) may occur with measles and encephalitis is estimated to occur in one or two in a thousand reported cases of measles.

Nowadays measles can be prevented by giving a child a dose of measles vaccine in infancy. This vaccine is usually offered early in the second year. The vaccine should not be given (or only with special precautions) if the child is ill, if he has ever had anything wrong with his nervous system – for instance, convulsions or meningitis, or if he is allergic to eggs, as the vaccine is made up in an egg medium. Some children react to the vaccine by developing a measles-like rash with a slight fever a week to ten days after being vaccinated, but this is not serious. Up to five per cent of vaccinated children subsequently get measles, though this is not usually severe. Encephalitis has been reported in one in a million vaccinated children. A baby whose mother has had measles is protected for the first four to six months of life.

See IMMUNIZATION

Meconium ileus   *See* CYSTIC FIBROSIS

Menarche   The first time a girl has a period. At PUBERTY the hormonal changes occurring in a girl cause her to develop her female shape and have periods. The age at which this occurs varies a lot from girl to girl, from family to family and from culture to culture, but in the UK the menarche occurs from between 10 and 17 years with an average at about 13. It's interesting that the age at which girls have their first period has come down over the last century in western countries. The menarche usually occurs two years after the first signs of change in the breasts.

Many parents worry if their daughters haven't started their periods along with all the

153

other girls they know, but this is unnecessary because children are all different and develop at different rates. If your teenage girl hasn't started her periods by the age of 17, it's worth asking for medical advice.

The first few periods a girl has are not usually accompanied by ovulation (the release of an egg).

See MENSTRUATION

Meningitis An inflammation of the meninges or outer coverings of the brain and spinal cord usually caused by viruses or bacteria.

Meningitis in babies is, fortunately, uncommon but is especially dangerous because it's so difficult to diagnose. The baby may simply be off his food and off colour and the parents think he's just starting a minor infection. Babies don't always have the classical signs and symptoms of meningitis that adults get, though a small baby may look pale, lie still and have a bulging soft spot (fontanelle) caused by the rise in cerebro-spinal fluid pressure. Convulsions or a squint are also fairly common in babies with meningitis.

Children over the age of two years have symptoms like those of adults – headache, irritability, neck stiffness, dislike of light, vomiting and fever – when they get meningitis. The child may also appear dazed and have glazed eyes. In one sort of meningitis, meningococcal meningitis, there is a rash. A child with these symptoms must see a doctor at once.

If there is no obvious cause for an infection, your doctor may have to arrange for a lumbar puncture. A child's spinal column is still forming and the gaps between the bones of the spine (through which the lumbar puncture needle is passed) are very large, so the procedure is easy to perform. Your child is laid down on his side and curled up so as to expose his back. The doctor disinfects the skin, puts a local anaesthetic into it and then inserts a needle into the fluid surrounding the spinal cord. He measures the pressure of the fluid and then withdraws some, which is tested for cells, bacteria and chemicals. By finding out exactly which bacteria are causing the infection, it can be treated at once and severe complications, or even death, prevented.

Treatment of bacterial meningitis is with antibiotics but there is no specific treatment for viral meningitis of which mumps meningitis is the commonest sort.

Possible long-term side effects of bacterial meningitis include brain damage, blindness and deafness. Complete recovery is usual from viral meningitis.

The secret of success for the treatment of meningitis and the best chance of avoiding complications lies in diagnosing it early, so if in doubt, ask your doctor. Once a child has recovered from meningitis, there is no need to over-protect him.

See CENTRAL NERVOUS SYSTEM

Menstruation The loss of blood from the uterus every month after puberty. The bleeding usually lasts for five to seven days within a cycle of about 28 days. Menstrual periods begin with the MENARCHE and end with the menopause.

Periods are an essential part of the body's preparation for pregnancy each month. During the cycle the egg-containing follicles in the ovaries ripen under the influence of follicle-stimulating hormone from the pituitary gland. Only one egg matures fully and all the others degenerate. Five to ten days after the bleeding has stopped, the mature egg is released from the ovary (under the influence of another

A diagram of the menstrual cycle, showing what happens if pregnancy does not occur.

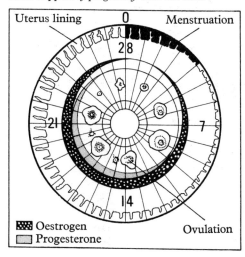

Uterus lining	0 Menstruation
	28
21	7
	14
▓ Oestrogen	Ovulation
▢ Progesterone	

hormone) and passes down the fallopian tube to the uterus. If the egg meets a sperm, it is fertilized and a pregnancy results.

Usually, the egg isn't fertilized and once the uterus realizes that the egg isn't going to need its thickened lining for a baby, the lining breaks down and a mixture of blood and lining matter is passed out through the cervix and vagina causing the bleeding of a period.

The first day of the menstrual cycle is taken as the first day of bleeding. If the egg isn't fertilized, bleeding usually starts about 28 days after the first day of the last period but this time varies both in any given woman (who may also have cycles of variable length) and in women in general.

Bleeding doesn't necessarily mean that ovulation has occurred – periods without ovulation commonly occur for one to three years after the menarche.

It's worth preparing your daughter so that she'll know what to expect long before her periods start. There's no harm in starting off with tampons from the very first period if your daughter wants to but you'll probably find that she'll prefer to use towels for the first few years.

Don't worry that your daughter will become anaemic or ill when she starts her periods. The majority of today's children eat well and don't become anaemic unless they have very heavy periods indeed. If your daughter ever has very heavy or very painful periods, see your doctor. However, some degree of cramp-like low abdominal pain, backache and leg ache at the beginning of a period is very common. Some girls find that a couple of hours rest with a hot water bottle over their lower abdomen helps, while others can carry on with whatever they are doing with no interruption. Nausea, vomiting, paleness and sweating normally occur in some girls at the beginning of their periods.

It's important not to forget that a girl may suffer from premenstrual tension for several days before a period, just as many older women do.

An absence of periods (once they have started) can be caused by hormone disturbances, psychological upset (many girls miss a period around examination time, for instance) or, rarely, by a condition called ANOREXIA NERVOSA.

Another reason for a missed period is, of course, pregnancy. If your teenage daughter misses a period, don't automatically worry that she's pregnant, because girls can have erratic periods early on. However, once her periods are well-established and she has settled into a normal cycle, missed periods must be taken seriously because she might be pregnant if she's been having intercourse. If ever you or your daughter are worried about her periods, don't hesitate to ask your doctor.

Mental retardation In Britain four in a thousand children are born with a severe mental handicap and many more with a mild degree of mental retardation. While those children who are only mildly intellectually handicapped will one day almost certainly be able to look after themselves in the community, have children themselves and perform a useful job of work, the severely handicapped will need care all their lives, though they too may work for their living in one of many sheltered workshops.

The causes of this condition are numerous and often it is impossible to diagnose the reason for any particular child's handicap. Much research needs to be done to help doctors find the causes, and prevent and treat those that are as yet either unknown or little understood.

A child may be affected even before birth by many factors. Genetic disorders include DOWN'S SYNDROME (mongolism), the commonest cause of mental retardation, affecting one in 600 babies; PHENYLKETONURIA (for which every child is tested soon after birth); many other metabolic disorders, some of which can be treated if diagnosed; and some types of HYDROCEPHALUS (water on the brain).

The foetus may be affected by an infection in the mother – German measles, cytomegalovirus and toxoplasmosis are some examples. It is very important for the pregnant woman to report any unusual symptoms to her doctor, as early treatment can sometimes prevent the foetus being affected. Today, schoolgirls are offered vaccination against German measles to prevent them from getting the disease later.

CRETINISM is still sometimes seen, and the commonest cause in Britain is absence of the THYROID gland. The baby often appears normal at birth because of the supply of maternal thyroid hormones in the uterus.

Other less well-defined causes of mental retardation are maternal malnutrition, placental abnormality and the taking of certain drugs or poisons by the mother during pregnancy.

A child may be affected at birth by such things as shortage of oxygen during or after delivery and injury to the head during delivery, which can cause bleeding inside the brain. However, factors occurring around the time of birth do not have a strong association with mental retardation. Severe jaundice due to rhesus incompatibility (or any other cause) may also lead to mental retardation if treatment is delayed. (*See* BLOOD GROUPS.)

Unfortunately, even a child who is perfectly normal at birth can be affected by a variety of factors after birth. Mental handicap can ensue at any time during childhood and many parents have said that it is even more distressing to look after a handicapped child who has been quite normal for a large part of his life than to look after one who has been handicapped since birth. Such factors include infection (for example, meningitis and encephalitis), road traffic accidents and other injuries, poisoning (with lead and carbon monoxide, for example) and the well-publicized, though very rare, damage after whooping cough immunization.

Mild mental retardation is sometimes increased, if not caused, by lack of stimulation, though once this problem is spotted, with adequate help the child will realize his full intellectual potential. Many handicapped children also suffer from other defects such as poor hearing, poor vision, language disorder, convulsions and CEREBRAL PALSY. The early assessment of such children is vitally important in order to be able to advise parents on the correct management, and initial and follow-up examinations should be done by a team of experts specializing in this field. With the facilities available today there is no excuse for any mentally handicapped child to have any unrecognized, and untreated, disorder.

Most retarded children will get the best start in life if they can be looked after at home. Parents will need plenty of practical and emotional support from relatives, friends, voluntary organization workers and professionals (health visitors, teachers, social workers and doctors) if they are to manage the child at home, as many retarded children can be exhausting and difficult to look after. Some areas offer places in playgroups or nurseries, and special schools for the educationally subnormal sometimes take children into a nursery class before the age of five years. (*See* EDUCATIONAL SUBNORMALITY.)

Short-stay facilities are available at some hospitals for mentally retarded children in order to give parents a break from their sometimes overwhelming burden. Some homes for retarded children suggest that they go home at weekends, and this can be a good compromise for many families.

Voluntary organizations exist to help parents cope with their children and some have meetings for parents to discuss their problems. Airing such problems often helps parents to view their children in a new light and prevents them from carrying the psychological burden of their handicapped child alone.

See INTELLIGENCE

Mesenteric adenitis *See* ABDOMINAL PAIN; LYMPHATIC SYSTEM

Migraine A disorder often starting in infancy, late childhood or early adolescence which may be preceded in early childhood by attacks of vomiting for no obvious reason. Boys and girls suffer from it in equal numbers.

Classically, the one-sided headache of migraine follows a short-lived disturbance known as an aura. The aura takes the form of scintillating zigzag lines moving across the field of vision and part of the visual field may be lost temporarily, causing partial blindness which recovers as the migraine attack goes. Occasionally a child may notice numbness or tingling of part of an arm or leg and sometimes even temporary paralysis or inability to speak.

The headache is usually on one side, though it may be bilateral and in children is usually at the front of the head. It is a throbbing pain which is usually relieved by sleep. Nausea or vomiting nearly always occur with the headache and the child may want to sleep.

The aura of migraine is thought to be caused by an abnormal constriction of arteries inside the brain, causing a reduced blood flow to the affected part. The headache itself is due to a dilation of arteries, especially those of the scalp, which is thought to stimulate pain fibres in the walls of the arteries themselves.

Two out of three children with migraine have a family history of the condition – often one or other parent is also a sufferer. What actually precipitates migraine is as yet unknown, though stress increases the number of attacks. Some people are prone to migraine after eating certain foods and there are probably 20 or 30 other precipitating factors. Foods which may precipitate migraine include wheat, orange, eggs, tea and coffee, chocolate, milk, beef, corn, cheese, alcohol, sugar and yeast. Most attacks are over within 24 hours.

Treatment should initially be with simple medicines such as aspirin. If this doesn't help, ergotamine preparations can be used.

There are several other associated conditions in childhood. RECURRENT ABDOMINAL PAIN and an episodic illness with loss of appetite, pallor, fever and pale stools are the two commonest.

Milia Tiny, yellowish or pearly white spots in the skin of newborn babies, most often occurring on and around the nose. Forty per cent of babies have milia which disappear spontaneously within a few weeks. The spots are little cysts caused by blocking of the openings of the skin's sebaceous glands.

They should never be squeezed and no treatment is necessary.

Milk A liquid produced by mammals in order to feed their young. It consists of proteins, fats, carbohydrates, minerals, vitamins, hormones, enzymes, anti-infective substances and live cells, all either dissolved or suspended in water. Each mammal produces milk of a highly specific nature, suitable for its own young. Not only are the proportions and concentrations of the various constituents

different but some are present in some milks and not in others.

We in the West chose cows' milk as an alternative to breast milk for baby feeding because herds of cows were already being reared for meat and dairy produce. Cows also produce large volumes of milk and are easy to milk. However, cows' milk differs greatly in its composition from breast milk and because some of these differences can cause serious medical problems if untreated cows' milk is given to a human infant, the baby milk manufacturers have ingeniously altered its chemical composition to make it more suitable for babies. The tins and packets of dried milk formula that are available at chemists are, however, still based on cows' milk and are not the same in chemical composition as breast milk.

In spite of all the modifications, cows' milk is still a poor substitute for breast milk, at least in the first four to six months, because breast milk contains every ingredient a baby needs and is the perfect baby food, which modified cows' milk can never be. Breast milk may look thin and even bluish compared with cows' milk formulae, but this is quite normal. Drops of milk expressed from the breast at the beginning of a feed contain more watery milk than those expressed at the end of a feed, though some mixing does occur.

Breast-fed babies are statistically healthier than bottle-fed babies. While this fact has been known for decades, doctors and nurses have been wary of telling the public for fear of making those mothers who couldn't or didn't want to feed their babies feel inadequate or guilty. Now that we know that nearly every mother is able to breast feed, provided she feeds on an unrestricted basis, doesn't reduce her milk supply by feeding on a schedule, and has enough informed advice, it is only reasonable to discuss the very real advantages of breast feeding.

Recent research has helped to show why it is that breast-fed babies suffer from fewer infections than bottle-fed babies. Milk contains antibodies which are destroyed by heating, so even if the antibodies in pasteurized cows' milk were effective against human diseases, which they aren't, they would anyway be destroyed before they ever reached the baby. There are also many other anti-infective substances in breast milk besides antibodies.

Among the infections a baby can be protected from by breast milk are tetanus, pneumonia, diphtheria, gastroenteritis, typhoid, dysentery, 'flu and polio. When he is older he is able to make his own antibodies but in the first few months he is dependent upon those in his mother's milk.

Another function of antibodies in breast milk is to coat the gut wall to prevent the entry of infective organisms into the bloodstream. They also prevent the entry of large protein molecules which could sensitize the susceptible baby and so cause an allergic response (such as eczema or asthma) later. Breast-fed babies are well known to be far less likely to develop allergies. (*See* ALLERGY.) Breast milk confers many other advantages, both in infancy and in later life, such as some protection against dental decay and cot death and possible protection against ulcerative colitis. Research is also being done into the suggested protective effect of breast feeding against multiple sclerosis and ischaemic heart disease.

Some children are naturally 'allergic' (intolerant) to cows' milk protein and this is increasingly recognized as a cause of symptoms as different as failure to thrive, eczema, nettlerash, runny nose, cough, wheezing, DIARRHOEA and vomiting. Studies suggest that up to seven per cent of bottle-fed babies are allergic to cows' milk. Goat's milk is sometimes given to children allergic to cows' milk but may itself cause allergy. It needs supplementation with vitamin D, iron and folic acid if used exclusively for a baby and should be boiled before use.

Milk made from soya bean protein is one example of the non-animal milks available for babies with cows' milk allergy.

Breast milk is always suitable for a healthy baby and most premature and ill babies need the nourishment and protection that only breast milk can give.

Children weaned from the breast don't need to drink cows' milk. All the nutrients present in cows' milk can be obtained from other foods so if your child doesn't want to drink it, there is no need to make him or to disguise it in other foods, provided he eats an otherwise balanced diet. However, cows' milk as part of a mixed diet is valuable for its protein, calcium and riboflavin content. It's important not to leave milk exposed to sunlight for over an hour because this destroys much of its riboflavin and vitamin C.

Lactase, the enzyme which digests lactose (milk sugar) may decrease in amount during adolescence, especially in black and oriental people, so producing diarrhoea, a blown-out abdomen, dehydration and vomiting within hours of drinking milk. Lactose intolerance may develop with, for example, gastroenteritis or coeliac disease in babies or older children and a lactose-free milk may be necessary for babies dependent on milk until lactose is again produced normally, within a few days or weeks.

See BABY FEEDING; BOTTLE FEEDING; BREAST FEEDING; DIARRHOEA; MALABSORPTION; SUGAR INTOLERANCE; WEANING

Milk intolerance *See* DIARRHOEA; MALABSORPTION; MILK; SUGAR INTOLERANCE

Mole (pigmented naevus) A flat, brown mark, a skin-coloured or brown swelling or a

A hairy (above) and a hairless mole.

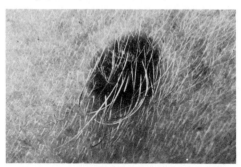

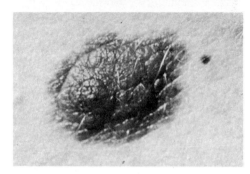

frondy tag of skin, each of which may be hairy or hairless. Many children are born with moles but they rarely cause any trouble or embarrassment. Moles can be removed surgically if they give trouble or are very unsightly, but most are completely harmless and are best left alone. If ever your child has a mole that bleeds, becomes larger, blacker or tender, take him to a doctor.

Some specialists advise that moles in areas of the skin subject to pressure (for example, on the soles of the feet) should be removed or observed from time to time.

Mongolism *See* DOWN'S SYNDROME

Moniliasis (candidiasis) An infection of the mouth (thrush), nails, vagina or body folds (armpits, umbilicus, between the buttocks or at the top of the thighs) caused by the fungus Candida albicans. The infection is occasionally generalized. Monilial infection is most common in babies who may otherwise be quite healthy.

The infection can start at birth, if the mother has vaginal moniliasis, when the baby comes down the infected birth canal.

Thrush (oral moniliasis) can be contracted via unsterilized bottle teats. If your baby gets thrush, don't be surprised if your doctor asks if you have vaginal moniliasis, as you may be passing it on to your baby. The inside of the cheeks, the tongue and the back of the mouth are the areas affected. The patches look remarkably like milk but, unlike milk, don't wipe off easily and leave a bleeding base when scraped off. A tongue infected with thrush is very white and furry. Thrush often presents itself as a feeding problem as the mouth lesions are actually painful.

There are two ways of clearing patches of thrush in the mouth, both needing a doctor's prescription. One is to paint over the patches with a watery solution of gentian violet (0.5 per cent) on some cotton wool. Painting should be continued for a week after the last patch has cleared. The other is to use a liquid drug called nystatin. The latter is placed in the child's mouth in drops. If left untreated, thrush can go through the child into his stools and cause a NAPPY RASH.

The fungus may cause an infection round the nail (paronychia) with redness and swelling of the surrounding skin and horizontal ridging of the nail if the infection has been present for several months. This is seen most often in finger or thumb suckers. Treatment of any thrush in the mouth should be carried out in addition to local treatment of the nail.

Older girls who are diabetic, on prolonged antibiotic treatment, pregnant or on the Pill may suffer from vaginal moniliasis. The resulting vaginal discharge is thick, white and curdy and the vulva is very itchy. Treatment is with nystatin pessaries and ointment.

Motion sickness (travel sickness) Motion sickness can occur with any form of rhythmical motion (including that of swings and roundabouts) but is most common in a car, coach, plane or boat. Some children are troubled by it to such an extent that travel becomes really unpleasant or impossible.

The child is pale, cold and clammy and feels sick or actually vomits. No one really knows what causes motion sickness but the innermost part of the ear that controls balance probably plays an important part. The eyes also play a part as has been shown in experiments in which people were shown film of aerobatics on a wide cinema screen. Some of them vomited although they were sitting still. Body position has some part to play as it has been found that if a person is lying down he is less likely to be sick.

Children seem to be especially prone to motion sickness and are also sick with quite smooth movements that don't affect most adults. Children as young as six months can suffer from motion sickness but it's important to remember that children can be sick in cars and trains for reasons that are nothing to do with the motion.

There are certain things that are worth trying in order to prevent at least some children getting sick. Make sure your child doesn't have a large, fatty meal before travelling but give him a small, easily-digested one instead. A combination of movement and an empty stomach can produce severe motion sickness. A small snack while travelling may help prevent sickness.

The most important thing is probably to stay calm and try not to anticipate trouble. A lot of travel sickness starts in the mind and if you start fussing about hours before you set off, your child will be keyed up and ready to be sick. Make sure he is occupied before and during the journey. Unfortunately, the safest seats in a car – the back ones – are also the most likely to induce car sickness but don't be swayed into letting your young child travel in front. The passenger seat in the front is the most dangerous seat in the car and adult seat belts will not save a small child.

Although there are lots of old wives' cures for travel sickness, few work for many children. The best thing to do is to give the child an anti-motion sickness tablet (most contain antihistamines) half an hour before starting out. Even if your child has taken a tablet, take a thick paper bag with you. Polythene bags are not a good idea because the sight of a bag full of vomit is enough to make all the other passengers feel sick, let alone the affected child! If you are travelling by car, keep a window open and stop at regular intervals to let your children out of the car to walk about.

To end on a happier note, children tend to be less travel sick as they grow older.

Mouth ulcers Small ulcers found on the lining of the mouth or on the tongue. Aphthous ulcers are small, harmless and acutely painful out of all proportion to their size. Why they appear no one knows, but they may be brought on by stress and are sometimes caused by allergies.

Children often get ulcers from biting their tongue or cheek and these, like aphthous ulcers, get better quickly on their own.

If the pain from a mouth ulcer is so severe that eating and drinking becomes painful, mouth washes, steroid tablets to suck, or special analgesic gels are useful and may help healing. If your child has an ulcer that lasts for more than a week, he should see a doctor.

If your child has mouth ulcers together with a white, curdy covering to the lining of the mouth, he probably has MONILIASIS.

The first infection with the virus HERPES SIMPLEX can cause mouth ulcers.

Multiple sclerosis An uncommon disease in children involving the breakdown of areas of myelin (nerve sheath) in the brain and spinal cord. One in a hundred adults with multiple sclerosis has symptoms that began before he was 15. The characteristic feature of the disease is that there are relapses and remissions for the rest of life. During a remission there may be no symptoms and it is impossible to predict when the next relapse will happen.

The signs and symptoms of multiple sclerosis vary according to the sites of the patches involved, but include unsteadiness of movement, weakness and stiffness of one or more limbs and some disturbance of sight. After many relapses, the child may eventually be left with a permanent disability, but this may not be for very many years.

Once the diagnosis (which is often difficult to make) has been made, physiotherapy, and steroid drugs if the symptoms are severe, may be advised and the prompt treatment of urinary tract infections is essential.

The underlying cause of multiple sclerosis is not known. A viral infection has been suggested but not proved, and some experts believe that it is a disorder of the immunity system. One survey showed that adults with multiple sclerosis were twice as likely to have been bottle-fed as normal people in a control group. This raises the possibility that breast feeding may be protective, though much more research needs to be done.

Mumps An acute infectious viral illness causing inflammation of the salivary glands. The disease is common in older children and young adults but rare under the age of five years. After an incubation period of two to three weeks the child may feel unwell, have a fever, muscular pains, especially in the neck, and a headache. These symptoms are uncommon in young children, however, and usually the first sign is a swelling in front of one ear (where the parotid salivary gland lies). The other side often but by no means always swells a day or two (or more) later and the mouth becomes dry. The child's jaw is painful, especially on movement, and this makes eating and talking painful. Sour liquids, in particular lemon juice and vinegar, cause pain. In a few children (10 to 15 per cent) with

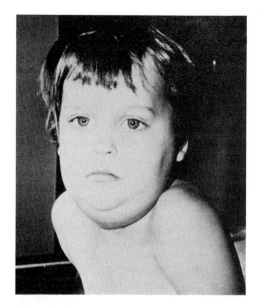

The typical swollen face of mumps is the result of the enlargement of the parotid salivary glands in front of both ears.

mumps, only the salivary glands beneath the chin swell. In some others, swelling is of the parotid and of the other salivary glands as well. However, in the majority only the parotid glands are affected. The condition usually resolves without specific treatment and the swelling usually subsides in three to seven days.

Over one third of children with mumps have a subclinical infection with no obvious symptoms or signs. Normally, a child is infectious from 24 hours before the swelling occurs to three days after it has subsided, but should be isolated, if necessary, for a minimum of seven days from the beginning of the swelling. Babies seem to be protected by antibodies transferred across the placenta from mothers who have had mumps.

Although there is no specific treatment, your child can be made more comfortable in many ways. Because it's so painful to eat solid food, give him fluids and soft, mushy foods. Keep his mouth clean with regular mouth-washes and tooth-brushing. This is important because GINGIVITIS is likely to occur.

About 20 per cent of boys who get mumps after puberty suffer from an inflammation of the testes caused by the same virus. Contrary to the old theories, this very rarely results in sterility but it is sensible to keep men and older boys away from children with mumps. About seven per cent of adolescent girls with mumps suffer from pelvic pain and tenderness due to inflammation of the ovaries but there is no evidence of impairment of fertility afterwards.

Mumps is probably the commonest non-bacterial cause of meningo-encephalitis (*see* ENCEPHALITIS). About ten per cent of children with mumps have symptoms of this condition and mumps can cause it even before the parotid glands have swollen. The mumps virus is spread throughout the body and can cause many other less common complications such as pancreatitis.

Because mumps can have such unpleasant side-effects, a vaccine has been developed but is not widely used in Britain. Mumps vaccine is used in the USA, where it is given to children of one year old. It is claimed to be useful and free from harmful effects in 95 per cent of children.

Muscular dystrophy A degenerative disease affecting the muscles. The type of muscular dystrophy depends on which group of muscles are involved.

The commonest form (Duchenne muscular

Abnormally large calf muscles are one of the signs of muscular dystrophy.

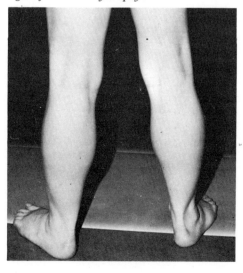

dystrophy) is most often seen in boys under five years old. It is rare and only occurs in one child in ten thousand. Half the affected children have a family history of the disorder (which is inherited by a sex-linked recessive mechanism) while the other half have none — in the latter, the disease is thought to be the result of a genetic mutation.

The disease is often not diagnosed before three years old, though on looking back, most of the children will have been slow to sit, walk and run. Early signs include a waddling gait with difficulty in climbing stairs and in getting up from the ground. The calf muscles may become abnormally large.

Unfortunately, many children with muscular dystrophy die before they reach twenty years as there is no specific treatment as yet. Physiotherapy is advisable, but bed rest and strenuous exercise are not.

Genetic counselling for the parents of these children is invaluable and a test to detect female carriers of the disease is available.

Myopia *See* VISUAL PROBLEMS

N

Naevus *See* BIRTHMARK; MOLE

Nail The tough, thickened plate of keratin at the end of a finger or toe. A nail consists of three parts: the root which is buried under the skin and from which the nail grows; the centre part; and the free edge that needs cutting. Nails, like hair, grow even before birth and continue to grow all the time except during certain illnesses or under the influence of certain drugs. Fingernails grow back completely in about six months if lost or removed surgically, whereas toenails take 12 to 18 months to regrow. This is why fingernails need cutting more frequently than toenails. If you have a low birth weight baby, you may notice that his nails don't reach the ends of his fingers or toes but grow within a few weeks.

Nails are normally pink, shiny and smooth but can be affected by disease. Severe iron deficiency ANAEMIA, MONILIASIS and PSORIASIS are three conditions that can cause changes in the nails in adults but these are rarely seen in children. Sometimes nails are ridged for some unknown reason. Occasionally a ridge appears that coincides with a previous feverish illness and may be caused by the death of some of the protein in the nail brought about by the high fever. Many parents worry that white flecks in their children's nails are caused by eating too little calcium. There is no evidence for this but they may be caused by hard knocks.

Babies scratch themselves easily and their nails can be kept short by the parent biting them off. Use blunt ended scissors for your older child's nails if he is reluctant to sit still.

The areas around the nail may become red or even frankly inflamed due to infection with bacteria or monilia. This is known as a paronychia. Any inflammation that doesn't

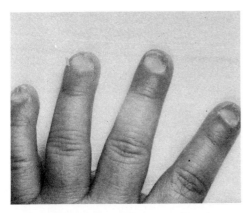

An example of koilonychia, spoon-shaped, brittle fingernails, which are sometimes a sign of chronic anaemia.

go within a day or two, or redness that goes pussy or causes real pain, should be seen by a doctor. Boils alongside a nail (whitlows), or splinters under a nail both need medical attention.

Nail biting A habit occurring in children of school age. If a child's nails are too long, this can start off the habit because he finds long nails unpleasant. Usually, though, it's a habit copied from other children or practised because the child gets enjoyment or comfort from doing it. Boredom, excitement, worry or embarrassment are all possible contributory factors. Nail biting is unpleasant because it makes the fingers look unsightly and makes infections of the skin around the nails more likely.

Cures for nail biting are mostly useless. The best way of handling nail biting is probably to ignore it. What might simply be a temporary habit will then stay that way and not become a focus for the family's gaze. Older children are most easily motivated to stop biting (especially girls) because they realize that it's unattractive. Some parents find that older girls will stop biting their nails if they allow them to use nail varnish.

Nail biting is so common that it would be ridiculous to label every child who bites his nails as neurotic or insecure. However, compulsive nail biting needs looking into to find out if the child is worried or anxious.

Nappy rash Most babies suffer from a nappy rash at some time and the commonest cause is the skin being left in contact with the urine in a wet nappy for too long. More frequent nappy changing should prevent the skin getting soggy and sore. One-way nappy liners may also help to keep the skin dry. Plastic pants create a warm, moist atmosphere next to the skin because of the lack of ventilation, and this can make the skin more liable to become sore if the nappy is not changed often enough.

A wet nappy is also likely to chafe the skin mechanically – think how sore you would feel if left in a cold, wet, rough nappy for hours on end.

Another common rash in babies with sensitive skin is caused by the irritant effect of stools on the skin around the anus. To prevent this, change the baby as soon as he is dirty and use a barrier cream after washing his bottom with soap and water and drying it well. A barrier cream simply acts as a thick protective layer, shielding the skin from the effects of urine and stools. To be effective, it needs to be applied frequently and liberally.

An ammoniacal nappy rash is caused by the irritant effect of ammonia on the skin. You'll be able to smell the ammonia when you change the nappy and it may even make your eyes water. There is no ammonia as such in urine but it is released from urine by the action of bacteria in the stools which split urea – a chemical naturally present in urine. These bacteria thrive if the stools are alkaline and if the baby has diarrhoea. Breast-fed babies have more acid stools and so are less likely to suffer from this sort of nappy rash than are babies fed on cows' milk. The rash is seen on the penis or vulva and can spread to the thighs and buttocks. It tends to spare the creases. The generalized redness of the skin then progresses to a tight, papery appearance and this is followed by red pimples which may turn into pustules (tiny boils) or shallow ulcers. The skin becomes very raw in bad cases and the baby obviously feels uncomfortable.

To *prevent* an ammoniacal nappy rash, wash your baby's bottom with soap and water every time he has a dirty nappy. This removes traces of stool from the skin. Rinse and dry well, then, if he has loose stools, put on a barrier cream such as zinc and castor oil. There is no need to use cream for fully breast-fed babies as it is normal for them to have loose stools. Nappies should be either boiled to kill the bacteria in the stools, soaked in a hypochlorite solution, or have a final rinse with a suitable antiseptic solution such as benzalkonium chloride. Simply setting your washing machine to the highest temperature is not enough to disinfect nappies. Some vinegar in the final rinsing water (one fluid ounce of vinegar to one gallon of water) also helps prevent (and treat) this sort of nappy rash.

To *treat* an ammoniacal nappy rash, change the nappy more frequently, stop using plastic pants, wash your baby's bottom with soap and water at every nappy change, then rinse and dry well. Either use zinc and castor oil cream as a barrier or use a suitable antiseptic cream (such as one containing benzalkonium chloride, a safe antiseptic). Cope with the nappies as above. (Steer clear of boric acid powder and hexachlorophene, as they can be harmful if absorbed through raw skin in large amounts.) Try to expose your baby's bare bottom to the air as much as possible: sunlight in particular will help.

If your baby has thrush (*see* MONILIASIS) in his mouth, he may develop a monilial nappy rash due to this fungus or it may appear even without an oral infection. The rash is usually around the anus and buttocks. Treatment involves clearing up the rash with nystatin ointment or cream. Gentian violet is also effective but is rather messy to use.

More unusual is a seborrhoeic nappy rash (seborrhoeic DERMATITIS) which tends to involve the creases at the tops of the thighs. The baby usually has signs of seborrhoea on the scalp (CRADLE CAP), behind the ears or in his armpits, and the rash is a brownish colour. It should be treated with a suitable cream (such as one containing sulphur and salicylic acid or, if this fails, one containing hydrocortisone) from your doctor and you should expose the baby's bottom to the air as much as possible. Cradle cap should also be treated, as otherwise it might cause a recurrence of the nappy rash.

Some babies with a tendency to allergic disorders develop allergic contact dermatitis to the dyes in some detergents or to plastic pants. Others are sensitive to a chemical present in nappy liners. Treatment involves accurate diagnosis followed by the avoidance of the offending substance. Steroid cream (from your doctor) will clear up the rash, but should only be used in small amounts and only if absolutely necessary. Nappy rash may be an early sign of atopic ECZEMA.

Finally, any rash can become infected with bacteria. If this happens, not only must the bacterial infection be treated with an antibiotic cream but the underlying cause of the original rash must also be treated.

Nephritis (glomerulonephritis or pyelonephritis – 'pyelitis')

Inflammation of any part of the kidney. The most common form of inflammation of the glomeruli of the kidney (acute *glomerulonephritis*) is precipitated by a sensitivity to an infection, usually of the throat but also possibly of the skin, by streptococci. While streptococcal infection is a common cause of nephritis, nephritis is rarely seen with streptococcal infection. The infection occurs nine to eleven days before the symptoms of nephritis appear. Twice as many boys are affected as girls. Prompt treatment of streptococcal sore throats with antibiotics reduces the chance of developing this sort of nephritis by half. The inflammation in the kidney is not caused by the streptococci themselves but follows an immunological response of the body to the infection, resulting in the deposition of antigen-antibody complexes in the glomeruli. A child with glomerulonephritis is not usually seriously ill. The onset of the illness is abrupt: the child passes small amounts of brownish-red (blood-containing) urine and has some slight swelling of his face. He may also have ankle swelling, high blood pressure, a headache, a fever and abdominal pain.

Treatment is non-specific and the decision on whether to send a child into hospital depends on the severity of the illness. Most children have fully recovered within three weeks.

If your child ever has bloody urine you must see a doctor, but don't be too alarmed because some red sweets, laxatives containing phenolphthalein, and beetroot can cause red urine in certain susceptible children. Your doctor will test the urine to see if blood is present.

Pyelonephritis (pyelitis) is an inflammation of the kidney caused by infection. The infecting organisms reach the kidney either via the ureter, following acute or chronic CYSTITIS or, less often, via the bloodstream. There may be a structural abnormality in the urinary tract which makes infection more likely.

The child with pyelonephritis may have no symptoms at all and the infection may be a chance finding when investigating abdominal pain. However, common symptoms are an urgent and frequent desire to pass urine, pain on passing it, dribbling, and perhaps day-time or night-time wetting in a previously dry child. The urine may be smelly and the child may have a fever, vomiting, abdominal pain and loss of appetite. In babies, urinary tract infection may cause jaundice, failure to thrive and apathy. Children rarely appear seriously ill. Girls are three to four times as likely to get urinary tract infection as boys (except in infancy) and during childhood one girl in 20 suffers from it.

In children, the finding of a urinary tract infection, whether pyelonephritis or cystitis or both, leads on to treatment with urinary antiseptics or antibiotics, depending upon the results of urine testing to establish the sensitivity to drugs of the infecting bacteria. Because urinary tract infections may recur, repeated testing and, if necessary, prolonged drug treatment should be carried out.

Many other diseases involve the kidneys, including the 'nephrotic syndrome', in which the child suffers from generalized swelling, has too much protein in his urine (and too little in his blood) and too much fat in his blood. In the commonest type of the nephrotic syndrome, the cause is unknown, one in fifty thousand children under 12 years is affected each year and children from two to seven are the ones usually affected. Spontaneous recovery may occur, through many children need expert treatment and a few have permanent kidney damage.

If your child is ever ill without an obvious reason, your doctor may test his urine to rule out nephritis.

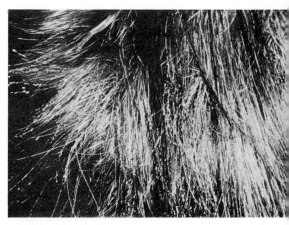

Nits in a child's hair.

Nephrotic syndrome   *See* NEPHRITIS

Nettle rash   *See* URTICARIA

Nightmare   A terrifying dream perhaps causing the child to wake. Some people find that certain foods precipitate nightmares, so it's worth looking at your child's diet to see whether there may be a dietary factor. Children who are ill, feverish or sickening for something often have nightmares.

Some children go back to sleep at once after a nightmare but others need comforting and perhaps taking into their parents' bed. If a child is so frightened that he cannot sleep in the dark, try keeping a night light on in his room for the next night or two. Repeated nightmares can be a sign of an anxious or disturbed child, so if your child suffers from them night after night, see your doctor.

See ANXIETY.; SLEEP

Nits   The eggs of lice. A louse is an insect about 2mm long which lays its eggs on the hairs of the head. The eggs or nits are tiny, pearly white, cigar-shaped objects firmly glued on to the hairs and they hatch into adult lice within two to three weeks. The adult lice feed on human blood and their bites at first cause reddish spots. Repeated bites can cause sensitization with severe itching of the inflamed spots, sometimes with secondary infection causing folliculitis (inflammation of the hair follicles), impetigo and enlargement of the lymph nodes at the back of the neck. If a child is found to have head lice, the whole family must be examined and treated if necessary. A child may pick up head lice from another child at school by using his brush or by touching heads. Nit infestation is so common that the old standard treatment is becoming ineffective for the newly resistant 'super' lice, but lotions containing malathion will kill the lice and nits. The lotion should be rubbed into the hair, which is then allowed to dry and shampooed 12 hours later with an ordinary shampoo. The wet hair should be combed with a fine-toothed comb. If the nits are firmly stuck to the hair, try combing with a fine comb dipped in hot vinegar. Repeat the treatment in a week's time.

It's easy to mistake small blobs of hair spray or flakes of scurf for nits and, if there's any doubt, your doctor will examine the 'nits' with a magnifying lens.

Nosebleed   Bleeding from the nose is usually caused by a knock or by picking, but can also occur with respiratory infections, hay fever and various childhood infections.

Children and adolescents are especially prone to nosebleeds and usually there is a perfectly simple and harmless cause. Children may push things up their noses and a bead or nut there can easily cause bleeding long after it has been forgotten.

If your child has a nosebleed after a fall on the head, he ought to be seen by a doctor because this can be a sign that the skull is fractured. Any child that gets repeated nose-bleeds for no apparent reason should also see a doctor because, rarely, it can be the first sign of leukaemia or a bleeding disorder.

The first aid treatment for a nosebleed is to loosen the child's collar and reassure him. It's often the first time a child has lost blood and he may be terrified. Get the child to sit down, preferably at a table, and lean him forward over a basin or bowl (so that he doesn't swallow the blood which can irritate the stomach and cause vomiting, thus raising the blood pressure and restarting the nosebleed). Squeeze, or get him to squeeze, the soft end of the nose firmly. This will stop the bleeding by giving the blood a chance to clot. He'll probably have to sit like this for ten minutes. If the bleeding hasn't stopped by this time, the chances are it won't stop and will need medical attention. The doctor may cauterize the bleeding area or pack the nose with a gauze ribbon.

Make sure that your child doesn't pick or blow the nose to see if it's clear as this will dislodge the clot and you'll be back to square one again.

Nystagmus   A condition caused by many diseases of the nervous system, characterized by involuntary, flicking movements of the eyeballs. One type of nystagmus however is quite normal and can be seen by watching someone's eyes as he stares out of the side window of a moving vehicle.

Most types of nystagmus have a slow and a fast component. In nystagmus secondary to certain brain conditions, the fast 'flick' of the eyeball is always seen most easily when the eye looks outwards, and the slow component when the eye looks in. An overdose of barbiturates can also cause this type of nystagmus.

Nystagmus can be congenital and it is usually associated with poor vision.

If ever you notice that your child has involuntary, rhythmical eye movements, you should seek medical advice.

O

Obesity Overweight, usually caused by excessive food intake. Anyone who is 20 per cent or more heavier than he should ideally be is defined as obese. Unfortunately, increasing numbers of children fall into this category.

Parents make endless excuses for their children's overweight but the truth of the matter is that 98 per cent of fat children simply eat too much. While it's true that some children burn up food better than others, and can eat more than others without getting fat, there is still an optimal calorie intake for each individual child which will keep him at the right body weight. It's important never to force a child to eat, as this may cause a child to eat too much to please his parents. The evidence about fat children becoming fat adults is confusing and more research needs to be done, but it does seem that obese adults are more likely to have been fat children than their thin brothers.

Obesity matters because it throws unnatural strains on the body and especially on the heart, gall bladder, knee joints and feet. Adults who are obese die younger than those who are slim and are more likely to suffer from many conditions including high blood pressure, infertility and hiatus hernia.

Modern research is showing that the main cause of obesity is that we eat too many refined foods and too much fat and added sugar. White bread, white flour and its products, and sugar in all forms seem to produce body fat very effectively. Foods rich in roughage (dietary fibre), including wholemeal flour products, bran-containing cereals and brown rice, containing exactly the same number of calories as their refined equivalents, are not so well absorbed by the bowel and so cause less obesity. They also fill up the

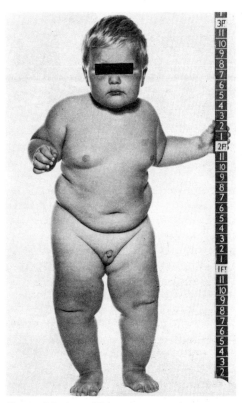

Overweight in a child may cause embarrassment and teasing at school, and may lead to many other, more serious, health problems if he remains obese as an adult.

stomach and satisfy the appetite more than refined foods. Refined cereals and sugar in a baby's diet are one of the main causes of obesity in infancy.

It's not true to say that babies don't get fat if they're breast-fed but studies have shown that fat children are much more likely than those of normal weight to have been bottle-fed. The mechanism behind this is complex but it seems that breast milk is supplied by the breasts in such a way as to slake thirst yet control the appetite. Also, breast milk is always exactly the right strength for the baby whereas some mothers make up bottle feeds that are too strong and so give the baby too many calories as he drinks to satisfy his thirst. Children usually get fat (if they're going to) either in the first year of life, around the age of five, or during adolescence. Some-

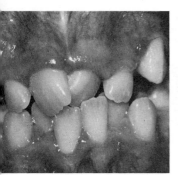
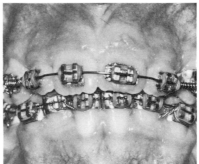
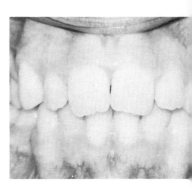

Straightening the teeth with a fixed appliance. This is usually done once the second teeth are established, at between 8 and 10 years. Left, the teeth at the beginning of treatment. Above, the brace in place, and right, the appearance of the teeth 24 months later when the treatment was completed.

times the child has a double chin and a boy may have such a heavy deposit of fat on his chest that it looks as though he has breasts. This causes great embarrassment at school. Fat boys may also appear to have very small genitals because their penises become 'lost' among the fat around the pubic area. Fat children are more likely to get knock knees and may suffer from a particular hip disease (slipped epiphysis) rarely seen in thin children. Some fat children are psychologically disturbed, but it's difficult to be sure which comes first, the disturbance or the obesity.

Ideally, all children should be breast-fed, weaned on to wholefoods and kept away from refined ones. Eventually a child will want to eat sweets and cakes like other children, but you may hope that by then he'll either have no desire for sweet things or will be sensible enough to eat them in moderation. Far too many parents use food as a bribe and their children soon become fat as a result. There's nothing pleasant about being fat, especially as a child. Fat children are teased at school, can't enjoy sports and games, have difficulty with clothes and stand a good chance of dying prematurely in adulthood. If you want to prevent your child suffering from all the problems of obesity, you can't start too soon, because once he has been educated to eat badly, it's a difficult job undoing the damage.

Obsessions Persistent or repetitious thoughts or actions which the child usually realizes aren't based in reality. For example, a child may be obsessed with the idea that his parents are going to die or that they're going to send him away somewhere. A child may also carry out repetitious acts that serve no obvious purpose. He will go through rituals that are meaningless to the rest of the family, straightening his shoes before going to bed, smoothing the bedclothes immaculately, going round the house closing doors, or walking along the pavement carefully avoiding cracks between paving stones, for example. This sort of behaviour is more common in adolescence than in younger children.

If obsessional behaviour occurs in a happy, well-balanced child, there is no need to worry but if it is present in a child who is worried or unhappy, then it is worth asking for the help of your doctor who will refer him to a child psychiatrist for therapy (either individual or family) if he can't help you himself.

Repetitive movements (tics) and HABITS such as THUMB SUCKING, hair pulling and HEAD BANGING are not obsessions.

Orthodontics The treatment of crooked teeth. Crooked teeth are usually caused by an imbalance between the growth of the jaws and the teeth because a child may inherit a tendency to a small jaw from one parent and big teeth from the other. The result is an overcrowded mouth.

Many parents worry that thumb or finger sucking harms the teeth but there is no evidence that this is so. (*See* THUMB SUCKING.)

Helping your child develop nice straight teeth starts with caring for his milk teeth.

Premature loss of the milk teeth can cause the second teeth to come through crooked or in the wrong place. Some children have too many teeth and others have teeth that stick out but it's useless for your dentist to push them back into place with braces unless there's room for them to move. This means that he may have to remove some teeth to make room for the others to move over.

Most dentists don't start orthodontic treatment until about the age of eight to ten years because the second teeth haven't developed fully until then. All dentists know about crooked teeth but orthodontists specialize in them.

When you take your child for treatment, the dentist will carefully examine his mouth, make models and take X-rays. If necessary, he'll then work out what sort of brace is suitable. Some are fixed and stay in for months and others can be taken out at night to be cleaned.

Braces work by putting slow, continuous pressure on badly positioned teeth to move them back into place. This takes a long time and you'll need to encourage your child to have patience.

Otitis externa An infection of the outer ear caused by fungi, bacteria or viruses which gives rise to inflammation, pain that worsens on moving the jaw, and enlargement of the lymph nodes around the ear and in the neck. Chronic infection causes itching in the ear and perhaps also a discharge. Unfortunately, this type of infection is very easy to pick up and parents who screw the corner of a towel or flannel deep into their child's ears to clean them risk infecting the canal in this way. Children may poke things into their ears and this too can cause an infection. Treatment is usually simple and should be carried out by a doctor who will clean out the ear canal and possibly put some drops in. He will also look with a special instrument (an auriscope) to see if there is a foreign body in the canal that could be causing the infection. A foreign body in your child's ear should be removed by a doctor – never poke about in the ear yourself. Occasionally an insect can get into the ear canal and cause the child great distress because of its

movement and buzzing. If the insect doesn't find its own way out, your doctor may have to remove it.

Keep your child's ears clean simply by cleaning the outer ear and the outermost part of the canal with a flannel and soap or a cotton wool bud. There is no need to clean the canal itself.

Otitis media An infection in the middle ear that is a common cause of EARACHE. This infection isn't visible to a parent and can only safely be diagnosed by a doctor using an auriscope. Middle ear infections are usually preceded by tonsillitis, the common cold, 'flu, scarlet fever, whooping cough or measles. Infecting bacteria travel up the eustachian tube to the middle ear. Otitis media is especially likely to be seen in children with infected ADENOIDS, tonsillitis, or sinusitis. Bottle-fed babies have more otitis media than breast-fed babies and children with a cleft palate are also prone to it. Otitis media is a common condition and is most often seen in children between five and seven years old.

Infection is more likely if the nose is blown forcibly when the child has a cold or if a sneeze is suppressed.

Any mild earache occurring during an upper respiratory tract infection should be treated with decongestant nose drops in an attempt (often successful) to abort an infection of the middle ear. The nose drops should be put in each nostril in turn with the child lying on his back and his head turned slightly to the side of the nostril being treated. Half strength ephedrine nose drops should be used for children under twelve years old.

Otitis media causes a bad, throbbing earache which keeps the child awake at night. Young children scream, shake their heads and may pull their ears because the pain is so severe. The child is ill, has a temperature, loses his appetite and becomes temporarily deaf to some degree. Sometimes the only signs of an ear infection are fever, vomiting, loose motions and irritability. The vomiting and loose stools are thought to be due to the effects of the infecting bacteria on the gut. Without treatment the build-up of pus in the middle ear may become so great that it cannot escape adequately down the congested eustachian tube, so the eardrum bursts, pus comes out of the ear canal and the pain is dramatically relieved.

If your child complains of earache and pulls his ears when he has a cold or any infectious illness, it's wise to see the doctor because infection is best treated early. No doctor will mind being asked to look at your child's ears, especially if he has recently had or is suffering from an infectious illness.

Treatment usually consists of antibiotics to clear up the infection; painkillers for the earache; and nasal decongestants to clear the nasal passages and allow the pus to drain down the eustachian tube into the throat. If the tension of the eardrum causes severe pain even after about 24 hours on antibiotics, a specialist may have to make a tiny incision into the eardrum to let the pus out: this produces dramatic relief.

The child's hearing may take several months to return to normal after an attack of otitis media. Your doctor may advise you to return for a check of your child's ears a few weeks after treatment.

Chronic infections of the middle ear can cause mastoid infection, a continued discharge through the perforated eardrum and hearing loss, all of which need expert advice and treatment. Some children have sterile (non-infected) fluid in their middle ear due to a poorly functioning eustachian tube and this may clear up on its own accord or become sticky or glue-like. (*See* GLUE EAR.)

See AUDIOMETRY; DEAFNESS; EARS; HEARING TESTS

Ovaries A girl has two ovaries, lying one each side of the pelvic cavity. The ovaries are responsible for producing the female sex cells (the eggs or ova), one of which is released halfway through each menstrual cycle. All the eggs are present at birth, each contained in a Graafian follicle, though only one matures each month under the influence of follicle stimulating hormone from the PITUITARY gland.

In the first half of the menstrual cycle (the two weeks following the beginning of MEN-STRUATION), the ovary produces the hormone oestradiol which thickens the lining of the womb ready to receive the egg. At ovulation,

the egg passes from the ovary, down the Fallopian tube to the womb. The follicle which released the egg turns into a 'yellow body' which produces the hormones oestradiol and progesterone. If the egg is not fertilized, the yellow body degenerates and menstruation follows.

See MENARCHE; PUBERTY

Overbreathing If a child makes himself breathe very rapidly for two minutes, then stops, he will faint. The temporary loss of consciousness is caused by the rapid removal of the carbon dioxide from the lungs. This occurs because carbon dioxide normally stimulates the breathing centre in the brain.

Overbreathing is occasionally practised for fun among groups of schoolchildren in the playground and its effects can cause great concern among onlookers.

Prolonged overbreathing can also cause temporary tetany with characteristic muscle spasm, numbness and tingling of hands and feet.

The female sex organs. a. fallopian tube, b. ovary, c. uterus, d. cervix, e. vagina, f. vulva, g. clitoris.

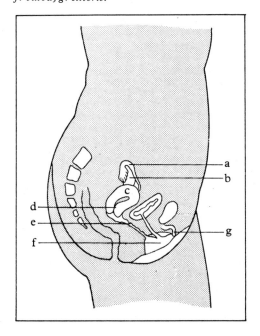

P

Pain   A protective mechanism whereby the body lets us know something is wrong.

However pain arises, it warns us that we ought to do something about it. The simplest way of doing something about it is the reflex withdrawal of the part of the body being hurt. When we burn ourselves, for example, the pain receptors in the skin send messages via nerves to the brain very quickly. As this is happening, some nervous messages go through a shorter link in the spinal cord and cause muscles to act in such a way as to remove the body from the source of the pain. This 'reflex arc', as it is called, is a very primitive protective mechanism and is one we use a lot in our everyday lives.

Pains are of many different kinds and the nature of a pain helps the doctor decide what the cause might be. For instance, throbbing pains may be caused by a disturbance affecting the wall of an artery; and dull, sickening pain with a feeling of faintness often results from deep organ trouble (as in diseases of the abdominal or chest organs). Pain may come in waves and disappear completely in between. This type is called colic and is caused by a hollow organ trying to pass something through. The uterus trying to pass a baby, the ureter trying to pass a stone, or the cervix passing a clot of blood during a period can all produce this type of pain.

Inflammation of tissues also causes pain. When the body's cells are damaged by physical, chemical or bacterial agents, they release chemical substances locally that cause pain. A recently discovered group of substances called prostaglandins is now known to produce pain at a cellular level in the body and much research is going on to see if this might lead to the development of better painkilling drugs. But while the prostaglandins seem to sensitize the cells to pain there are other naturally occurring substances – the endorphins – that are *nature's* painkillers. It has recently been discovered that the brain produces natural kinds of opiate painkillers. These are probably responsible for our not feeling pain most of the time. Their levels are raised in pregnancy, after any painful stimulus, such as when acupuncture needles are used, in opiate addicts, after taking a dummy tablet (in some people), and in gross obesity. Our knowledge of these remarkable substances is still in its infancy but it is likely that we'll be able to understand pain and its relief better once we learn how nature herself deals with it in the body.

Some children have pain when there is no apparent physical cause. Many of these are suffering from psychogenic pain – a condition in which the brain believes there is pain, when there is none. Some of these children respond to treatment of underlying depression or a similar illness.

The problem for parents with a child complaining of pain is to know how seriously to take it. Young children complaining of headaches should be taken seriously and seen by a doctor. Any pain severe enough to make a child vomit or faint must be reported and a child with any really severe pain with no obvious cause must be seen at once by a doctor. Never ignore severe pains, wherever they occur, as they always mean something. Most parents get to know when their child is putting it on and can deal with the problem accordingly, but will still need medical advice from time to time. Some children go through patches of complaining of odd pains, repeated tummy aches and all sorts of other pains that can alarm parents. Try not to show your concern because sometimes these pains are simply in the child's mind, though no less real for that. If you're in any doubt about the cause of a pain, ask your doctor. Sorting out pains can sometimes be a difficult business and needs expert help.

See ABDOMINAL PAIN; ANALGESICS; AR-THRITIS; GROWING PAINS; HEADACHE; RECUR-RENT ABDOMINAL PAIN

Pancreas   A long, thin gland that lies in the

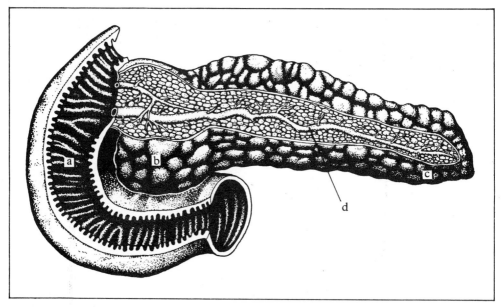

The pancreas, and part of the duodenum.
a. duodenum, b. head of pancreas, c. tail of
pancreas, d. pancreatic duct.

upper part of the abdomen behind the stomach. The right part of the gland is rounded and called the head and the left is long and thin and called the tail. The head of the pancreas lies close to the duodenum (the first part of the intestine after the stomach).

The pancreas has two functions. First, it is a digestive gland, producing enzymes that are passed through a duct into the duodenum. Second, it produces two hormones vital to the working of our bodies. Throughout the body of the gland are small cell groups called the islets of Langerhans. These produce the hormone insulin which lowers glucose levels in the blood by encouraging tissues to take it up. They also produce glucagon which releases sugar into the bloodstream. These two hormones act with other substances to control the balance of the body's sugar – its vital energy source. Incidentally, this has very little to do with actually eating sugar. Nobody needs added sugar in their diets – indeed the vast majority of people in the world never eat it at all and are perfectly healthy. The sugar in the blood is glucose, a sugar produced in the intestine by the breakdown of all the car-

bohydrates we eat in any form. Although the level of sugar in our blood is critical, it is *not* essential to eat added sugar to provide blood sugar for energy.

The only major diseases in children that affect the pancreas are DIABETES and CYSTIC FIBROSIS.

Paracetamol   *See* ANALGESIC

Paralysis   A temporary or permanent loss of muscle power affecting one or many muscles depending upon the nerve or nerves damaged. This loss of power can be complete or partial and is caused by various conditions affecting the brain, the spinal cord or the peripheral nerves.

The commonest causes of paralysis originating from the brain in adults are bleeding from or clotting in its blood vessels but these are uncommon in children. CEREBRAL PALSY is the commonest form in children. Brain tumours can also cause paralysis.

POLIOMYELITIS, a disease once common in children and young adults, may affect the nerves in the spinal cord so as to produce paralysis. SPINA BIFIDA can cause paralysis of the legs.

If a peripheral nerve is accidentally severed (for instance in a car crash) it can regrow and

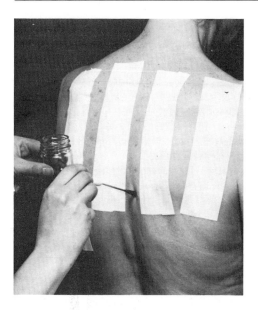

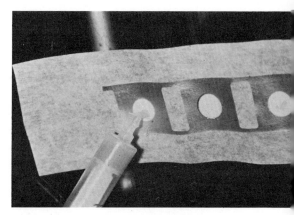

Patch testing for allergens. Suspected substances are put on to small pieces of gauze (above) which are brought into contact with the skin, or they may be applied directly to the skin (left) to see if an allergic reaction develops.

eventually perform normally again. Nerve cells themselves cannot regrow, once destroyed, but the nervous processes that make up the peripheral 'nerves' (in our limbs, for example) can regenerate.

A child with severe pain (as in inflammation of the hip joint or scurvy) may appear to be paralysed because he does not move his limbs.

Treatment of paralysis depends very much on the underlying cause. If the paralysis is caused by pressure on a nerve, that pressure can be relieved, but sometimes the muscles of the affected area are so weak and wasted that the person never regains good use of them.

Managing a child with paralysed legs is a time-consuming and trying business. Much can be done today with hand or electrically propelled wheelchairs, calipers, crutches, orthopaedic care and physiotherapy to help these children lead a relatively normal life. Also, many aids are available to help parents lift children in and out of the bath, on and off the lavatory and so on.

See CENTRAL NERVOUS SYSTEM

Paronychia *See* NAIL

Patch test A test used by doctors to try to find substances to which a child may have an ALLERGY so that they can then be eliminated, when possible, from the child's environment.

Suspected culprit substances are put on the skin on small pieces of gauze or blotting paper and held in place with sticking plaster. The areas usually tested are the skin on the arms, thighs and back. The patch is left in place for 48 hours unless severe irritation occurs, in which case it is removed sooner. Many different substances can be tested at once.

A person who is allergic to one of the substances develops reddening of the skin in contact with the test substance. Some highly sensitive individuals react very strongly and develop blisters and lots of reddening.

The interpretation of the tests is not always easy: there may be false positive results and a negative result doesn't necessarily mean that the child is not sensitive to the substance tested, partly because the test doesn't necessarily reproduce the conditions under which the allergy occurs. Nevertheless, the patch test is widely used and can be very helpful in isolating the allergenic substances that cause some children so much trouble.

Penicillin *See* ANTIBIOTICS

Penis The erectile male sex organ through which urine and semen can be passed. Some mothers worry about the smallness of their son's penis, but many babies have a pad of fat over the pubic bone which makes the penis

173

look shorter than it really is.

The penis is composed of a shaft, full of spongy tissue able to fill with blood to produce an ERECTION, and a top (glans) which is wider than the shaft. On the top of the glans there is a small slit-like opening through which urine is passed from the bladder. In some boys there is an abnormality in which the opening is not in the top at all but on the undersurface of the shaft (hypospadias). If your baby has this condition he must see a doctor. The only serious danger lies in having the child circumcised before the hypospadias is noticed, as this can cause troublesome scarring. The majority of boys with hypospadias need an operation to remedy it and some will need more than one operation.

Baby boys may suffer from soreness and even ulceration around the urethral opening as a result of an ammoniacal NAPPY RASH.

See BALANITIS; CIRCUMCISION; MASTURBATION; SEX EDUCATION; TESTES

Perinatal mortality A term used to cover babies stillborn after 28 weeks in the womb, and those babies who die within a week of birth. It is expressed as the number of babies that die for every thousand babies that are born.

The average rate for Britain is about 18 in every thousand, and the rate of babies dying when born to mothers living in very poor social circumstances is significantly greater than that for babies born to people living in good conditions. Babies born to older mothers (those over thirty) and firstborns are at increased risk. Because of these and other variables, perinatal mortality rates differ in various parts of the country.

The two major causes of babies dying at or near birth are congenital abnormalities and babies being born too small (either because they are born early or because they have failed to grow normally inside the uterus). Again, these two factors are more common amongst socially disadvantaged people.

Many countries, especially some in Europe, now have a lower perinatal mortality rate than Britain's, but the reasons for this are complicated. Britain has a higher rate of congenital abnormalities (especially spina bifida and anencephaly) and also a high rate of babies born too small. Why this should be is not known but environmental factors may well be involved. It seems that antenatal care plays an important part in keeping mortality figures down – perinatal mortality amongst women receiving no antenatal care is five to ten times higher than average, though this may partly reflect the type of woman who chooses not to have antenatal care.

Improving the social circumstances of many people by providing better housing, education, and nutrition might be a helpful factor in reducing the number of babies who die or are born handicapped.

Periodic syndrome *See* RECURRENT ABDOMINAL PAIN

Peritonitis An inflammation of the lining of the peritoneal cavity. It is an acute and potentially dangerous condition tending to affect newborn babies and older children more than those in the middle age range.

In older children, peritonitis is usually caused by a ruptured appendix following APPENDICITIS. In the newborn, peritonitis can follow twisting or perforation of the bowel or can be caused by an infected UMBILICUS. In both age groups, blood-borne infection (septicaemia) can cause peritonitis even in previously healthy children but this is more likely if the child is suffering from liver or kidney disease.

A child with peritonitis is very ill. He looks pale, usually has a high temperature and a tender, swollen tummy and may vomit.

An exploratory abdominal operation (a laparotomy) may be necessary to establish the diagnosis and to repair the bowel if it has ruptured (perforated).

Perthes' disease A softening of the upper end of the thigh bone (the femur), causing pain in the hip and a limp. It affects boys more often than girls and can occur at any age between three and ten years. The cause is unknown, though there is often a history of injury to the hip. Perthes' disease usually affects only one hip.

The pain is not severe and is dramatically relieved by bed rest. It may come and go and the child is otherwise well.

Over a period of one to three years, X-rays show that the bone gradually returns to normal. During this time, weight-bearing on the affected leg must be avoided, because pressure on the soft bone can cause squashing of the bone and osteoarthritis later in life brought on by this deformity in the joint. As this can be a very long process the child may have to have special arrangements made for his education to continue while he cannot attend a normal school.

Treatment usually takes the form of bed rest with traction for several months, followed by the use of a caliper which allows walking without weight-bearing on the affected side.

Pertussis *See* WHOOPING COUGH

Pets Pets can spread disease, especially if children kiss and cuddle them or crawl on the ground and then put dirty hands in their mouths.

To control FLEAS, groom and disinfest the pet regularly and don't let the hair become matted. Make sure its bedding is clean. If you can't get rid of the fleas, the house probably needs treating as well.

If your pet scratches a lot or has any skin disorder, or if any of the family has a skin disorder (such as ringworm or scabies) that your doctor thinks might be caused by an animal, take it to a vet. All animals, including birds, mice, tortoises, and terrapins, carry germs or worms of one kind or another, so be as hygienic as you can and don't let animals lick children's faces. Tortoises and terrapins can spread salmonella infection, causing gastro-enteritis.

Worm your dog or cat regularly, and train

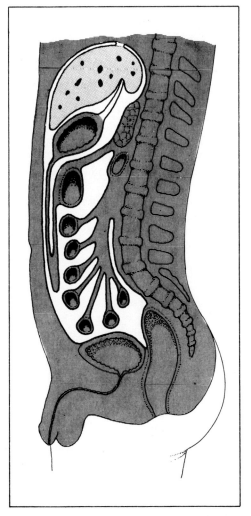

A vertical section through the abdomen showing the continuous line of the peritoneum enveloping the liver, stomach and intestines. Most of the abdominal organs are contained in its folds.

pets to defaecate in areas set away from where children play. Keep animals' plates separate and don't let them lick or eat off your plates. Be scrupulous about clearing up your pet's faeces. If necessary, wash the area with disinfectant, and wash your hands thoroughly.

Toxocariasis is an infestation with the worm Toxocara canis or cati. It is usually caused by putting dirty hands in the mouth. Infested animals pass worm eggs in their bowel motions so any area where they defaecate is hazardous. In some children migration of the larvae causes a variety of symptoms, including blindness and brain damage (both rare). No treatment is satisfactory, though recovery is usual within 6 to 12 months if there is no reinfestation. Roundworms and whipworms may be passed on in the same way.

Some children are allergic to certain animals and the allergy (asthma, hay fever, or eczema, for example) may be due to mites in their coats. The animal may need to be washed with a suitable solution up to six times to get rid of the mites.

Toxoplasmosis is a protozoan infestation which can cause congenital abnormalities in a baby born to a mother who has the condition in pregnancy. It is spread by diseased cats and poorly cooked meat. A pregnant woman should eat only well-cooked meat, and should avoid handling her cat's litter, especially if it eats fresh, uncooked meat.

Rabies is a killing disease which has been eradicated in Britain by means of strict quarantine regulations.

When buying a pet, either deal directly with an accredited dealer or breeder or go to a pet shop where the animals are healthy-looking and well kept. If you are at all unsure how to choose a pet, ask for your vet's advice.

A new pet should be seen by a vet for a thorough physical examination and any necessary vaccinations. Vets also advise regular checkups to ensure that a pet is as healthy as possible.

Pharyngitis Pharyngitis (sore throat) is one of the commonest reasons for taking a child to the doctor. The tonsils are almost invariably affected as well as the pharynx (the back of the mouth) except in babies under one year, who have very small tonsils.

There is usually some degree of pharyngitis with any infection of the upper respiratory tract (nose, ears and sinuses) as all of these passages communicate with each other. It may also be seen with some generalized infections and is a prominent feature of diphtheria and glandular fever.

Children between four and seven years old are particularly likely to suffer from pharyngitis. The younger the child, the less likely he is to complain of a sore throat: he is more likely to say that his tummy hurts, because of concurrent enlargement of the lymph nodes of the abdomen (mesenteric adenitis). Older children may also complain of pain in the ear and while this may be due to OTITIS MEDIA (a middle ear inflammation), it is just as likely to be due to referred pain from the inflamed throat. This is why a doctor will always examine the throat of a child complaining of tummy ache or earache, or of a child who is generally unwell.

The size of the tonsils is not a reliable indicator of the severity of infection as it is normal for children of a certain age to have large tonsils.

Sore throats may be caused by viruses (about 80 per cent) or bacteria (about 20 per cent). The streptococcal sore throat is the most usual of the bacterial infections and may be caused by a special type of streptococcus called the β-haemolytic streptococcus. Unfortunately, this bacterial infection can lead on to unpleasant conditions such as rheumatic fever and glomerulonephritis (*see* NEPHRITIS) in a few children, which is why it is a good idea for streptococcal sore throats of this type to be treated with penicillin to prevent such complications. Some children with a streptococcal sore throat develop SCARLET FEVER.

However, it is extremely difficult to distinguish a viral sore throat from a streptococcal sore throat just by looking. Both infections can also cause a fever, general malaise, loss of appetite, hoarseness, a cough, runny nose and enlarged neck nodes. A streptococcal sore throat may cause vomiting and also tends to produce pain in the throat more quickly than the viral one, but as a child seldom complains of a sore throat anyway, it is not a very useful feature.

For this reason, many doctors routinely give antibiotics, usually penicillin, to children with sore throats. Others take a throat swab to send for bacterial culture and only give an antibiotic if the culture is positive for β-haemolytic streptococci. This is perhaps better medical practice but takes time for the test to be done and it would be extremely expensive for the health service if every child with a sore throat had a swab taken. What is more, it has been estimated that between 10 and 20 per cent of healthy children normally carry β-haemolytic streptococci in their throats, so culture in these children would not prove that the illness was due to this organism. Yet other doctors give antibiotics at the same time as taking a swab if they are fairly sure of the diagnosis.

Other treatment includes bed rest, tepid sponging to lower the child's temperature, cool, soothing drinks and a light diet if the child wants anything to eat at all.

Complications of pharyngitis include otitis media, SINUSITIS, QUINSY (an abscess occurring in or around a tonsil) and LARYNGITIS, besides those already mentioned – nephritis, rheumatic fever and scarlet fever.

If the child has a streptococcal sore throat and is treated with antibiotics, he will be non-infectious within a few hours. However, if, as is most likely, it is a viral sore throat, he will remain infectious for several days.

See TONSILLITIS

Phenylketonuria A condition affecting one in ten to fifteen thousand babies, due to a defect of the enzyme that converts the amino acid phenylalanine to tyrosine. Harmful breakdown products of phenylalanine in the first weeks of life harm the developing brain and usually cause mental retardation and cataracts.

Because it is not possible to diagnose phenylketonuria by looking at the child until the damage has been done, all newborn babies are tested for the disease with the Guthrie test, done on a sample of blood from a prick in the baby's heel on about the sixth day after birth. If the test is positive, the blood level of phenylalanine is measured to confirm the diagnosis.

Affected babies are often fair-haired and blue-eyed, may have a tendency to seborrhoeic DERMATITIS and have musty-smelling urine. About a third have convulsions. They also tend to suffer from irritability and vomiting.

Treatment involves putting the baby on a diet low in phenylalanine. A specially prepared brand of milk is available. From time to time a trial of a normal diet can be given, monitored by blood tests to see whether the chemicals are rising to harmful levels again. Many children, however, have to stay on the diet for a long time. Early treatment by strict dieting

lessens the risk that the brain will be affected.

The disease is passed on by a recessive gene from each parent, about one in 50 of the normal population being symptomless carriers of this gene. Unfortunately there is as yet no reliable test to identify carriers of the disease. (*See* INHERITED DISEASES.)

Phobia An irrational fear of a thing or a situation. The fear is irrational in that it is not caused by what the child outwardly fears but is due to unconscious factors. It is no less real because of that and a child with a phobia may suffer greatly if he is forced to try to overcome it.

Some fairly commonly encountered phobias are a fear of the dark, a fear of tigers (for example) in the bedroom, a fear of robbers and a fear of going to school. Unconscious worries producing these phobias may be many. School phobia, for instance, may be due to a suppressed fear of leaving home and mother or to a fear of another child or a teacher at school.

There is no need for parents to worry unless the fear is incapacitating to the child. School phobia has to be dealt with very carefully and a thorough discussion of the possible causes should be undertaken by parents, teacher, school doctor and any other concerned party. If necessary, a child psychiatrist can help with either individual or family therapy. (*See* TRUANCY.)

Physical handicap Some children are born with a physical handicap while others acquire one later in life. The most common types present at or soon after birth are CEREBRAL PALSY and SPINA BIFIDA, but there are many other conditions that can disable a child. Some types of physical handicap are caused by an inherited defect while others are due to problems arising during pregnancy or labour. Yet others can arise as a result of illness or injury at any time.

As medical science advances, some babies with a very severe physical handicap are kept alive at birth, whereas without intervention many of them would have died. In some areas, parents are given a chance to discuss how much active medical intervention should be carried out, but any decisions are, of course,

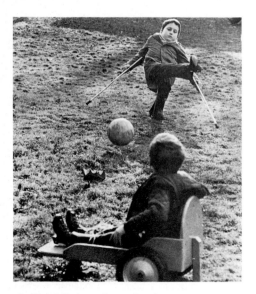

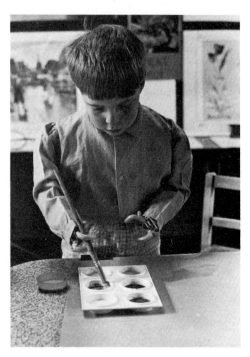

Artificial limbs and crutches do not prevent these children from pursuing the normal occupations of childhood, despite serious physical handicaps.

appallingly difficult, especially for the parents of a newborn baby.

Conditions such as MENINGITIS, ENCEPHA-LITIS and road traffic accidents can cause a permanent physical handicap in a child who was quite well before. In the past, POLIO-MYELITIS was responsible for disabling many previously fit children.

Physically handicapped children should be under the care of a paediatrician to ensure that they have the best possible treatment. Physiotherapy is often useful and the parents can usually learn enough from the therapists to carry out some treatments themselves at home. Thorough assessment of physically handicapped children is essential, partly because of their relatively increased likelihood of having visual, hearing, intellectual, emotional and social problems in addition to their physical handicap. If your hospital cannot offer this sort of assessment, your family doctor or paediatrician can refer your child to a specialist centre. It is not always easy to diagnose certain physical handicaps, such as cerebral palsy, in the first year, and accurate prediction of the future extent of the handicap may be especially difficult, for instance with spina bifida.

However, diagnosis as early as possible is important so that enough expert help and counselling can be given to the parents, as well as medical help to the child.

The physical care of the young handicapped child is relatively easy: problems are more likely to arise later as he grows heavier and becomes less easy to lift and carry. There are many aids available to make it easier for parents to manage such children at home. Wheelchairs of several types, including electrically operated ones, can be issued from special wheelchair centres. The council can install mechanical lifting devices to help lift the child into the bath; they can also carry out structural alterations to the house to make it easy for a wheelchair to enter every room; they can install handles by the lavatory and help in many other ways too.

Schooling for physically handicapped children varies according to the facilities available in each area and according to the child's general ability and need for special medical supervision, nursing care and various forms of therapy. Special schools for physically handicapped children usually cater for those who are disabled but of normal intelligence. They have special treatment rooms and other facilities not found in ordinary schools. Some children are unfortunately not only physically handicapped but mentally handicapped too, in which case they may have to be placed in schools for the educationally subnormal. (See EDUCATIONAL SUBNORMALITY.) Yet other children have associated visual, hearing or speech defects and need even more specialized schooling. A few disabled children are placed in ordinary schools and manage well. Their success is based on the enthusiasm of the staff and other children, the suitability of the building and the availability of extra care to help with the lavatory, dressing and so on.

Pica See DIRT EATING

Pigeon toe (intoeing) Pigeon toe or intoeing is commonly seen as a child starts to walk. The child may simply walk with his toes turned in, he may throw one leg around the other as he walks, and he may actually fall over his own toes.

There are three basic causes for this condition. The most common cause of intoeing is an inward turning of the foot itself. Mild cases correct themselves with the help of good, well-made shoes. Twisting of the tibia, associated with bow leg and usually with an inward turning of the foot itself, corrects itself as the child grows. Some degree of twisting of the leg above the knee may cause pigeon toe, but almost always corrects itself spontaneously with time – usually by the age of six years. Looking at a child with some twisting of the femur, the knees can be seen to point inwards or even face each other. In a very few children this condition does not resolve and, if the child is upset by it, an operation can be done to untwist the femur or leg bone. This, however, leaves a scar, so should only be done if absolutely necessary.

See FEET

Pituitary The 'master' gland of the endocrine system. It is an organ about the size of a pea, situated in a bony shell within the skull just behind the back of the nose. It has three parts: a front, glandular part, an intermediate part and a back part. It is connected to the brain by a stalk through which there is a considerable two way traffic of information.

The front part produces hormones which control body growth, milk secretion and thyroid function. Its hormones also regulate the development of ova in the ovary and sperms in the testes and regulate hormones produced by these organs. Lastly, it produces the hormone (ACTH) that controls the functioning of the adrenal gland.

Overactivity of the front part of the pituitary gland can make a child grow into a giant. Other conditions produce various symptoms including precocious puberty, masculinization of females, loss of periods, obesity and high blood pressure.

The back lobe of the pituitary produces the hormone oxytocin which makes the involuntary muscles of the uterus and breast contract. Another hormone regulates the body's water balance and is known as anti-diuretic hormone.

Pityriasis A mildly infectious disease, possibly transmitted by a virus, mainly affecting young adults but also seen in children.

There is usually no sign of illness apart from a rash, though occasionally the child has a sore throat, a raised temperature and swollen lymph nodes. The first sign of the rash is the so-called 'herald patch' which appears on the trunk or on an upper limb between 5 and 14 days before the main rash. This patch is flat, red and scaly and heals from the centre outwards. The rash proper is composed of smaller, pinker, scaly patches, often arranged in line with the ribs, giving a fir tree pattern on the trunk. It is not usually itchy and takes six to eight weeks to clear up.

No treatment is necessary for pityriasis and there is no need to isolate the child.

Pneumonia An inflammation of the lungs which may be caused by infection with bacteria, viruses, or other organisms; irritant substances; inhaled matter (such as vomit or a foreign body); or allergy. Two main types are seen in children. Lobar pneumonia affects a small area of a lung, while bronchopneumonia affects larger areas and can be generalized in both lungs. BRONCHIOLITIS is a type of pneumonia.

Lobar pneumonia comes on suddenly in a healthy, older child while bronchopneumonia usually affects children under five years who already have a cold, an ear infection or gastroenteritis. Measles and whooping cough can also lead on to bronchopneumonia.

Lobar pneumonia starts with a high temperature but in bronchopneumonia there may be no fever. Both produce rapid, shallow breathing often accompanied by grunting, a cough and sometimes diarrhoea and vomiting. Children rarely cough up sputum – they swallow it instead, so the isolation of the organism causing the infection can be difficult and a sample may have to be obtained from the stomach via a tube.

Some children with pneumonia get a stiff neck which can be so severe as to make the doctor think of meningitis. No one knows why this occurs but it can happen in other infections of childhood too. If the temperature is high, there may be convulsions. Pneumonia can also produce abdominal pain and pain in the chest.

The diagnosis of pneumonia is often difficult in children because appendicitis, meningitis and tonsillitis can all produce similar clinical pictures.

Antibiotics are the best treatment for bacterial pneumonia. Some children need to be given oxygen. Many children can now be treated very well at home without admission to hospital. The child may like to be propped up in bed so as to ease the difficult breathing but, apart from this, a nourishing diet if the child wants to eat, plenty of fluids and possibly some physiotherapy will be all he needs.

It's important to avoid overheating the child, especially if he has a FEVER.

Poisoning A poison is a substance which, when taken into the body in sufficient quantity, is capable of impairing health or even causing death. Poisons can be solids, liquids, or gases and some usually harmless substances or valuable medicines, taken in excess, can be poisonous.

Every year thousands of children poison themselves, sometimes fatally. Usually the poison is a common household cleaner or medicine. Gas poisoning used to be relatively common when domestic gas supplies contained carbon monoxide, but natural gas only produces carbon monoxide when the appliance burning it is poorly serviced or badly ventilated and burns the gas incompletely. Clothes just returned from the dry cleaner, if left in a closed car (especially on a warm day), can give off fumes of residual cleaning fluid and poison a child left in the car, so always keep a window open in these circumstances.

Research has shown that many households contain dozens of different medicines at any one time. Many of these are old and possibly dangerous. Tablets and capsules are brightly coloured and look very similar to sweets, so it's scarcely surprising that children find them attractive. The trouble is that they see adults swallowing them and think they can too. Drugs are prescribed in small doses for children, because their bodies are smaller than those of adults. This means that the normal adult dose of a drug can be dangerous or even lethal to a child, so don't be complacent if your child eats only one or two tablets or capsules.

Because of good medical care, the average child who eats tablets ends up staying in hospital only overnight, but the anxiety his parents go through is enormous, partly because they feel guilty at having let it happen. The answer is prevention. Make time to go all around the house and remove or make safe any poison hazards there may be. Start by thinking whether there are any poisonous berries or shrubs in the garden. Laburnum and laurel can be deadly and children should be taught never to eat any berries. The dangers of poisonous plants have been overstressed however, as they rarely cause death.

Next, look in the kitchen, laundry room, shed, and outhouse. Take all the bleaches, disinfectants, weedkillers, lavatory cleaners, and similar fluids and put them high up out of reach. Never transfer one liquid to the container of another. Many children have been poisoned because their parents used an old lemonade bottle for a poisonous household chemical. Household cleaning liquids are almost all very dangerous and may damage the skin as well as the child's stomach if he swallows or spills them. Remember that small children and babies are not put off as adults would be by the noxious smell of some caustic fluids.

The third place to look in is your bedroom. Cosmetics or nail varnish remover, for instance, can be lethal. Put these things into a lockable drawer or very high up. It's certainly more inconvenient but it's a small price to pay for safety.

The medicine chest is, of course, the most dangerous place. Medicine cabinets should not be in the kitchen or bathroom where steam and heat can get to drugs and damage them. Wherever your cabinet is, keep it locked at all times and place it high on a wall. If you're taking tablets regularly and can't keep locking them away, keep them high up and out of reach. Take out the tablets you need and consume them immediately, returning the container to its safe place. The kitchen table is no place for tablet containers. Never leave sleeping tablets by the bedside.

Never pretend that tablets or medicines of any kind are sweets – even to encourage your child to take his medicine. This encourages the wrong attitude entirely and may backfire on you one day. Don't get large quantities of drugs from your doctor if you have little children about. It's better to go more often for a repeat prescription than to have a poisoned or dead child.

Unfortunately, some of the commonest tablets are the most dangerous. Iron tablets (seemingly harmless and looking very much like sweets) can kill children; vitamin tablets are harmful in overdose; and paracetamol is extremely dangerous. Whenever possible, buy tablets in child-resistant containers or buy these containers to put your tablets in. Many manufacturers now sell potentially dangerous, commonly used tablets (such as the Pill or painkillers) in foil or other unit packaging. This makes them much safer from a child's point of view.

If your child has consumed any poison you must phone a doctor or call for an ambulance. Don't put off going to the casualty department just because you think one or two tablets won't hurt him. You won't necessarily know exactly how much he's taken and anyway the effects may not come on at once.

Always ask a child what he has eaten if it isn't obvious. It might be the last chance you have to find out what's been taken before he loses consciousness, and knowing could be helpful in the treatment. Always take the container of whatever the child has eaten along to the hospital – it could help them in treating him. If the child has stopped breathing, do artificial respiration (*see* KISS OF LIFE) and in any event don't leave him until expert help comes. If he's vomiting, keep him on his side in the recovery position, so he doesn't inhale any of the vomit (*see* SHOCK).

Until recently, first aid experts always taught that you should give fluids to poison cases. This is probably not a wise thing today. If you are sure that your child has taken a highly caustic or corrosive chemical, try washing round the mouth with water and give the child milk to drink but don't under any circumstances make him vomit. Apart from this, it's probably wiser to give the child nothing to drink but to get him to a hospital as quickly as possible.

Poliomyelitis (polio)   An infectious disease affecting the cells of the brain and spinal cord (*see* CENTRAL NERVOUS SYSTEM).

Polio viruses are usually swallowed. An attack may be unnoticed and the child then builds up an immunity to the virus. In about two-thirds of all cases there are 'flu-like symptoms and in such cases recovery is complete and there is no paralysis.

In some children the nerve cells are affected but recover, causing only temporary paralysis. If the nerve cells are seriously affected, the child has a fever, stiffness and pain in the back and limbs, muscle tenderness and general weakness. Paralysis then follows. Lower limbs are most commonly affected but higher levels of the body can be affected, perhaps also causing difficulty in breathing, needing treatment with a respirator (an artificial lung). If PARALYSIS occurs, without proper care the affected limbs can become deformed, and physiotherapy may be needed for several years.

Today's children should be fully immunized against polio by having three doses of oral vaccine in the first year, followed by booster doses at five years and then on leaving school. If a baby or child has diarrhoea or is otherwise unwell he should not receive the polio vaccine.

Breast-fed babies are protected against

polio early in life by antibodies in breast milk, especially if their mothers are immune. There is, though, no need to delay polio IMMUNI- ZATION in a breast-fed baby as the dose of virus given is large enough not to be neutralized by these polio antibodies.

Because polio has been kept at bay by im- munization, many people have forgotten how horrible it can be and are not bothering to have their children immunized. This means that it is now possible that polio might rear its head again, and only recently there was a suspected outbreak which led to a mass immunization programme. This attitude is partly a by- product of anti-whooping cough immuni- zation propaganda. There is no reason to think that all immunizations are potentially danger- ous and anyone who has seen a polio victim will make very sure that his children are immunized against this potentially crippling infection.

Because polio is still common in some countries, it is sensible to make sure that your children are adequately immunized before travelling anywhere except Northern Europe, Canada and the USA.

Port wine stain   *See* BIRTHMARK

Possetting   *See* REGURGITATION

Posture   The way your child holds himself is principally determined by heredity, though some children can alter and improve their habitual posture by continual concentration.

If your child is round shouldered, no amount of nagging will correct his posture unless he is really keen to stand up straight himself. A better way of improving the way he looks is to compliment him when he does stand up straight. This works better with an older child who is more conscious of his appearance.

Tall or fat children sometimes stoop in an attempt to make themselves look smaller or shorter than they are, as most children are very wary of being different in body build from their peer group. Try if you can to point out tall or fat people who hold themselves attractively and proudly, so that the child can see that these people really do look better than they would if they stooped.

See BACK

Potty training   The golden rule for parents potty training their children is to be relaxed and treat the process as something normal and spontaneous, which it usually is. Parents who have a rigid approach to training expect too much of their child in their anxiety to get him dry and clean, become emotionally involved, perhaps angry, threatening and even punishing. This may only delay the desired control.

All normal children eventually become dry and clean. If you decide you want to train your child early, you may be lucky but you make him take a dislike to the whole idea. Mothers are sometimes successful in catching bowel motions when their babies are under one year old, by putting them on the potty after a meal. However, this is purely the result of a reflex bowel movement and is not because the child can voluntarily open his bowels and empty his bladder in the right place at the right time. Only when he does this can he be said to be trained.

If you wait until your child shows signs that he is ready to control his bowel and bladder, you are more likely to succeed in training with no problems. Wait until your child tells you (or signals by pointing or some other sign) that he wants to open his bowels; this may be any time from 18 months to round about two years old. You can then take him to the potty or put him on the lavatory – either on a special child's seat or on the adult seat. A potty allows the child to sit in a more natural way, with his feet on the ground, but you might like to make or buy a box to put in front of the lavatory for the child to rest his feet on. Obviously you will need to do some ground work beforehand – let your child see other children using the potty or lavatory and let him see you doing it as well. Buy a potty and let him play with it for a few months or weeks, telling him every so often that that is where he should sit to do a 'pooh' or 'wee-wee' or whatever words your family uses for a bowel motion or urine. Some mothers find it helps to play a game with a doll sitting on the potty.

When you change his nappy, if it is dirty, you can say that one day he will be able to do a pooh in his potty, like a big boy (or like his brother or sister or friend). He will gradually associate potty with pooh, until the golden day

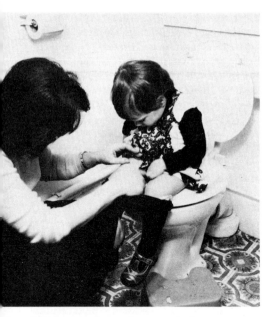

Children can be taught to use the lavatory rather than a potty, with a box to support their feet and a special child's seat fitted over the adult one.

arrives when he tells you he wants to use the potty and does so.

You are bound to have messes and puddles on the floor, in his nappy and around the lavatory and potty seat at first, and it's worth accepting this calmly and not getting upset. Young children have a relatively small bladder capacity and need to pass water frequently if they drink a lot. They may be so engrossed in what they are doing that they don't reach the potty quickly enough. By the time the full bladder makes its demands felt, the need to go is urgent. Sometimes a child may tease you by saying he wants to go and then doing nothing. Don't be too cross because, if you are, he will have found a good way of annoying you in the future. Reminding him to use the potty every so often may help prevent wet pants.

Similarly, while you should praise him for using the potty, don't be over-emotional – after all, it's a normal function.

Bladder control usually comes a little later than bowel control and day-time wetting may continue well into the third year, even if only by accident. Night-time dryness usually comes

between two and three years, though a few are dry before this and many are still wet after this. Between 10 and 15 per cent of normal children wet the bed at the age of five years, and one per cent at the age of fifteen.

Like bowel control, bladder control can only happen when the child is physically mature enough, so there is no point in trying to train before he is ready. When you notice that he is dry for periods of two hours or so during the day, and if he is already showing signs of gaining bowel control, then is the time to start putting him on the potty or lavatory every so often to see if he wants to empty his bladder. If he can tell you he wants to go, so much the better, though children usually start off by telling their mothers *after* they have wetted their nappy.

Trainer pants (terry towelling-lined plastic pants) are helpful while potty training as they can be pulled down more quickly than a nappy and also soak up quite large amounts of urine if the child has an accident. If you are training your child in summer, let him run around with no pants on. The sensation of urine trickling down his legs will help make him more aware of the need to sit on the potty.

See BED WETTING; CONSTIPATION; ENURESIS

Premature baby   *See* LOW BIRTH WEIGHT

Prolapse of the rectum   A protrusion of the rectum through the anus (back passage). This usually occurs in a child under five years old who has strained too hard to open his bowels. It also occurs in children with cystic fibrosis. There's no need for concern because the rectum always goes back, though when parents see the bright red protrusion for the first time it certainly looks alarming.

Treatment is simple. First, do your best to prevent constipation. Keep the child's diet rich in dietary fibre (roughage) and make sure he drinks enough. Should a prolapse occur, lie the child down and raise the end of the bed on blocks or books. To push the rectum back in, wrap your finger in some tissue, insert it into the centre of the prolapse and push it back in. If you do this without paper your finger will pull the rectum right back out again as you withdraw it. The paper is passed with the next stool. If you can't get the rectum to go back – call the doctor.

If your child has this condition, try to reduce the 'doubling up' of his body as he squats to open his bowels. Encourage him to use a lavatory rather than a potty and if necessary get him a smaller lavatory seat.

See CONSTIPATION

Psoriasis A chronic and recurrent skin disorder tending to run in families. The cause is unknown and it is uncommon in children under six years of age.

The first sign in a child may be a sudden eruption, often following an acute infection such as tonsillitis, of small, red, raised spots on the skin. These become scaly after one or two weeks and usually disappear completely. Eventually the child develops the more typical skin lesions of psoriasis seen in adults – one or more well demarcated areas of red, scaly, thick skin on the fronts of the knees, backs of the elbows, ears, chest, lower back or scalp. The nails may be finely pitted. The scales of psoriasis are silvery and dry and the patches may itch and flake. Rarely, psoriasis causes nappy rash in babies. It may flare up at times of stress and emotion, or after an injury.

Treatment is basically with ointments containing dithranol, coal tar and salicylic acid, or steroids. A newer treatment, suitable for some severe cases, involves taking the medicine psoralen together with a course of ultra-violet light treatment.

Puberty The stage during which a child becomes capable of sexual reproduction. The changes that bring this about are caused by hormones that are produced in increasing amounts around the ages of 11 years in girls and 13 in boys. These hormones cause the child to grow rapidly and to develop secondary sexual characteristics (body hair, body shape, deeper voice, breast development etc.).

Girls need preparing for their first period and boys for their first emission of semen. However, it is not only physical changes that occur during puberty. The emotional changes of ADOLESCENCE often need patience and understanding by parents. An increased awareness of the opposite sex brings its own pleasures,

problems and fears as the years go by.

Many parents wait until their children have emotional (or even physical) problems before they discuss sex, VD, contraception and love. By then it may be too late. Adolescence is a time when a child needs protection not only from outsiders but also from himself. Emotions can easily become mixed, there are many social pressures today that are more powerful than they used to be and mistakes made now can mar a child's development and enjoyment of sex for ever.

See MENARCHE; MENSTRUATION; OVARIES; SEX EDUCATION; TESTES

Pyelitis, Pyelonephritis *See* NEPHRITIS

Pyloric stenosis A narrowing of the outlet from the stomach by muscle tissue. The condition affects five times as many boys as girls. The narrowing doesn't cause symptoms until about two to three weeks after birth, when the child starts VOMITING without any change in feeding, becomes constipated and weight gain slows or stops. Classically, the vomiting is projectile – a jet of fluid shoots out of the mouth and lands a few feet away. The child is very hungry yet soon vomits any milk he drinks. The vomit contains curds and that of a bottle-fed baby smells unpleasant.

The condition can be serious because, by repeated vomiting, the child loses so much fluid that he becomes severely dehydrated, and in the end, too feeble to suck. The doctor makes the diagnosis by feeling for a lump in the abdomen over the pylorus, which hardens and softens while the baby is feeding.

Doctors can give a medicine to help relax the muscles at the outlet of the stomach but the usual treatment is a simple operation. This cures the condition permanently.

Five stages in the development of the breasts.
1. The nipples protrude slightly before puberty.
2 and 3. Breasts and nipples protrude and the nipples become larger. 4. In most girls, the nipples and areolae form a second semi-circular mound. In others, the breasts go straight from stage 3 to maturity (stage 5), when the areola is again flat and only the centre point stands out.

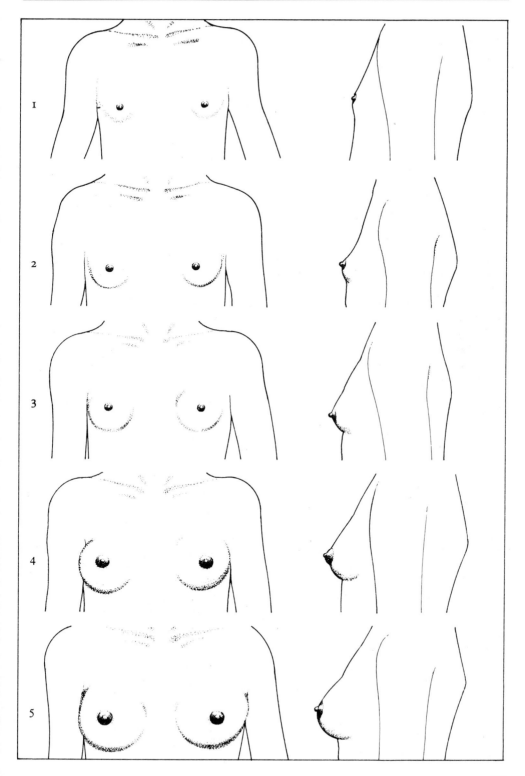

Q   R

Quinsy An abscess of the tonsil and surrounding tissue, uncommon in childhood. The infecting organism is usually a haemolytic streptococcus, which first causes acute TONSILLITIS. The pain of quinsy is severe, especially on swallowing or speaking, and the child's temperature may be high. Treatment is with antibiotics, painkillers and, if necessary, incision of the abscess, which will otherwise rupture spontaneously.

See TONSILS

Rash An eruption of the skin. Rashes are of different types and can help doctors diagnose a disease if they look typical. A *macular* rash is one in which the affected reddened areas are flat, cannot be felt, and are separate. A *papular* rash is one in which these areas are raised, can be felt, and are separate. A *vesicular* rash is composed of blisters and a *pustular* rash is one in which these blisters have become infected. Many common childhood rashes are a mixture of two or more of these types.

Rashes can also occur on the inside linings of the body. For example, in measles, little white spots called Koplik's spots are found on the inside of the cheeks (on the mouth lining). Not all rashes are itchy, and not all are infectious.

Apart from childhood infections, children can get rashes from food they have eaten to which they are allergic; drugs (especially antibiotics); certain plants and fungi; chemicals; stings and bites; excess heat; sweating; the ammonia released from wet and dirty nappies and various generalized illnesses.

If your child has a rash, telephone the doctor before going to the surgery as he won't thank you for taking an infected child into the waiting room where there may be other children or pregnant women. Describe the rash to your doctor and see what he says.

Never ignore a rash – it's the body's reaction to a stimulus or insult. If the answer is obvious (HEAT RASH, drugs, bites, stings etc.) then there's no need to worry. Remove the source of the problem and try to avoid it in the future. If there's no obvious answer, seek your doctor's advice.

Rectum, prolapse of *See* PROLAPSE OF THE RECTUM

Recurrent abdominal pain A condition affecting 10 to 15 per cent of schoolchildren in Britain.

There are many causes of recurrent abdominal pain in children although the vast majority of these children (95 per cent) have nothing seriously wrong. Often the child says 'I've got my pain' but continues whatever he is doing without interruption. If there are no other symptoms there is unlikely to be any recognizable cause. Any unusual symptoms or signs during an attack should lead to investigation being carried out to exclude conditions such as a urinary tract infection, tuberculosis, sickle cell anaemia, tonsillitis and inflammation of the lymph nodes in the abdomen (mesenteric adenitis). Even if your child has had several attacks of ABDOMINAL PAIN with no apparent cause, his next attack could be due to an acute condition such as acute appendicitis or a twisted bowel, so a severe pain should never be ignored. The doctor should be consulted if you are at all worried, especially if the pain makes the child double up.

There may be a family history of recurrent abdominal pain or MIGRAINE and indeed the child's pain may be diagnosed as being a form of migraine. He may vomit repeatedly, eventually only retching once the stomach is emptied, and this may go on for about a day. Unexplained recurrent attacks of abdominal pain plus vomiting are often labelled as the periodic syndrome, or even abdominal migraine, cyclical vomiting or 'bilious attacks'.

In the 95 per cent of children with no obvious physical cause for their pains, the pain may occur daily or at frequent intervals of a few days; it is usually vague, constant, felt in the centre of the abdomen and is momentary or lasts for minutes only. Often it happens before school in the morning and some children say that opening their bowels relieves it. The child may be pale, feel sick, be off his food and have a headache during an attack. Some doctors consider it worthwhile to exclude all foods of cows' milk origin for a time to see if the symptoms are caused by an intolerance to cows' milk protein or to an intolerance of lactose (milk sugar). If the child is constipated, attention must be given to his diet (*see* CONSTIPATION).

Sometimes the pains are provoked by emotional troubles at home or at school, such as the stress in a family from marital, financial or housing problems. If there is no way of avoiding such situations, the child should be helped to come to terms with them so that he is better able to cope with his stress. His pains should then stop.

Regurgitation Most normal, healthy babies bring up food from their stomachs into their mouths at some time or other and this is known as regurgitation. A baby can bring up a large volume of stomach contents but it is more usual for a small amount to be regurgitated. Regurgitation (possetting) usually occurs a short time after a feed and may occur as the child brings up wind, but may happen hours after a feed or may be continual. It is uncommon after the first year. Occasionally regurgitation is explosive, but it is never projectile (*see* PYLORIC STENOSIS).

Regurgitation alone does not suggest that the baby is ill, even if the whole feed is occasionally brought up. An *ill* baby who regurgitates or vomits is also unhappy: he may cry, have a temperature, diarrhoea or some other sign of illness. An ill baby may keep little food down and eventually loses weight if he continues to bring up his food. The normal, fit baby who regurgitates, thrives, even though he may bring up part of each feed.

The main practical problem with regurgitation is keeping things sweet-smelling and clean, as the baby tends to bring up partially-digested food over not only his clothes but his mother's clothes, the carpet and other furnishings. Protection is better than cleaning up, so always keep a spare nappy handy to drape over your shoulder or under the baby's chin and lie the baby with his head on a nappy on the cot, sofa or carpet. The fully breast-fed baby's vomit smells much less unpleasant than that of the bottle-fed baby or the baby on solid food.

Babies sometimes regurgitate when they burp after a feed. To try and prevent this, it's sensible not to move the baby around quickly or jog him up and down too soon after a feed. Holding him upright after a feed may also decrease the amount of regurgitation.

A baby who has brought up some of his

milk into his mouth may ruminate (chew the cud). This can become a habit but there is no need to stop him from doing it.

See VOMITING

Respiratory distress syndrome A condition which causes difficulty in breathing, affecting about one in ten of all premature babies. It is most commonly seen in babies weighing less than 5½lb (2500g), affecting 70 to 80 per cent of them. Besides small and premature babies, larger babies may suffer from it, such as those born to diabetic mothers; those born near term by caesarean section; and when there has been bleeding before birth. The disease rarely occurs in full-term infants. Respiratory distress syndrome is the most common cause of death in the first week.

The cause is a lack of a substance called surfactant, normally present in the full-term infant's lungs which keeps them expanded after the first breath has sucked air into them. Without surfactant the condition of the lungs prevents the blood from collecting oxygen efficiently. Breathing becomes distressed, rapid and shallow, causing the rib cage to be drawn inwards and upwards instead of expanding with the breath. Without treatment the baby cannot survive for long. In mild cases, the symptoms reach a peak in three days.

The baby is treated in an incubator with oxygen-rich air and may often need mechanical assistance in breathing. He may also need intravenous feeding with a special solution to regulate his body's acid-base balance, which becomes altered because of the lung trouble. These rather complex treatments are difficult outside specialized units. The aim of treatment is to keep the child alive until he makes enough surfactant. Most babies with respiratory distress syndrome survive with proper treatment.

It is possible to find out whether foetal lungs are making surfactant by testing amniotic fluid (*see* AMNIOCENTESIS). If we could prevent babies from being born prematurely, the respiratory distress syndrome would no longer be a problem.

See LOW BIRTH WEIGHT

Retinoblastoma *See* BLINDNESS

Rheumatic fever A relatively rare disease caused by a sensitivity to certain streptococcal bacteria. Many thousands of children get streptococcal sore throats but few develop rheumatic fever. Any streptococcal infection of the upper respiratory tract or ears, including TONSILLITIS, SCARLET FEVER and OTITIS MEDIA, can cause rheumatic fever. Although the disease is more common in certain families it is not known whether this is due to an increased exposure to streptococcal infections or to genetic factors.

Rheumatic fever is uncommon today, but as recently as 1928 it filled one quarter of all the beds in a London children's hospital. The improvement has come about because of better public health, improved living conditions, better food and the control of streptococcal infections with antibiotics.

Rheumatic fever has fairly typical signs and symptoms and begins from one to four weeks after a streptococcal infection (usually tonsillitis). There is often an acute FEVER with headache and aches in several joints, usually the big ones (knees, ankles, elbows and wrists). The joints become painful, swollen and tender and then get better after a few days. As several joints can be affected one after the other this leads to the sensation that the pains are flitting from joint to joint. Moving the affected joints is extremely painful.

There is a rash in about one fifth of cases and the pink, irregular circles or crescents are quite typical of rheumatic fever. Some children get nodules or lumps under the skin, especially on the knuckles, elbows, knees and spine.

The most serious effect of rheumatic fever is on the heart muscle and the heart valves, causing enlargement and heart murmurs. Death can occur (though rarely) from heart failure. The damage to the heart valves can last into adulthood. Today, with good treatment, the chances of a child getting heart disease after rheumatic fever are very small indeed.

Rarely, the brain is involved, and jerky, inco-ordinated movements of the limbs and face occur (St Vitus's dance).

A child that gets rheumatic fever today should take penicillin by mouth daily (or by injection monthly) for several years to prevent further attacks. If your child has had rheumatic fever he should be 'covered' by penicillin every time he has dental treatment or any operation, however small.

Aspirin is the best treatment for acute rheumatic fever and is used in very high doses to relieve the pains and fever. Steroid drugs are sometimes used.

Thanks to penicillin, streptococcal infections are killed off if caught early, and so rarely go on to produce rheumatic fever. If ever your child has a sore throat or earache, and complains of joint pains or doesn't seem to be recovering as you would expect after about ten days, see your doctor.

The arthritis of rheumatic fever does not last like the joint swelling of rheumatoid arthritis.

Rheumatoid arthritis   An illness including not only inflammation of joints but also involvement of many other parts of the body. About five per cent of adults with rheumatoid ARTHRITIS first had symptoms during childhood. Some children have an acute form of the disease known as Still's disease, the cause of which is unknown.

In 40 per cent of children with rheumatoid arthritis, the main symptom is arthritis of many joints, including the small joints of the hands. There is a sudden or gradual development of joint stiffness, swelling, and a loss of range of movement. The stiffness is most pronounced after a night's sleep or any other period of inactivity. In some children, only a few joints are affected. In 25 per cent of affected children, the main symptoms are a high fever and a rash, though many other symptoms may occur and arthritis eventually develops, usually within a few months.

Three out of four children with rheumatoid arthritis eventually become symptom-free, but some develop crippling joint deformities, including severe hip disease. An associated chronic inflammation of the eye (iridocyclitis) can produce pain, redness, dislike of light and loss of vision.

Treatment is with drugs and physiotherapy and needs expert and long-term supervision, usually by a team of specialists. Rheumatoid children should be encouraged to lead as normal a life as possible and should not be treated as invalids. Their need for education is as great as that of any other children.

Rickets   A disease caused by a deficiency of vitamin D. Such a deficiency is most harmful during periods of rapid growth and this is why rickets is seen in children.

The skull may be asymmetrical and the fontanelles (soft spots) take a long time to close. The teeth erupt late and there is a

A child suffering from rickets, which is relatively common in coloured children living in a temperate climate. The softening of the bones results in such signs as bow legs.

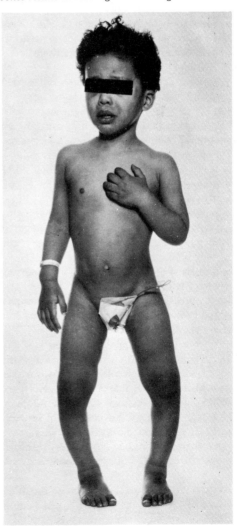

tendency for the child to develop dental caries. The chest has a row of prominences at the junction of the breast bone and the ribs. The back may be twisted or bent, there may be knock knees or bow legs and the child is weak and constipated.

Rickets is uncommon today in Britain but still occurs in crowded urban areas, especially among coloured children who don't spend much time in the sunshine. These children are especially susceptible because they are often kept indoors out of the sun, and eat a traditional diet low in vitamin D-containing foods. The sunlight is weaker than in their native countries, and the ultra-violet light is screened by polluted urban atmospheres and by glass, so that it reaches the skin only in very small amounts, and much longer exposure is therefore needed to produce significant levels of vitamin D in the skin.

Vitamin D is normally formed in the skin by the action of ultra-violet light from the sun. Even a few hours' sunlight a day on a baby's face is said to supply him with enough vitamin D. Research has shown that vitamin D produced in the skin in the summer months lasts to some extent into the winter. The vitamin is also present in some foods, for instance fish oils, herrings, kippers, tinned salmon and sardines, eggs, butter, margarine, liver and cheese, but exposure to sunlight is more important than any dietary source of the vitamin.

Bottle-fed babies get enough vitamin D from their fortified cow's milk formulae, and wholly breast-fed babies don't need vitamin D added to their diet if the mothers themselves aren't short of the vitamin.

Vitamin drops containing vitamins A, C and D, given to all children from weaning to the age of five years especially in the dark winter months and in such areas as the North of Britain, will prevent rickets from developing. However, if your child gets plenty of sunlight and eats a well-balanced diet he doesn't need extra vitamin D, and, indeed, excessively high doses of vitamin D can cause damage.

Ringworm A fungal infection of the outer layers of the skin, hair or nails which most often affects the scalp, feet and groins.

Ringworm of the feet is known as ATHLETE's FOOT.

Ringworm is highly contagious and can be transferred via infected animals (cows, cats, dogs and various other small mammals) by infected objects such as combs and scissors (scalp ringworm) or by the floors of swimming baths (athlete's foot). The fungi live deep in the horny parts of the skin and nail and so are very difficult to eradicate by local treatment. Fortunately, a drug, griseofulvin, when taken internally, can kill ringworm.

Body ringworm produces circular rashes which spread by enlarging at the edges as the centres heal. Treatment with anti-fungal ointment is useful.

Ringworm of the scalp causes round or oval bald patches. The centre heals (as on the body) but the patch is covered with stumps of broken-off hairs. Griseofulvin cures the condition in about three weeks as the infected layers of skin are shed. During this stage the child should stay away from school because the shed skin cells, brushes, combs, towels and so on are infectious. Other members of the family can pick up the infection, so great care must be taken to wash all the child's belongings well.

See BALDNESS

Roseola A mild disease occurring in children between six months and two years of age, also called sixth disease or exanthem subitum. There is an incubation period of nine to ten days. Children with roseola are well until they have a sudden fever which may rise to 103–105°F (39·4–40·5°C) and which lasts for three to five days. Although the child usually seems well, convulsions occasionally occur. When the fever drops, a rash appears on the chest and back, spreading to the neck and limbs. The rash is made up of small, flat, pink spots which remain separate and soon disappear.

Roseola is caused by a virus infection, often in small epidemics. It may come and go unnoticed, which doesn't matter as there is no special treatment other than controlling the temperature (*see* FEVER).

Rubella *See* GERMAN MEASLES

Rupture *See* HERNIA

S

Safety Home can be a dangerous place and many thousands of children a year are injured or even killed in or around their homes. As parents we have to strike a balance between being overprotective and being careful. The following checklists will help you prevent unnecessary injury or suffering around your own house.

In general, buy only furniture and equipment that conforms to a recognized standard of safety. Safety at home means always keeping one step ahead of your adventurous child.

Never leave saucepan handles sticking out like this for a child to pull down, and don't leave things cooking unattended when there are children in the kitchen.

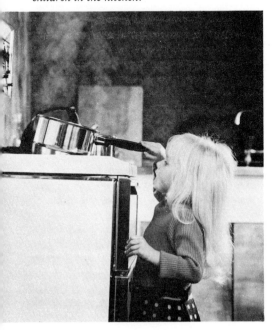

In the car
Always secure your carry-cot with properly anchored straps.

Always use a car seat of an approved design, properly bolted to the car.

Never leave things lying on the back shelf that might fall on to a child in a carry cot.

Never leave a child in a closed car in the summer – it can easily get very hot.

Never leave freshly dry-cleaned clothes in a closed car with a child – the cleaning fluid continues to evaporate from the clothes and the vapour could poison the child.

Make sure that children don't travel in the front of the car unless they are old enough to wear an adult seat belt safely.

Use specially made child seat belts for the back seats.

If your car has child locks on the back doors, ensure that they are always in the locked position.

Always lock your car so that children can't get in and release the handbrake.

Check that a child isn't hidden behind your car when reversing.

On the road
Teach your children to respect roads from an early age.

Teach your child the Green Cross Code, when he is old enough to understand it, and help him to adhere to it.

Show your child how to use the various types of pedestrian crossings and help him understand traffic lights.

If he has a bicycle, ensure that it is kept in a safe condition and that the brakes are checked regularly.

In the kitchen
Be careful what you keep in cupboards within easy reach of children.

Turn handles of saucepans sideways, away from the edges of work surfaces or the stove.

Keep poisons, cleaning fluids and disinfectants high up and preferably locked up.

Don't prise open cans with your fingers.

Never leave fat heating in a pan on the cooker unattended.

Wipe up spills at once.

Avoid highly polished floors.

Keep sharp things in drawers.

Make sure plugs and wiring on domestic appliances are safe.

Don't overload sockets.

Don't leave teapots or any containers of hot fluid near the edge of a table – they can easily be pulled off.

Sweep up broken glass or china at once.

Have a fire extinguisher or fire blanket handy and learn how to use it.

Never put water on a fat fire – put a lid on the pan or cover with a fire blanket.

Keep matches out of reach.

Teach children to respect kitchen machinery.

Have a first aid kit handy.

Never leave children alone in the kitchen when things are cooking.

Never leave a flex overhanging from an electric kettle.

In the bathroom

Keep all drugs and medicines well out of children's reach, preferably in a cupboard that locks.

Flush all old medicines and those without labels down the lavatory.

Have your gas water heater serviced annually.

Never block ventilation holes.

Never leave children alone in the bath.

Use a non-slip mat in the bath.

Put in cold water first when filling the bath.

Don't use portable, mains-operated electric appliances in the bathroom.

Place an electric heater high up on the wall or ceiling, but not over the bath.

Have a pull cord for the light switch.

Have a razor socket only – no other power outlets.

Keep razors well out of children's reach.

Have non-slip flooring.

Have a bathroom mat with non-slip backing.

In the shed, garage and workshop

Make sure that your garden gate has a safe fastening.

Use ramps for cars, not piles of bricks.

Keep garden tools hanging safely on walls.

Keep weedkiller and other chemicals high up and out of reach. *Never* use domestic containers (e.g. lemonade bottles) for weedkiller.

Check your child's bike for safety at least twice a year.

Keep a child at a safe distance when sanding, grinding or spraying. In one third of do-it-yourself accidents, it is the watching child who is hurt.

Keep petrol in metal cans only (plastic degenerates and leaks). No more than four gallons may be stored at home.

Never run an engine in a closed garage.

In gardens

Make sure ladders have a firm footing.

Don't be over-protective to older children.

Supervise small children on swings all the time.

Keep ponds fenced or covered if you have young children.

Keep water butts safely covered.

Keep the pram covered with a cat net if you leave your baby in it in the garden.

Teach children to recognize poisonous trees and shrubs.

Teach children to respect swimming pools.

Put out fires before going to bed.

Never throw inflammable liquids or aerosol cans on to fires.

Never leave a lawn mower unattended when the engine is running or when an electric mower is still 'plugged in'.

Don't leave garden tools lying around.

Keep septic tanks properly covered.

Check deckchairs and garden furniture for safety after the winter.

In the living room

Keep fires guarded. It is illegal to leave a child under 12 in a room with an unguarded fire.

Keep pins, needles and scissors away from young children.

Make sure bookshelves can't be pulled over.

Put electric flexes where people won't trip over them, but don't put them under carpets.

Replace flexes immediately if they are at all chafed or worn.

Unplug the television when going to bed or leaving the house.

Never take the back off the television or obstruct the ventilation slots.

Keep all plastic bags away from children. This includes the inner linings of record sleeves.

Never leave windows open without a safety catch where a child plays.

Never put mirrors over the mantelpiece: clothes could catch fire while looking in the mirror.

Don't leave small objects lying around with small children about – they'll swallow them or put them in their ears or noses.

Beware of catching fingers under sash windows and in doors.

Examine toys regularly to see that no loose buttons, eyes etc. are likely to come off and be swallowed and that there are no sharp edges that could cut the child.

In bedrooms, hall, stairs and passages
Never move an oil heater when it is alight. Position it where it cannot be knocked over.

Fit safety catches to all windows above ground level.

Electric convection heaters are safest for children's bedrooms. When using paraffin heaters ensure that there is adequate ventilation.

Close medicine containers and return to medicine cupboard at once after use.

Don't smoke in bed.

Disconnect an electric underblanket before going to bed.

Return electric blankets to the manufacturer for regular servicing.

Never use electric blankets for children who wet the bed.

Check that your cot bars are close enough together so that your baby can't trap his head between them.

Loose mats should have non-slip backing strips.

Use safety gates on the stairs with very young children about.

Make sure the stairs are well lit.

Fix stair carpet securely.

Don't store rubbish or anything inflammable under the stairs.

Never leave things lying on the stairs.

Never meddle with gas or electricity installations. Call in an expert.

Repair holes and worn patches in carpets so feet don't catch.

Scabies Scabies or 'the itch' is an infectious skin disease caused by the mite Sarcoptes scabiei. The mite is transferred from person to person by close skin contact or indirectly from infected clothing or bedding. It can live up to a week away from the human body.

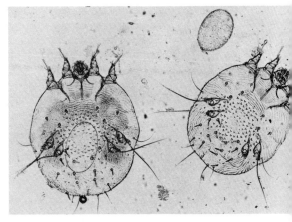

The scabies mite, Sarcoptes scabiei.

The female mite burrows into the skin – usually between the fingers, on the palms, in front of the wrists and elbows, in the armpits or round the waist – and lays her eggs over a period of a month. The eggs hatch into larvae which either make new burrows or go back to the skin surface and down hair follicles.

The skin invasion causes intense itching, especially at night, with consequent scratching. The rash is made up of little blisters where the mites entered the skin, fine, zig-zag, discoloured lines representing the burrows beneath the skin, and pimples – the inflamed follicles containing the larvae.

Some people have an allergic reaction with URTICARIA, while others have a secondary bacterial infection of the skin.

The rash usually spares the face, though a breast-feeding mother may transfer the infection to her baby's face if the skin around her nipples is infected.

The diagnosis can be difficult to make as the mite itself is only just visible to the naked eye as a white speck, and the characteristic burrows may be distorted by scratching. If there is any suspicion of scabies, mites and eggs are looked for by a doctor in scrapings or needlings from the rash, either under a microscope or with a hand lens.

Treatment is a thorough scrubbing in a long, hot bath followed by the application of benzyl benzoate or other recommended solutions all over the body (avoiding the eyes).

When this is dry, a second application is made. The next day, two more applications are put on, and on the third day another long, hot bath is taken. After this course of treatment all clothing and sheets should be washed.

The whole family must be treated at the same time in case the disease has spread and the person who infected your child should also be treated.

Canine scabies may be transferred to humans. Treatment of both child and dog is as above.

Scar If an injury to the skin involves more than the superficial layer, a scar results. If the severed edges of the skin are widely separated or if the wound is very deep, the scar may be wide and unsightly because of the large amount of fibrous tissue formed to bridge the gap. In order to minimize scarring, the edges of the skin should be brought close together during the healing process, either with stitches or sticking plasters. Scar tissue is connective tissue but lacks the elastic nature of normal skin and tends to remain pale in colour for a long time.

Over a period of six months or so a scar fades, though in some people (especially negroes) the scar becomes raised, red and hard (a keloid scar). Scars are hairless but scalp wounds are quickly covered by the growth of surrounding hair and eyebrows can be pencilled in if necessary.

Keloid scarring at the site of an operation – a phenomenon especially common in negro skin.

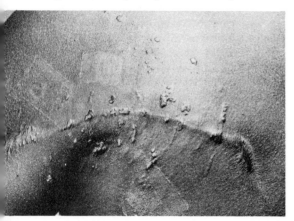

Whenever possible, surgical incisions are made along the natural lines of the skin, so giving the best chances of minimal scarring.

If a scar lies across a joint, contraction of the tissues may impair movement of that joint. Such a contracture can be relieved by plastic surgery, which can occasionally improve the appearance of unsightly scar tissue elsewhere. Keloid scarring is unfortunately very difficult to reduce, as surgery is usually followed by more keloid formation.

Scarlet fever A relatively mild disease caused by infection with β-haemolytic streptococci spread by droplets from infected people. Many strains of streptococci produce

The distribution of the scarlet fever rash (in its early stages).

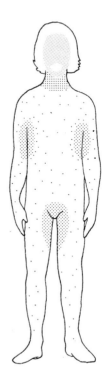

only a sore throat. Scarlet fever (a rash and a sore throat) is produced by strains making specific toxins that are carried round the body in the bloodstream to create the characteristic signs and symptoms and which stimulate the body to make antibodies. Later re-infection with the same strain of streptococcus is counteracted by these antitoxins.

The incubation period is between two and five days, then there is a sudden onset of fever, headache, swollen lymph nodes in the neck, loss of appetite and vomiting. Although the throat is sore and TONSILLITIS develops, the child often does not complain of a sore throat. He may however have a tummy ache and this is usually due to mesenteric adenitis (inflammation of lymph nodes around the bowel). The rash appears the next day and consists of slightly raised red spots on a flushed skin, beginning on the neck, armpits and groins and spreading to the rest of the body. From a distance the child simply looks red, hence the name scarlet fever. The skin around the mouth is not affected and looks pale. After a week, the skin flakes over the spots and especially on the fingertips and in the skin creases. The tongue, previously furred with red projections like a white strawberry, becomes red and shiny, like a red strawberry.

Rare complications are RHEUMATIC FEVER and acute NEPHRITIS. Inflammation of the middle ear is more common.

Treatment is with a course of antibiotics which have revolutionized the outcome of an attack of scarlet fever. When the child looks and feels better, he can go back to school.

School phobia *See* TRUANCY

Scurvy A disease caused by a deficiency in vitamin C intake, most often seen in Britain in babies from six months to two years old. It is rarely seen in its classical form today though many experts believe that we in the West are chronically short of vitamin C.

Vitamin C is necessary for proper bone formation. Its lack causes tenderness and

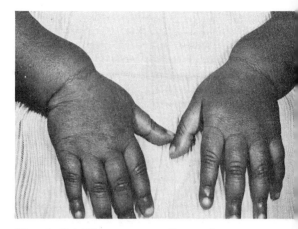

Vitamin C deficiency causes swollen, tender joints, as in the wrists and fingers of this child.

painful swellings in the bones, with bleeding beneath the membrane that covers them (the periosteum). It can also cause swollen, painful joints; loosening of the teeth; swollen, bluish gums; delay in the healing of cuts and other wounds; bruising of the skin and mucous membranes; fever; lack of energy and slowing of the child's growth, both because of poor appetite and because of the delay in the growth of the long bones.

A baby with scurvy cries on moving or being picked up because of pain in his joints and bones. This is especially likely when his nappy is changed. He tends to look apprehensive and he may begin to cry when an adult approaches for fear of this pain. To minimize the pain caused by movement, he lies in a frog position, with his thighs splayed open, and so still that he may seem paralysed.

The diagnosis is made from this history, from a medical examination, and the finding that his diet has been deficient in vitamin C. Bone X-rays show characteristic changes that can be recognized in the earlier stages before any symptoms have appeared. Laboratory tests are available but seldom needed.

The final proof is the disappearance of the pain within two days of giving vitamin C.

Prevention of scurvy is easy – make sure that your baby takes enough vitamin C. The breast-feeding mother should eat plenty of vitamin C-containing foods to ensure that her milk contains enough.

Bottle-fed babies should be given vitamin C supplements because not enough of the vitamin is present even in modified cows' milk. Vitamin C can be given in vitamin drops (available at the clinic), as non-sweetened orange juice or tomato juice. Rose hip syrup and sweetened orange juice are rich in vitamin C but can cause tooth decay. Remember not to boil vitamin C-containing drinks, or to add boiling water to them, as heat destroys the vitamin. Older children can get enough vitamin C from their diet but if they don't like vitamin C-containing drinks or foods, you can give it in the form of vitamin drops. You can also give it by crushing a 50mg tablet and adding it to the child's drink once a day.

Seborrhoeic dermatitis *See* CRADLE CAP; DERMATITIS

Sex education Learning about sex is part of a child's general education and shouldn't be separated into a neat little box only to be brought out when the child is 'ready'.

The wise parent answers his child's questions as they arise, in the same way that he answers questions on any other subject. There is no need to give a lecture on sexual intercourse when a child asks where babies come from. Simply say that a baby grows in his mummy's tummy. If he is not satisfied but wants to know more, explain further. For instance, that the baby gets there because daddy puts a seed into mummy's tummy; or that the baby gets out between mummy's legs through a special hole. As he grows older, he will ask more specific questions and you can give correspondingly more detailed answers.

Your child may ask the same questions over and over again; he may ask them in front of almost complete strangers; and he may even ask whether he can have a baby. Have the patience to talk to him sensibly and without embarrassment, as the way you answer will reflect your views on the subject and will inevitably colour his own attitudes.

The child who grows up in a family whose members are openly loving and physically demonstrative to each other is lucky. Unfortunately, many children learn their sexual attitudes in families which are rather embarrassed about sex. These are the children who may have trouble later in adjusting sexually and emotionally to a partner.

Sex education in school should ideally only complement what has been taught over the childhood years at home. That it's essential is in no doubt, as some children are taught practically nothing by their parents and the knowledge they pick up from other children is likely to be incomplete and sometimes wrong.

Contraception and morality are subjects that must be discussed, and if you feel that you are unable to present a rounded view, then it may be best left to the school. Whatever your views, remember that your child may not necessarily agree with you, though what you say will have an important bearing on his attitudes. In order to protect your child from the possibility of becoming an unmarried mother or father before she or he is ready to face up to the problems of bringing a child up alone, you must make sure that the topic of contraception is well and truly aired.

A special danger today is that a child will be taught all about sex but nothing about the emotional commitment that goes with it. Both boys and girls should be taught how important it is to bear the other person's feelings in mind during any relationship.

Finally, it's wise to warn your child against going for walks with strangers, though there's no need to frighten him unduly. Subjects such as homosexuality may crop up in your discussions with the older child, so be prepared to talk about them.

Sexual feelings colour much of our lives. If you make sure that your child develops a well-balanced, positive attitude to sex early on, you will help him enjoy life to the full.
See PUBERTY

Shock A serious condition which threatens life because the circulation of the blood to the tissues is so bad. Many people confuse it with grief or surprise. In the medical sense it means something much more specific. Emotional shock can make a child feel faint or even actually faint but this is not like true shock which can be brought on by many different things. Severe loss of blood is the commonest cause of true shock; loss of body fluid from

BURNS or from severe diarrhoea and vomiting; serious internal loss of blood, electric shock, severe infections (a burst appendix for example), and even allergies can all cause true shock.

Although there are so many causes of shock the most obvious is that in which there is such a severe blood loss that the body cannot sustain normal life. Damage to a large artery or vein can cause the loss of very large volumes of blood. A fractured bone can cause a very large bleed, yet there may be no visible blood at all if all the bleeding has taken place inside the tissues. A fractured shoulder can cause a loss of one to two pints of blood, while a fractured thigh can lose two or three pints in an adult.

A failure of the heart to pump blood around the body can also cause shock and it's this type that is produced when an adult has a heart attack. Heart failure is a rare cause of shock in children. Overdoses of certain drugs, especially barbiturates, and certain bacterial infections can also cause the heart to function poorly and so produce shock.

A severely burned child will be in a state of shock because of the loss of plasma from the blood, which reduces the blood volume and means that the tissues become starved of blood. Fluid escapes from the burnt area for up to five days, so fluid replacement via a drip is most important in treating severe burns.

When a person becomes shocked, his body tries to maintain its vital functions. Blood is diverted from the less vital organs (such as the intestines) to the brain. The blood vessels in the skin contract so as to allow blood to be used more valuably elsewhere and it's because of this that a person in shock looks so pale.

Except in the case of very severe haemorrhage, shock takes time to appear. This gives parents or first aiders plenty of time to call for help. Don't leave things so long that the victim becomes seriously ill. Most shocked people show the following obvious features. Their skin is pale or grey and the lips and nose tip are blue. The victim is often in a cold sweat and feels cold and clammy to the touch. The pulse is rapid and weak and may be very difficult to feel. The breathing is shallow and fast but in really serious cases may be gasping and deep – this is known as air hunger. The victim thinks and reacts slowly and may be

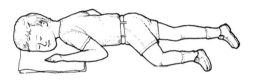

The recovery position.

irrational. He may, of course, be unconscious, as eventually the blood supply to the brain becomes very poor.

If ever your child is like this, for whatever reason, get an ambulance at once and lie him down in the recovery position. Loosen tight clothing; stop obvious bleeding by pressing over the bleeding point; restart his breathing and heart beats if these have stopped (*see* KISS OF LIFE; HEART MASSAGE); keep him warm but not hot; and keep him calm until professional help comes.

Lastly, never give anyone you suspect is shocked any form of liquid. If you do, he may inhale the fluid if he vomits (and shocked people do vomit).

Short sight   *See* VISUAL PROBLEMS

Sickle cell anaemia   *See* ANAEMIA

Sickness   *See* VOMITING

Sinusitis   Air-filled spaces in the facial bones lined with mucous membranes are called sinuses. They are all connected with the inside of the nose and are liable to become infected. They are still developing in children. Obviously a child cannot get inflammation in a sinus that hasn't developed.

The cold virus affects the mucous membranes lining the sinuses. A watery discharge is produced which drains into the nose and trickles down the back of the nose to the throat forming part of the post-nasal drip. This tickles the back of the throat and is a common cause of a cough.

Usually the sinuses return to normal after a cold but occasionally one or more sinuses can become acutely infected by bacteria. The symptoms produced by this secondary infection depend upon which sinuses are involved.

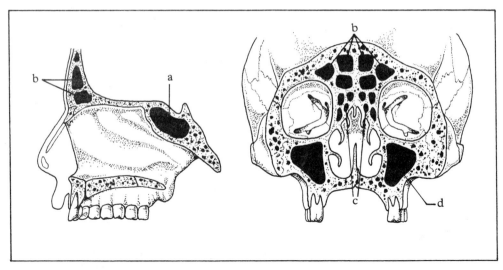

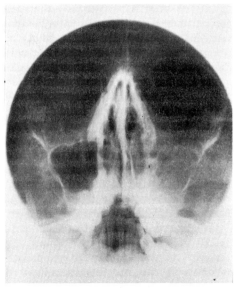

The paranasal sinuses. These develop gradually during childhood – the frontal sinuses are not completely developed until the age of 10 years. a. sphenoidal, b. frontal, c. ethmoidal, d. maxillary.

pain in the face and a fever. The roots of the teeth, if infected, can also cause this sort of sinusitis, as can a foreign body in the nose, blocking the drainage of the sinus.

The frontal sinuses in the forehead are not well developed until the age of ten. Symptoms of acute frontal sinusitis include pain, tenderness and swelling above the eye.

Treatment of acute sinusitis is with antibiotics, painkillers if necessary and decongestants (either as nose-drops, inhalations or medicine). Sometimes, if there is no improvement, a drainage operation is necessary.

See MASTOIDITIS

X-ray showing infection in the child's left maxillary sinus.

Under two years of age, the ethmoids in the bridge of the nose are the only sinuses large enough to become infected. Acute ethmoiditis is rare but serious. It causes a high temperature with pain and swelling around the eye. Infection can spread to the brain and to the eye itself if there is no treatment.

The maxillary sinuses in the cheekbones are usually well developed by the age of four years. Symptoms of acute maxillary sinusitis are

Skin The external covering of the body. The skin consists of two layers, the outer, thicker one called the epidermis and the inner one, the dermis. On the soles of the feet and the palms of the hands the epidermis is thickened and horny and this is essential because, with so much friction, cells are constantly being rubbed off and having to be replaced. The skin grows from below upwards, the lower layers regenerating and replacing the epidermal layer as it gets shed. The dermis is composed of connective tissue and is rich in blood vessels.

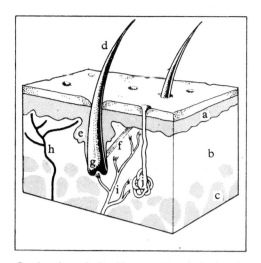

Section through the skin. a. epidermis, b. dermis, c. subcutaneous fat, d. hair shaft, e. sebaceous gland, f. erector muscle, g. hair follicle, h. nerve, i. blood vessel, j. sweat gland.

Hairs are found everywhere except on the palms and soles and parts of the external genitals. They vary considerably in length, being shortest on the eyelids (where they don't project above the skin surface) and longest on the scalp. Each hair consists of a root and a shaft. The root is embedded in a hair follicle (a sort of deep dip in the epidermis) into which one or more sebaceous glands empty their secretions. Sebaceous glands keep the skin 'oiled' and soft.

Sweat glands are of two types. Eccrine glands are very numerous (there are probably about two million all over the body) and are found everywhere except for the lips, ear canals and nails. They produce a thin, watery sweat. Apocrine glands are very much larger, fewer in number, and are localized to the armpits, pubic, genital and anal areas, and to a lesser extent around the navel and breasts. These glands produce thicker sweat which is responsible for sweat odours. The WAX glands in the ear canals are modified apocrine glands.

The skin performs many functions but basically it is a barrier that protects us from the outside world. The skin surface is covered with bacteria that are harmless to us and in fact positively help us by keeping down infections with other potentially harmful bac-teria (rather as ground cover plants keep down weeds in a flower bed). The skin acts as a filter for certain harmful rays of the sun and makes vitamin D in large amounts when exposed to ultra-violet light (*see* RICKETS).

The skin also bears many nerve endings specialised to sense heat, cold, pain and touch. This keeps us 'in touch' with our environment because our skin feeds information into our brain all the time about what's going on around us. But one of the skin's most vital functions is to control temperature. When it is warm around us the tiny blood vessels of the skin expand, bringing more blood to the surface and allowing heat to be lost to the air. Sweat glands become more active and the sweat cools the body as it evaporates. When it is cold, the blood vessels contract and conserve heat.

Because skin covers our bodies, many different things can happen to it which give us clues to underlying problems. It can become reddened, blue, pigmented, swollen, puffy, discoloured, hot, cold, dry or wet, pale, or covered by a rash. The skin to a great extent mirrors what is happening in the body and can be a great help when a doctor is making his diagnosis.

See ITCHING; JAUNDICE; MILIA; RASH; SUN-BURN

Sleep Sleep in the rural societies of most non-western countries is very straightforward. A child sleeps when he is tired, for as long as he needs, wherever he is most comfortable – usually near the rest of the family.

Most of us spend one third of our lives asleep and babies and young children spend even longer sleeping. While we sleep, our brains are still very active, as EEG (electro-encephalograph) recordings can show. Although we are not usually aware of it, we dream four or five times a night for a total of nearly an hour. While we're dreaming the brain produces unusual electrical signals, and the body undergoes certain physiological changes. We become totally relaxed and our eyeballs move about rapidly under closed eyelids. Because of this particular body activity, this type of sleep is called Rapid Eye Movement (REM) sleep. Babies spend a much greater proportion of their sleep in REM sleep than do adults, and the proportion slowly becomes less as they grow.

In our high-technology, western society, children are expected to sleep for certain lengths of time, to go to bed at the same time each night, to wake up at the same time each morning and to sleep alone. No wonder then that little children so often have sleep problems.

However, living in our complex society inevitably makes certain demands. Children have to get to school on time, so in order to get enough sleep, a fairly regular bed-time is advisable. Parents may have to go to work in the mornings, so they too must have enough sleep. The most important thing is that most parents – especially parents of very young children – expect to have their evenings alone, with their children in bed. If you feel that it's important to have some time alone, then you should try to encourage an early, regular bed-time for your children from early on. Remember that your children may not need as much sleep as you would like them to have, so they will either wake up early or not go to sleep for some time even when they are in bed. The older child can read in bed or in the morning but the young child will expect to be amused when he wakes early in the morning.

The amount of sleep different children need is very variable and some children, especially very bright children, need less sleep than their parents. Charts of hours of sleep a child needs at each age are based on average figures; but as they rarely give the range, they are not much use for the individual child. If your child needs very little sleep and is bright and cheerful during the day, and if you want him to go to bed early so that you can have the evening alone, you could have a problem. Books and persuasion work wonders for the older child. A regular bed-time ritual and a busy day-time schedule with plenty of fresh air and exercise may encourage the younger child to go to bed willingly.

Babies vary in their sleep requirements right from the day they are born, so don't make the mistake of judging how good a baby is from the amount of sleeping he does. A crying baby may not be hungry or uncomfortable; he may just be awake, lonely and bored with staring at the sides of a cot.

A baby will sleep anywhere, provided he is warm, sleepy and fed. In hospitals babies are sometimes wrapped securely to make them sleep better. Rural peoples in developing countries often carry their babies close to their bodies all day and the warmth, rhythmical movement, proximity to the mother's breast and sound of her voice and heartbeat make these babies very contented – much more so than the average western baby. We can take a leaf out of their book and carry our babies more to make them feel more secure. The best sort of baby sling is the one which leaves both the mother's arms free. The baby can be carried in a sling from the day he is born, and a sling allows a busy mother to get on with her shopping, housework and so on with her baby quite content.

If you are breast feeding your baby, the most convenient place to have him at night is in your own room. Some mothers have their babies in their own beds all night. The dangers of smothering or crushing the child have been greatly overstressed. There is no evidence to suggest that babies are in danger in their parents' bed unless either parent is extremely obese or likely to go to bed drunk or drugged, when it is wise not to have the baby in bed. In our society it is normal for children to sleep apart from the parents but in many other societies children and parents sleep together. Certainly far fewer children would be frightened of the dark if they slept in their parents' room. Perhaps an acceptable plan might be to have your baby in your room for the first year or two or until he has stopped having night feeds, then to move him into his own room or into his brother's or sister's room.

Don't keep the house quiet when your child is asleep – life will be easier for you if normal household noise is continued, especially during the day. Many children need a day-time nap for several years. Cutting this out in an attempt to make him sleep longer at night will probably only make him irritable during the day.

Ideally, sleep problems should be completely avoidable. If, however, your child doesn't sleep well and your own lack of sleep is making you irritable, get some help from your doctor. Children need rested parents and pacing up and down in the middle of the night is going to do you – and them – no good.

See BABY CARE; ENURESIS; NIGHTMARES; SLEEPWALKING

Sleepwalking Some children get out of their beds at night during their sleep, walk around, and then return to their beds. The child's eyes are open but he looks at familiar people unseeingly, because he is actually asleep. The child does not walk with his arms stretched out in front of him, as is commonly pictured.

Such children are often subconsciously worried about something and may also walk in their sleep during the course of a bad dream.

Don't wake a sleepwalking child but gently lead him back to bed. There is no point in telling him the next day that he walked in his sleep as that may only worry him more. Also, if you mention it in front of brothers and sisters, he may get teased.

Sleepwalking is most common in early adolescence. Talk over any problems you are aware of with your child and try to find out whether he has any that you don't know about. You could have a word with his teacher (without the child knowing) to see if he or she can throw any light on the problem. Children of this age often worry unduly about their parents' rows, so try to make home life as loving and secure as possible.

Small children A child may be small either because he is *underweight* or because he is *short* for his age.

The *underweight* child is one who is either not eating or not absorbing enough food for his metabolic needs, remembering of course that there is a wide variation in normal weight for a healthy child of any given height. The thin child whose weight is outside the normal range may not be having enough to eat. Alternatively, he may not want to eat enough, perhaps because he is ill and has lost his appetite (this can happen with chronic kidney, chest or heart disease); or perhaps because he is rejecting food (as in the condition known as ANOREXIA NERVOSA). In other thin children, the bowels do not absorb enough of the food that the child eats because of an abnormality such as COELIAC DISEASE or CYSTIC FIBROSIS.

The baby who is not growing at a normal rate is labelled as 'failing to thrive'. There are many causes of FAILURE TO THRIVE and hospital admission may be necessary in order to make the diagnosis.

If a child is medically investigated because he is abnormally small, it may be helpful to the doctor if the parents have kept any previous measurements of their child. Causes of a recent loss in weight differ from the causes of small size at birth, though there is some overlap.

The *short* child may be so for a variety of reasons. One or both parents may be short, in which case it is likely that he has inherited their height. He may have been poorly nourished over a long period – either through not eating enough or because of a chronic bowel disease. He may have a chronic kidney, liver, heart or chest disease. His pituitary or thyroid glands may not be working properly or his skeleton may have been affected by, for example, rickets or (rarely, now) spinal tuberculosis. Many mentally retarded children are abnormally short, some because of feeding difficulties.

Dwarfism can be caused by an inherited disorder of the cartilage (achondroplasia). This condition affects the long limb bones most severely, so that the child becomes shorter in comparison with his peers as he grows older. The head is relatively large, the forehead prominent, and the bridge of the nose flattened. There is no cure for this condition.

Finally, a child may be lacking in height because of long-term treatment with certain drugs or, surprisingly, because of emotional deprivation. Investigations should be made to find out the cause when a child is short for no obvious reason.

Being short is said to affect boys emotionally more than girls, just as being extra tall is said to affect girls more. Parents of a boy who is likely to grow up into a short man should try, over the years, to help him understand that height is no index of masculinity or happiness.

See ANOREXIA; GROWTH; HEIGHT; WEIGHT

Smallpox A generalized and serious viral infection producing a characteristic skin rash.

The viruses are spread by person to person contact or by infected bedding or towels. Infection occurs when the victim inhales the virus. Smallpox is highly contagious and can occur in epidemics.

The rash first shows on the palms of the hands and the soles of the feet. The trunk is usually spared completely. It starts as red areas which become blisters and then crusts. In mild cases the rash can look like that of chickenpox but the areas of the body affected are different in chickenpox. Smallpox begins on the arms and legs while chickenpox is first noticed on the body and face.

As a result of vaccination, smallpox has now been virtually eradicated from the whole world so that routine vaccination of babies is no longer recommended. Some countries still require all visitors to produce certificates of vaccination, so if you are travelling abroad both you and your children may need to be vaccinated if you have not been vaccinated in the last three years. Any travel agent, your doctor, or the embassy of the country to which you are travelling will tell you whether a certificate is required.

Modern vaccination techniques do not leave such bad scars as used to follow smallpox vaccination. An area not usually seen, such as the inside of the thigh, can be used.

The vaccine is a living virus and some children get a fever about a week after the vaccination when there is a reaction on the skin. Lymph nodes draining the area of skin may swell and become painful. You should allow at least two weeks between vaccination and departure abroad so that any possible side-effects are over before your holiday.

It's important to tell your doctor if your child has eczema or a nappy rash at the time he's due to be vaccinated, because vaccination is potentially dangerous for children with these conditions. It's also important to tell him if anyone else in the family has eczema at the time of the vaccination, because the viruses can spread on to this person's skin too. Your doctor will also put off vaccination if your child has recently had an infectious illness, has certain other serious conditions or has had a vaccination against something else within the last three weeks.

Smoking According to the statistics, more young people and children smoke today than ever before.

Most children start to smoke out of curiosity and to go along with their peer group or because it is a 'grown-up' thing to do. Among 16-year-olds, 43 per cent of boys and 36 per cent of girls do not smoke even one cigarette a day. However, four out of five young people who smoke more than one cigarette take up the habit seriously later on.

Whilst we as parents encourage our children to find out for themselves about most things, smoking is different and too risky because nicotine is addictive. On the other hand, forbidden fruit always tastes best, so somewhere between the two extremes every parent has to find a formula that works for him and his children.

One way of putting your child off the idea is to tell him the facts. 1) Smokers never enjoy full health. 2) Smokers are never as good at games and sports as their non-smoking friends of similar sporting potential. 3) Smokers can develop a smoker's cough as soon as their early twenties. This can progress to lung damage which could damage their career and social life. 4) Smokers die younger than they should. 5) Smoking, rather than making a boy seem more 'manly' in the eyes of his girlfriends may actually put them off. Smokers smell, their clothes and breath smell, their teeth and fingers are stained by nicotine and their whole body isn't as pleasant as it could be.

For girls there are additional hazards. 1) Babies of mothers who smoke during pregnancy are on average smaller than those of non-smokers and are more likely to be premature with all the dangers associated with prematurity (see LOW BIRTH WEIGHT). 2) One or two babies out of every ten that die at birth could have been saved if their mothers hadn't smoked during pregnancy. 3) Worst of all, even seven years later, the children of mothers who smoked heavily during pregnancy are still undersized for their age and are retarded on measurable parameters for abilities such as reading.

As parents we can set a good example to our children by not smoking ourselves; by not condoning their smoking; by watching for signs of pressure on a child that might lead him to take up the habit; and by pointing out what else he could get out of life if he didn't smoke. Cigarette smoking has been proved beyond any doubt to be a killer and a wrecker of people's lives. It is up to every one of us to help our children to keep clear of such a health hazard as best we can.

If you as parents smoke, you are definitely increasing the likelihood that your child under one year old will suffer from pneumonia and bronchitis.

Snake bites *See* BITES AND STINGS

Soft spot *See* FONTANELLE

Sore throat *See* PHARYNGITIS; TONSILLITIS

Soiling The uncontrolled or untimely passage of bowel motions, which may take the form of a slight staining of the pants or actual defaecation. The young child who soils his pants may simply not yet be ready to come out of nappies into pants.

A child potty-trained at the right time and in a relaxed way may have the odd accident but should quickly become reliable. Sometimes, when a new baby is born, an older child may soil his pants – the secret here is to put him back in nappies for a while and then to start again when he has got over his need to seek attention or to be like the baby. If he doesn't become reliable, you must accept that he is not yet old enough to control his bowels. Leave him in nappies and try again in a few months. (*See* POTTY TRAINING.)

The older child, previously reliably clean, who starts soiling out of the blue, has a real problem. The most common cause of soiling in this case is CONSTIPATION. This may seem surprising, especially as the soiling is usually semi-liquid, but it is because the bowel contents leak around the hard, craggy, constipated stools in the rectum. The chronically constipated child may not be able to control his anus, and so soils his pants as a kind of 'overflow' problem. The answer is to treat the constipation.

Soiling can produce behaviour problems, because of embarrassment, but it is rarely

caused by such problems.

Mentally retarded children frequently soil because of poor bowel training and a lack of awareness but almost all can be trained to be clean. Children with spina bifida may soil because of incontinence of their bowel motions due to inadequate nervous control of their anal sphincter muscles.

See ENCOPRESIS

Spastic *See* CEREBRAL PALSY

Speech *See* LANGUAGE

Speech delay, Speech therapy *See* LANGUAGE PROBLEMS

Spina bifida A defect in one or more vertebral arches forming part of the bony wall of the spinal canal encircling the spinal cord.

Spina bifida is one of the most common serious congenital abnormalities in Britain today and every year up to three thousand babies are affected, more girls than boys. Spina bifida and ANENCEPHALY both represent defects of the neural tube (from which the brain and spinal cord develop) and show similarities in their geographical distribution.

In the most usual type of spina bifida there is a skin defect and part of the spinal cord (usually covered by a transparent membrane representing the meninges) is exposed on the newborn baby's neck. The exposed nervous tissue is called a meningomyelocele. The extent of the disorder produced depends upon the level of the spinal cord exposed, as this determines which nerves are affected. Usually the defect is in the lumbo-sacral region (the lower back).

Spina bifida may cause paralysis of the legs, incontinence of urine and bowel motions, club foot, and dislocation of the hips, depending on the level of the spinal cord affected. Nine out of ten children with spina bifida have HYDROCEPHALUS, owing to a defect of the brainstem and cerebellum. One in two is mentally retarded to some degree.

The cause of spina bifida is unknown, though many theories have been suggested. Because it tends to run in families, it is thought that a genetic factor is involved. However, for a number of reasons (one that it is so common in certain areas such as South Wales and Northern Ireland; another that in some pairs of identical twins, one has been affected with a neural tube defect, while the other has been normal), it seems likely that there is an environmental and therefore perhaps a preventable factor involved as well.

An operation is usually carried out within 48 hours of birth to close the skin defect and prevent meningitis and the production of, or worsening of paralysis. This saves the lives of many children. Unfortunately, most children with spina bifida have severe problems all their lives and many need permanent care. A variety of treatments is available, including operations to divert the flow of urine into the bowel or on to the abdominal skin surface, and orthopaedic operations to correct hip and foot deformities. An organized plan of management by a team of various medical experts is conducive to optimal treatment.

A mother who has had a child with spina bifida or anencephaly has an increased risk of a subsequent baby being affected by either disorder. GENETIC COUNSELLING is available for families considering another baby. Tests have recently been perfected which enable the serum or amniotic fluid of a pregnant woman to be tested early in the pregnancy for the level of alpha-fetoprotein present. In this way, spina bifida and anencephaly can be detected and the parents may decide to ask for an abortion if the foetus is known to be affected. An ultrasound scan early in pregnancy can detect anencephaly. (*See* AMNIOCENTESIS.)

Spinal cord   *See* CENTRAL NERVOUS SYSTEM

Spleen   A large organ that lies in the left upper part of the abdomen between the stomach and the diaphragm. The spleen is spongy, filled with blood and can contract to squeeze blood out into the circulation when necessary. It performs four functions yet is not essential to life – many people have their spleens removed and live healthy lives. In early foetal life the spleen actually makes blood but blood is only produced by the spleen in children with certain diseases. The spleen is the main centre for disposal of old red blood cells.

It also acts as a reservoir of blood for severe emergencies such as haemorrhage, though people without spleens seem to cope well enough in these emergencies so it seems to be simply an additional back-up system. Lastly, the spleen produces antibodies and white blood cells to fight infection. In fact, in acute infections the spleen can enlarge to produce more of these protective cells.

Sometimes the spleen has to be removed surgically. Most usually this is done because it has been ruptured in a car accident or by another traumatic event. Some rare blood diseases can be cured by removing the spleen.

Sprain   The joints of the body are held together by tough, fibrous bands called ligaments. A sprain involves the tearing of these, with local bleeding.

Sprains are common injuries especially among older children playing violent games. The main feature of a sprain is acute pain. There is usually also swelling around the joint and an unwillingness to move the affected joint.

It may be difficult to decide whether a child has a sprain or a fracture and an X-ray may be necessary. There is no way of distinguishing the two for certain without an X-ray, so if you find that your child is getting worse rather than better, take him to your local hospital casualty department.

The treatment of sprains is a matter of controversy. Some experts think that exercise helps prevent the joint from stiffening and others think rest helps it heal. In children the answer usually suggests itself.

In the period immediately following a sprain, the best thing to do is to rest the affected part, support it and bandage it firmly with an elastic bandage or adhesive strapping. Be careful not to put these on too firmly – any sign of whiteness or blueness in the limb beyond the strapping means you've done it too tightly. If this or any 'pins and needles' occur, undo the strapping and reapply it less tightly. Never use elastic bandages around joints directly without first applying a thick layer of cotton wool or similar material because the tight bandage could damage a superficial nerve.

Painkilling drugs may be necessary and surface-acting rubs can give temporary relief as can local heat, cold, or infra-red lamp treatment. Real relief comes only as the blood that has seeped out of blood vessels when the ligament was torn is absorbed and the ligament itself heals. This can take a surprisingly long time – a sprained ankle for example can take weeks (and, rarely, even months) to heal.

Squint (strabismus) A condition in which the eyes are not directed together to the object the child is looking at. If a child over three months old squints for much of the time, he probably has an imbalance of the muscles that move the eyeball. This is more likely if either parent squinted in childhood. In a younger baby normal eyes do not always move together.

It is important to take a squint seriously as a child with a persistent squint may in time lose the sight of one eye. This is because the brain cannot cope in the long term with double vision (the two images produced when the eyes are not working together) and so suppresses one image, eventually permanently. The child with an 'alternating' squint – one in which both eyes squint from time to time – is less likely to lose the vision of one eye but should still be examined by an ophthalmologist or ophthalmic surgeon.

Treatment varies from simply covering the good eye, so encouraging the squinting eye to work properly and thus exercising and strengthening the eye muscles, to surgical operations to reduce or increase the length of the muscles. Visual defects may also have to be corrected. Sometimes several operations are necessary before a satisfactory result is obtained.

A squint may arise because of poor vision – short sight, long sight, or astigmatism – that is inadequately treated. Measles, meningitis, and other diseases can also cause a squint.

Wise parents take their children for routine development checks by their clinic or family doctor. Tests include looking for squints and testing the eyesight in both eyes. If there is the slightest suspicion on the part of the parents or the doctor, a specialist opinion should be sought. Young babies frequently appear to be squinting because of the wide folds of skin over the inner corners of the eyes but a specialist

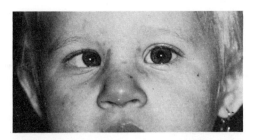

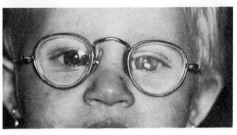

A right convergent squint, top, *and* above, *the squint controlled by spectacles which also correct the child's hypermetropia (long sight).*

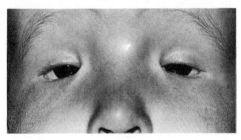

A slight squint in a young child. The exaggerating effect on the squint of the wide folds of skin over the corners of the eyes can be clearly seen.

can eliminate the possibility of a squint in such cases.

See EYES; VISION TESTING; VISUAL PROBLEMS

Stammer Interrupted or hesitant speech. With a stutter, sounds are repeated before the word or phase is eventually spoken properly.

Stammering and stuttering can be normal as speech develops in young children and they are most common between two and a half and six years. Stammering usually occurs because the child's mind is running ahead of his ability to get the words out. This type of stammering needn't cause concern because 99 per cent of children grow out of it. The best thing to do is not to mention the child's stammer to him and certainly not to discipline him to make him speak properly. Give him plenty of time to speak and never laugh or show signs of impatience as he struggles to get his words out. If you are concerned about your child's stammer, see your doctor or speech therapist for advice on what to do. Some experts believe that excessive parental discipline and fussing over early transient stammering are the causes of more permanent stammering. Unfortunately, this early stammering, if mishandled, can go on to become a more serious affair with the child only too conscious of his speech problem and his poor efforts to correct it. A stammering child may contort his face and tongue and his whole body may even become twisted and contorted as he tries to get the words out.

Stammering seems to run in families – no one knows why but it may be because the affected families are more conscious than most of the defect and tend to worry about it more, however subconsciously. Why stammering occurs, nobody knows for sure. Some psychiatrists think that stammering is a sign of disturbed parent-child relationships but this is difficult to prove in all but the most obvious cases. One study showed that the parents of stammering children were much more strict with them and demanded higher standards than did those of a control group of families. But such evidence should be interpreted with caution because, as we've seen, stammering is so often a perpetuation of a transient fault in otherwise normal speech development.

See LANGUAGE PROBLEMS

Starvation Today in the West no child need starve, but the world problem of starvation and its damage to health and life remains because of insufficient available food. The tendency in the West is to overeat greatly and to eat too much meat at great cost in animal feed grain. It has been calculated that if every American cut out one meat meal a week it would release enough grain to feed 60 million people!

Older girls (usually in their teens) may starve with a condition known as ANOREXIA NERVOSA.

Many parents worry if their children don't eat for some reason and believe that they might even starve. The worry is unfounded if the child continues to grow in height and weight. A child can go off his food for many days with an infection, or the taking of antibiotics and certain other drugs. Children are remarkably hardy and can go without much to eat for some time. During these times, however, a child's intake of fluid must be kept up and this provides an opportunity to give him some nourishment.

Very young children and babies need more careful handling. If your baby or young child goes off his food completely, even for a short time, get medical advice.

See ANOREXIA; DEHYDRATION

Sticky eye A type of CONJUNCTIVITIS that may occur soon after birth. The baby has a yellow discharge from one or both eyes which may make the eyelids stick together. A sticky eye is usually caused by blood or amniotic fluid getting into the eye during or immediately after birth. A swab should be taken from the eye and sent for bacterial culture but as the discharge is usually not infected, regular wiping of the closed eye with saline solution on cotton wool usually clears it up. In case the discharge is infected, it's sensible to wipe the eye from the inside outwards so as to avoid the transfer of infection to the other eye, and to lie the baby with the affected eye nearest the mattress so that infected fluid doesn't flow across the bridge of the nose and infect the other eye.

Sticky eyes caused by infection usually occur after the first two or three days of life and are treated with an antibiotic eye ointment. If the infection is due to GONORRHOEA contracted from an infected birth canal, treatment is with penicillin medicine as well as local antibiotics.

If the infection doesn't clear up, or if it recurs, this may be due to a blocked TEAR DUCT.

Stillbirth The birth of a dead foetus after the age of 28 weeks. Until recent years the stillbirth rate in the UK was comparatively low but today it compares rather badly with many other western countries. The commonest of many causes of stillbirth are toxaemia of pregnancy, too early a separation of the placenta, and abnormalities of the foetus itself such as SPINA BIFIDA and ANENCEPHALY, which are relatively more common in Britain than in many other countries. Caesarean section and induction of labour save many babies who would otherwise have died, but these methods of delivery can produce their own problems if the baby is premature. (*See* RESPIRATORY DISTRESS SYNDROME.)

Meticulous antenatal care for all women, improved social conditions and nutrition, less smoking and continued research will play an important part in reducing the stillbirth rate further.

The parents of a stillborn baby need a lot of sympathetic support as they grieve for their unknown child. Some need to see the baby and most say that they need to discuss their feelings instead of putting on a brave face and suffering in silence. Having a photograph of the baby and knowing where the grave is may help the parents in their mourning.

See PERINATAL MORTALITY

Stomach A J-shaped muscular tube in the uppermost part of the abdominal cavity into which food goes after it is eaten. The gullet (oesophagus) opens into the top end and the food leaves via the other opening – the pylorus. These two openings are normally kept firmly closed to ensure that food doesn't come back into the mouth or go onwards into the intestine until it has been properly digested.

The stomach is about the size of a fist but is capable of enormous distension. It stores food for up to four hours as digestive juices produced in its walls get to work.

PYLORIC STENOSIS, a narrowing of the pylorus, is caused by a thickening of the muscles surrounding the outlet from the stomach.

Young children sometimes swallow beads, pins or other dangerous objects. An object which becomes lodged in the oesophagus on its way to the stomach is especially dangerous because it can perforate the wall. Once a foreign body reaches the stomach safely, nine out of ten times it will pass safely onwards and emerge the other end. There are sophisticated instruments that can be passed into the stomach down the oesophagus to remove these foreign bodies if necessary.

VOMITING is a sign that the stomach is rejecting its contents for one reason or another. In children vomiting may be caused by things that are not strictly to do with the stomach.

A baby may be born with a hiatus hernia – a knuckle of the stomach displaced into the chest. Gastric ulcers, while uncommon in childhood, may occur.

See GASTROENTERITIS; REGURGITATION

Stork's beak mark, Strawberry naevus
See BIRTHMARK

Stings *See* BITES AND STINGS

Stutter *See* STAMMER

Stye (hordeolum) An inflammation of the eyelid, often caused by a staphylococcal infection in one of the sebaceous glands along its edge.

Styes rarely occur in normal, healthy children but are fairly common in ill or weak children. Some children get them in repeated crops for several months for no known reason.

Should your child get a stye, apply a hot, wet pad of cotton wool or lint to the eye. This increases the blood supply which soothes the pain and helps get rid of the infection. You could also pluck out the eyelash at the centre of the stye with a pair of fine tweezers as this sometimes releases the pus. Most styes respond to this sort of treatment within a few days.

Occasionally, repeated styes are caused by dandruff and will clear up with treatment of this seborrhoeic scalp condition. Because styes

A stye.

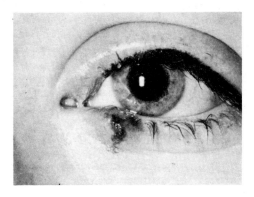

are infectious, try to keep the child's face flannel to himself and make sure he uses only his own towel. Styes are not highly infectious but these are reasonable precautions to take, especially if there are babies in the house.

See BLEPHARITIS; DERMATITIS

Suffocation *See* ASPHYXIA

Sugar intolerance A sugar is simply a sweet carbohydrate and there are several kinds of sugar apart from sucrose, the one we use as table sugar. Simple sugars (monosaccharides) include glucose (the sugar found in blood), fructose and galactose. Disaccharides include sucrose (a combination of fructose and glucose), maltose (made up of two glucose units), and lactose (a combination of glucose and galactose).

Sugar intolerance occurs as the result of a deficiency in one or other of the digestive enzymes which normally break down the disaccharides into single unit sugars in the gut. Lactase, the enzyme which breaks down lactose, is rarely deficient from birth. More usually, lactase deficiency arises during adolescence, especially in black and oriental people, when it causes abdominal pain, abdominal distension and diarrhoea within a short time of drinking MILK. A 'secondary' lactase deficiency can develop in normal children after any intestinal damage, for example after gastroenteritis. The motions may be watery or fatty; there is cramp-like abdominal pain, abdominal distension, nausea and noisy tummy rumbling. Secondary lactase deficiency can last from a few days to several weeks; if it lasts for several weeks there is also likely to be intolerance to other sugars.

A deficiency of the enzymes sucrase and isomaltase can be present from birth (inherited via abnormal, recessive genes) and produces watery diarrhoea, possibly with abdominal distension and cramps, from a few weeks after birth if the baby is fed on a cows' milk formula containing sucrose or maltodextrin. A susceptible breast-fed baby develops symptoms when weaning is begun. Treatment is with a low sucrose diet, and dextrose has to be used for cooking.

Lastly, glucose and galactose may not be properly absorbed because of a recessively inherited defect. Watery diarrhoea develops after the baby's first feed, whether this is breast milk or cows' milk. Treatment involves severe carbohydrate restriction. Secondary glucose-galactose malabsorption can occur after infectious gastroenteritis or as a result of cows' milk protein intolerance. Intravenous feeding is necessary until the gut returns to normal.

Suicide *See* DEPRESSION

Sunburn Some exposure to the sun is useful because ultra-violet light helps the skin to make vitamin D. Too much ultra-violet light, though, can cause reddening of the skin or even blisters. Fair or red-haired children tend to burn more easily than those with a darker complexion, so it's sensible to give them adequate protection from the sun.

Because sunburn only begins to hurt several hours after exposure, parents have to be especially wary and prevent trouble from occurring. A sunburned child cannot enjoy a holiday and can spoil it for the rest of the family.

Only let a child go out in bright sun for half an hour on the first two days of your holiday unless his skin is covered. A hat will give protection as well, particularly for babies. Remember that the sun doesn't have to be very bright to cause sunburn. Sun is also reflected off water and sand (making it even more powerful), so be careful at the seaside even if you think the same amount of sun wouldn't harm your child in the garden at home.

Good quality sun lotions and creams, applied frequently, especially after swimming, help prevent burning. They don't, however, prevent HEAT STROKE. Calamine lotion helps soothe burnt skin. The itching of sunburnt skin may be due to its dryness or to an urticarial reaction.

T

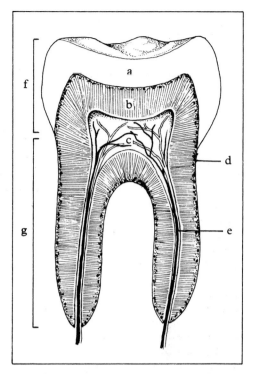

Diagrammatic cross-section through a molar tooth. a. enamel, b. dentine, c. pulp containing veins and nerves, d. cement, e. root canal, f. crown, g. root.

Tapeworm   *See* WORMS

Tearduct   The channel that takes tears from the eye into the nose. The surface of the eye is kept moist all the time by tears which are normally produced continuously. Small particles of dust and grit are washed down into the inner corner of the eye where they pass down the tear duct into the nose.

If the tear duct is blocked in a baby, the eye may be sticky. Most blocked ducts open on their own before the age of six months but if this doesn't happen it may have to be opened up by probing by an eye surgeon under a general anaesthetic.

See STICKY EYE

Teeth   The protruding part of a tooth is the crown and the part embedded in the jaw is the root. Teeth are composed of two main substances – enamel, the hard, outer coating, and dentine, the softer, living interior. The teeth appear in two sets – primary (milk) teeth and secondary (adult) teeth.

Babies are occasionally born with a tooth (or teeth), but most children start teething at between five and seven months. Some perfectly normal children do not have any teeth by the age of one year but they appear in time and nothing can be done to hurry them up. Girls tend to produce teeth earlier than boys and boys tend to lose milk teeth before girls.

The 20 milk teeth are all formed under the gums before birth and by the age of about two they have usually erupted. The incisors appear at about 6 to 13 months, the first molars at 12 to 15 months, the canines at 16 to 18 months and the second molars at 20 to 30 months.

The first permanent teeth to appear are usually the big back teeth (molars) at about six years old and the last to come through are the wisdom teeth (also molars). These come through at anything up to the age of 25, or may even never appear at all.

Although teeth are so hard on the outside (much harder than bone, for instance), they are vulnerable to decay because of the foods we eat.

Parents should not feel that as the milk teeth are going to be lost it doesn't matter if they decay. Badly decayed milk teeth that are lost earlier than they should be can mean that the second teeth come through in the wrong place or are crooked.

Teeth need protecting and looking after at home, and also need the expert attention of a dentist. He should not be a bogey man that a child is threatened with when he's naughty but should be treated as a friend and ally in the fight against tooth decay and crooked teeth.

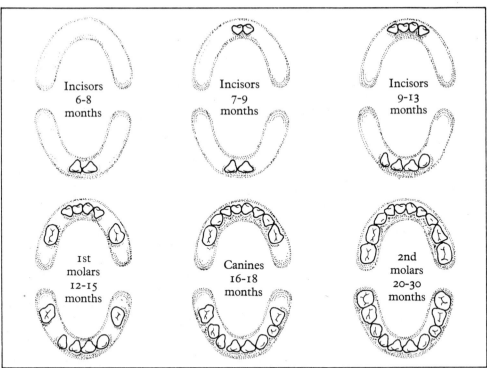

Primary teeth, above.   Second teeth, below.

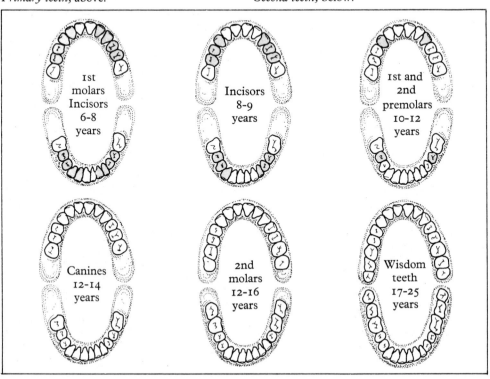

The way you handle those first few crucial visits to the dentist will colour your child's whole attitude to dentistry – possibly for life. Even if you don't like going to the dentist, don't frighten your children by telling them your horror stories or even by retelling dental stories in front of them. Remember, with today's knowledge and skill, with proper tooth cleaning, careful diet, and extra fluoride if necessary, your child need never lose a tooth because of decay. Parents tend to accept dental decay and a mouth full of fillings as 'normal'. For our children this need not be the case.

It's a good idea to take your younger child to the dentist when you go or when you're taking one of your older children so he gets used to the place and the people. Ideally, his first proper visit should be at about three years old. If possible choose a dentist who likes children and is used to treating them.

The worst part about going to the dentist with your children is the agony you go through for them even if they don't care at all about what's going on. Do try not to transmit your emotions to your child. Remember dentistry has come a long way since you were a child and causes much less pain. Some small fillings can even be done without any drilling at all.

The school dentist will see your child when he starts school and throughout his schooldays at various times, but this is no reason for not having your own dentist as well.

Even if you look after your children's teeth very well and they clean them every day, regular visits to the dentist are still essential. There may be early decay that isn't visible to the naked eye or the teeth may be starting to grow crookedly and need early help.

Remember – nearly 40 per cent of people in Britain over the age of 16 years have no teeth of their own. Surely it's worth taking trouble to see that your children don't join this group?

See DENTAL CARIES; FLUORIDE; ORTHODONTICS

Teething The process during which teeth break through the gums. Teething starts in infancy and goes on until the child has all his adult teeth, but when most people talk of teething they are referring to the eruption of milk teeth.

In babies it's tempting to put almost any minor ailment down to teething, but this is wrong. Many children are more irritable as they teeth especially as the very first teeth come through. Babies also produce more saliva than usual and sometimes the wetness and dribbling on to the cheeks causes a 'teething' rash. This can be prevented by applying a barrier cream to the baby's face and cheeks to protect the skin by making it more waterproof. Most babies like to be cuddled more than usual while they're teething and may like to chew on hard things or even on their own fingers for comfort.

There are many old wives' tales about teething but babies are likely to suffer from all sorts of minor illnesses during their teething time which are nothing at all to do with teething. It certainly doesn't cause bronchitis or convulsions, for example. If you're in any doubt about your child's health while he's teething, ask your doctor. Most ailments are nothing whatever to do with teething and mustn't be ignored.

While he's teething, a child may refuse his food, especially if it's hard or lumpy, so don't force food down because you think he's crying from hunger.

As babies teethe for a long time, it is unwise to use medicines at all. If things get really bad you could use junior aspirin (over the age of six months) or paracetamol, but these should not be given routinely or repeatedly.

A soothing analgesic gel to rub onto the gums can be very helpful and is available from a chemist.

Temper tantrums Sudden displays of uncontrolled rage are sometimes (or in some children often) seen under the age of four years. The behaviour takes the form of screaming, crying or lying on the floor with head banging and heels drumming. A tantrum is disruptive and demands the immediate attention of people around. It may last from a few seconds to many minutes, partly depending on how the child is managed.

Children of this age have temper tantrums because they are not yet able to control their emotions and have to release their anger or frustration at certain situations in the only way they know how. An inability to tell their parents what is upsetting them, because of lack of fluency with speech, makes some children annoyed, while others have tantrums simply because they cannot get their own way. Often when speech has developed well enough for the child to be able to express himself in any situation, tantrums become a thing of the past.

How should you cope with them? First of all, and perhaps this is most difficult, keep calm. Any undue emotion on your part will make the child worse. Find out why the child is frustrated and if it's something you can put right, do so. If it's because you won't let him do or have something, don't give in. If you do, you'll create a precedent and he'll know he's only got to throw a tantrum for you to give in next time. Quietly tell him why he can't do whatever it is, then, if he's still upset, give him a cuddle and try to divert his attention to something he likes doing. Physical punishment is not a good idea as it will only enrage him more. Remember that a child may be frightened by his rage and so needs you there to help him cope with his emotions.

See BEHAVIOUR DISORDERS

Temperature The temperature of a healthy person's body is kept remarkably constant whether that person is in the desert or on the North Pole. There is a range of normal temperatures in different people, so a normal temperature may lie anywhere between 97° and 99.5°F (36 and 37.5°C). Body temperature is usually measured in the mouth; if measured under the arm, it is 1°F lower; if in the rectum (back passage), it is 1°F higher. A large meal or exercise both alter body temperature slightly but on average, in a person at rest, the temperature taken in the mouth is around 98.4°F (about 37°C).

Children suffer from many minor illnesses and infections, some of which produce a high temperature. There is a very good case to be made for not having a thermometer in the house at all because a child's temperature can be an unreliable guide to how ill he is. Most parents can tell whether their child is feverish or not simply by touching him.

If you do have a thermometer and want to take your child's temperature, make sure you

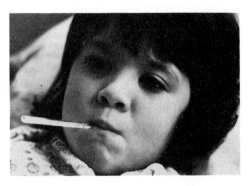

When taking the temperature by mouth, make sure that the child's mouth is kept closed and that you leave the thermometer in long enough to give the correct reading.

do it accurately and safely. Very young children bite a thermometer in their mouth and so temperature-taking by mouth should be avoided. Before you use the thermometer, shake the mercury level down with short, sharp, jerking movements of your wrist and look to see that it is right down at the bottom.

To take the rectal temperature, lubricate the end of the thermometer with petroleum jelly, then lay the child across your knee, face down, and gently put the thermometer into his back passage. Don't push it in too far and don't hold on to it too tightly because it might snap if the child moves. The best thing is to hold the thermometer between your fingers with the palm of your hand flat over the child's bottom and the thermometer coming through between your fingers.

Take the temperature of an older child by placing the bulb end under his tongue and leaving it there for the required time.

When you've finished, shake the mercury down, wash the thermometer in cool water and store it somewhere safe ready for next time.

One last point. Don't treat a child's temperature – treat the child. Just because he's got a temperature doesn't necessarily mean that he's ill. It's more sensible to judge by his general appearance and behaviour. If you're worried about him, call the doctor, no matter what the thermometer says.

See FEVER

Testes The male sex glands that are suspended in a sac (the scrotum) between the legs, under the penis. The testes produce hormones and sperms.

While a baby is in the womb, his testes move down from the abdomen into the scrotum. In some cases, their descent is interrupted, causing undescended testes. If your baby is born early, his testes may not yet be down but will probably come down within a few days. It's important for both testes to be down, particularly from the age of five or six years, because an undescended testis may have a lowered potential for producing sperms. However, there's no need to be too anxious if your baby son's testes cannot be felt because the vast majority of such testes are retractile and lie in a pouch above the scrotum. A doctor can gently push the retracted testis down into the scrotum, though it may pop back again. If both the testes have ever been felt in the scrotum there is little need to worry.

An undescended testis can be brought down

The male sex organs. a. vas deferens, b. seminal vesicles, c. prostate gland, d. urethra, e. penis, f. epididymis, g. testis, h. scrotum.

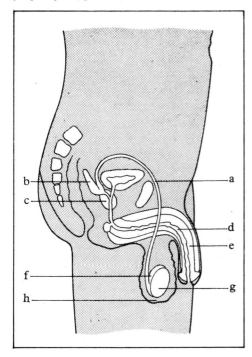

into the scrotum by an operation at about the age of five to six years.

At puberty the testes start producing male hormones which make the hair and beard grow, enlarge the testes and penis, deepen the voice and produce sperms.

Sperms are produced in a series of very long, fine tubes called seminiferous tubules. They pass from here to the epididymis, where they are stored. Another tube, the vas deferens, then carries these sperms to the penis and thence to the outside world.

The testes are very sensitive to temperature and need to be two to three degrees lower in temperature than the rest of the body to function properly, which is why the scrotum is outside the body.

Soon after puberty, boys may ejaculate sperms spontaneously and because this most often occurs at night, these events are called 'wet dreams'. As the boy masturbates or starts having intercourse, these spontaneous emissions stop and anyway are nothing to worry about.

If your son ever complains of pain in a testis, or if there is swelling or a change of colour, it's wise to go to see your doctor, especially if the pain can't be traced back to an accident. Very rarely the testis gets twisted on itself and has to be operated on in hospital.

Most boys' testes are not symmetrical: the left testis usually hangs lower than the right and they may be of different sizes.

See HYDROCELE; MUMPS

Tetanus (lockjaw) An infection with a bacterium called Clostridium tetani that produces spasm of the muscles, especially of the jaws and neck.

Although tetanus is very uncommon, several hundred people get it each year in the UK, and some die. Tetanus starts as an infection of a wound or cut and is more likely to occur if the wound is deep and the bacteria have little access to oxygen in the air. Skin abrasions suffered on the road surface are a relatively common source of tetanus infection – though less so since horse dung, a major source of the tetanus bacilli, has become less common on the roads. Gardeners who use horse manure are especially at risk and can die from even a tiny, unnoticed rose thorn prick if it is infected with tetanus. Middle-aged housewives are the greatest single 'at risk' group as many have never had protective injections and house dust can contain tetanus organisms.

Once in the body, the bacteria produce toxins which travel in the blood to the brain. The symptoms start a long time after the original cut or infection (twelve days to six months later) and this makes the diagnosis difficult. A sore throat may be the first symptom; pain in the neck and muscles follows; and then spasm of the mouth and jaw muscles sets in. The rest of the body, especially the neck, is then affected in severe cases and the patient can die if not treated.

Any large wound, or a deep puncture of any size, is an indication for reviewing your child's immunity to tetanus because these are the wounds that are particularly susceptible to tetanus infection.

The best way to handle tetanus is to prevent it, because even good treatment does not guarantee survival. Prevention starts during infancy when a baby receives tetanus toxoid for the first time as part of the triple vaccine. Three doses are given during the first year. A child should receive a BOOSTER at five years old, on leaving school and thereafter as necessary. (See IMMUNIZATION.) If your child is not immunized and gets a deep wound, your doctor may suggest that he has an immediate injection of anti-tetanus globulin which gives immediate protection against any toxins the invading bacteria may produce. An immunized child is given a booster dose of vaccine if necessary. There are two commonly held misconceptions: 1) that you can *only* get tetanus by cutting yourself in the web between the thumb and the forefinger; and 2) that tetanus is somehow caused by getting rust into a wound. Neither is true.

See BITES AND STINGS

Tetracycline *See* ANTIBIOTICS

Thalassaemia *See* ANAEMIA

Threadworms *See* WORMS

Three-month colic *See* COLIC

Thrush *See* MONILIASIS

Thumb sucking A normal activity for many babies and young children, sometimes seen even before birth, while the baby is still in the womb. During the first few weeks of life, the thumb only gets into the mouth by chance and doesn't stay there long. However, as the baby becomes better able to control his movements and explore things with his mouth, he can put his hand to his mouth on purpose. Some babies suck one or more fingers instead of the thumb.

A baby's instinctive urge to suck ensures that he will be able to get milk from his mother's breast. Thumb sucking helps satisfy this need to suck and also seems to give him enjoyment and comfort, sometimes occupying him for many minutes at a stretch. Some babies never suck their thumbs.

Is thumb sucking bad? Generally speaking no, and no attempt should be made to stop it. On the other hand, if the baby is not growing and gaining weight, it may be a sign that he is not allowed to suck long enough at his mother's breast to stimulate a large enough milk supply.

It may also be a sign that the baby needs extra physical cuddling and love from his mother or 'comfort sucking' time at an empty breast. If you are relying on natural breast feeding (that is, completely unrestricted breast feeding by day and night) to space your family, as many women in underdeveloped countries still do, though it is an unreliable method, your baby should be doing his comfort sucking at your breast, instead of at his thumb. This stimulates the nipples and so maintains the level of hormones in your blood which prevent the return of ovulation. Worldwide, prolonged breast feeding is the most commonly used method of contraception.

After seven years old thumb sucking should be discouraged as a child's permanent teeth may be pushed forwards at the top and backwards at the bottom. Ask your dentist for his opinion as to whether the teeth are being affected – if they are not, there is no need to stop your child sucking his thumb. There is no evidence that thumb sucking alone makes a child's teeth stick out but if there is a predisposing inherited likelihood that his teeth will protrude, then the thumb sucking may en-

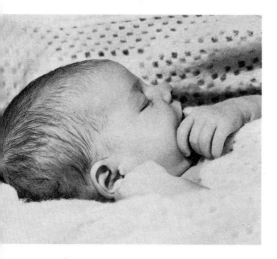

One of the best ways of helping a child to stop thumb sucking is to praise him when he's not doing it rather than going on at him when he is.

See HABITS

Thymus A mysterious organ that lies, in children, in the chest under the breastbone. It consists of two flattened lobes, each contained in a capsule.

The thymus grows rapidly during the first two years, then slows down, and at puberty begins to get smaller. At puberty the cells of the gland are replaced with non-functioning tissue.

It is not known exactly what the thymus does, but it seems to play an important role in the development of a baby's immunity system.

Leukaemia and certain other forms of cancer can cause an enlargement of the thymus.

Thyroid One of the endocrine GLANDS. It is found in the front of the neck and is made up of two lobes joined together across the front of the voice box (larynx) by another piece of the gland. The two main lobes lie on either side of the voice box and the windpipe (trachea).

The gland produces two hormones – thyroxine and triiodothyronine, both of which contain iodine. They are produced in the gland and then carried around the body in the blood, mostly bound to proteins. Thyroid hormones regulate the rate at which the body functions – the speed of the body's chemical reactions. When the thyroid fails or functions poorly, the body slows down, and when it is overactive, the body's workings speed up.

There are several sophisticated tests of thyroid function that can be carried out in specialized centres. When the gland enlarges, the enlargement is called a GOITRE.

See CRETINISM

Thyrotoxicosis *See* GOITRE

Tics *See* HABITS

Tongue furring Although many parents think they can tell a lot from the condition of their child's tongue, this is not really the case. Even very experienced doctors learn little from the tongue except in specific diseases that

courage this to occur. Malocclusions such as those seen in thumb suckers are almost entirely inherited.

If your baby sucks his thumb so hard that he develops sores or blisters, just keep the skin clean to prevent infection. Bandages will become soggy and fall off, while creams and ointments will simply be licked off.

In most babies, thumb sucking is quite harmless and there is no need to try to stop it. Some babies just enjoy the habit and some may need more sucking time than their peers. Thumbs are usually cleaner than dummies, give 'feedback' sensations which a dummy doesn't and are always there. Attempts by parents to stop thumb sucking can bring problems: a baby will be frustrated and cry and a toddler may start using some other comforting habit such as sucking a blanket. An older child will simply suck his thumb in secret and, worse still, may become resentful of your efforts to stop him. This resentment can then show up as a behaviour problem.

Children usually stop sucking their thumbs between the ages of three and six years but may revert to it when they are tired, unwell, bored or worried.

If your baby sucks his thumb, first make sure you are allowing him enough time at the breast. Second, make sure you are giving him enough attention and stimulation so that he isn't bored. If you are doing both these things and he still sucks his thumb, don't worry. Just accept it for the habit it is.

affect it. Almost all of these diseases are rare or unknown in children.

THRUSH is the only common condition to affect the tongue though small ulcers (aphthous ulcers) occur in children from time to time. Young babies get a white tongue from milk but this is easily distinguished from thrush. Dehydration and low grade fevers can produce a furred tongue, but constipation does not.

See MONILIASIS; SCARLET FEVER

Tongue tie A condition in which the tissues under the tongue bind part of its under surface to the floor of the mouth. In the past, doctors and parents alike used to worry a great deal about this condition but we now know that it does no harm and rarely presents any speech difficulty. Operation to free the tongue is rarely necessary.

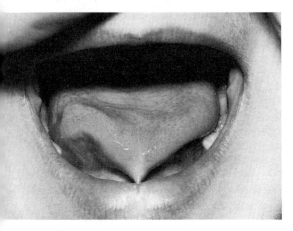

Tongue tie.

Tonsillitis Infection of the TONSILS. Tonsillitis is rare in babies under one year old in whom the tonsils are still very small. In older children, tonsillitis is frequently seen as part of a generalized infection of the throat (PHARYNGITIS) but it can also occur in isolation. Most cases are caused by a viral infection, for which there is no specific treatment. However, some are caused by streptococci. Antibiotics (usually penicillin) are valuable in treating streptococcal tonsillitis and in preventing the occasional development of associated illnesses such as rheumatic fever, nephritis and middle ear infection.

It is difficult to distinguish between the two types of tonsillitis unless a throat swab is taken to the hospital laboratory to be cultured, though children with a streptococcal infection are more likely to have a headache, tummy ache, vomiting and enlargement of the lymph nodes in the neck than are children with a viral infection. The size of the tonsils is not a reliable indicator either of the type of infection or its severity. Large tonsils that meet in the middle may well be quite healthy. The presence of whitish or yellowish deposits on the tonsils is not important either, as these can be present in viral as well as streptococcal tonsillitis, and may even be present on completely healthy tonsils.

Ideally, every child should have a throat culture if he has a sore throat, though it's important to remember that few young children complain specifically of a sore throat. If this reveals streptococci, a ten day course of penicillin should be given. If the culture is negative, no specific treatment is necessary. Either way, bed rest is only advisable if the child wishes to rest. Antibiotics should relieve the fever of streptococcal tonsillitis within 24 hours. The child is rendered non-infectious within a few hours of taking the first dose. There is no point in taking antibiotics for a viral tonsil infection: they will not cure the infection nor make the child non-infectious. Your doctor may be sure enough of his diagnosis to decide to prescribe antibiotics on clinical grounds, without doing a throat swab culture, or while waiting for the result of one.

If the tonsils become chronically infected, causing recurrent tonsillitis, bad breath, difficulty in eating and chronic swelling of the nodes in the neck, then tonsillectomy should be considered. However, this is rarely necessary before the age of four years, and may be avoided after that. If the tonsils are still active in defending the body against infection, the child will receive no benefit from tonsillectomy. If, however, they are so chronically infected that they no longer have a useful role to play, in which case they are likely to be small, fibrous and obviously infected, or if they are so large that swallowing is difficult, then they are best removed. Remember that tonsillectomy will bring with it no decrease in the number of upper respiratory infections the child has, no decrease in the frequency of chest infections and laryngitis, and no decrease in the amount of middle ear infections, sinusitis or nasal allergy. Your child will still get sore throats after tonsillectomy but may feel better in himself, eat more because of being able to swallow more easily, and will possibly lose his bad breath.

To sum up, unless your child is having very frequent attacks of tonsillitis, has had frequent attacks for several years running, is missing a lot of schooling and seems to be eating less than usual, don't bully your doctor to refer your child to hospital for an operation. Although necessary tonsillectomy will bring an improvement in the child's health, unnecessary tonsillectomy will make no difference and besides making him more susceptible to infection (by removing the natural defence of the tonsils), will also mean that he has been hospitalized for no good reason and subjected to an anaesthetic and an operation, both of which have their dangers, however small.

See ADENOIDS; LYMPHATIC SYSTEM; QUINSY

Tonsils   The two knobs of lymphoid tissue lying one each side of the back of the throat and forming part of the ring of lymphoid tissue round the back of the throat.

The function of the tonsils is to help provide a defence against infection. When harmful foreign bacteria are breathed in, healthy tonsils enlarge and lymphocytes (protective white cells) are formed in them. When the defence mechanism of the tonsils is overcome, they may become a site of acute or chronic infection. (*See* TONSILLITIS.)

The tonsils are relatively small in the first year and increase in size as a child grows older. They are usually at their largest between the ages of four and seven years.

Even tonsils so large that they meet in the middle may be quite healthy. Only rarely is swallowing difficult and the airway from the nose to the windpipe is unaffected.

See LYMPHATIC SYSTEM; QUINSY

Toothache   A pain produced by irritation of the soft, sensitive, inner part of the tooth, the pulp. There are several causes of pain in and

around the teeth but DENTAL CARIES (tooth decay) is by far the commonest.

The outer, hard, enamel surface of the teeth is not sensitive but the soft, inner pulp contains nerves that are sensitive to the acid produced by dental decay. Once toothache occurs, you'll know there's something seriously wrong with your child's tooth because, as the inner part is the sensitive part, the tooth must be decayed right through the enamel in order to be painful.

Toothache is usually of a stabbing nature and may be brought on by hot or cold foods in the mouth. It always seems worse at night.

In the short term, all you can do is to give the child the correct dose of aspirin or paracetamol and place a warm face flannel or hot water bottle over the area of the face that's affected. Never place an aspirin tablet in your child's mouth against the gum as this can cause ulceration. Avoid giving hot or cold foods and give him lukewarm drinks. Oil of cloves can be very soothing when placed on the tooth and it's probably worth keeping some in your medicine chest. However, it is only useful for large cavities or if your child has lost a filling.

If your child falls over and breaks a tooth, bathe the edge in alcohol (such as whisky). This kills off the surface cells and makes it less painful while you await dental help.

Make an appointment with the dentist quickly if your child has toothache. Most dentists keep some spare appointments so they can fit in cases like this. The best way of tackling toothache is to prevent it in the first place and the way to do this is to prevent tooth decay.

Once a tooth is so badly decayed that it produces pain, it will usually need either filling or removing completely.

Toxocariasis   *See* PETS

Toxoplasmosis   *See* CONGENITAL ABNORMALITIES; PETS

Travel sickness   *See* MOTION SICKNESS

Truancy   The child who plays truant from school is not usually the same as the one with school PHOBIA – a fear of going to school usually associated with stress within the family, with bullying, poor academic progress or lack of friends at school and which may show itself as tummy ache or vomiting in the morning before leaving home. (*See* RECURRENT ABDOMINAL PAIN.)

The truant is much the same age as the child with school phobia – 10 to 12 is the commonest age – but is likely to be less intelligent and to have other behaviour problems such as lying and stealing. He may have little respect for what school has to offer, considering it a waste of time. The truant may be reacting against the rules of the school and the authority of the teachers or may simply be led by friends that he wants to 'keep in with'. Usually the truant does not stay at home, whereas the school phobic does. Often the truancy is not discovered for some time, as the school thinks the child has a good reason for being away and the parents think he is at school.

For whatever reason the child is not willing to attend school, careful counselling of him and his family is often necessary. Initially this can be attempted by the teacher and head teacher, but later, help from a child guidance clinic may be advisable.

Tuberculosis   A disease caused by infection with the bacterium Mycobacterium tuberculosis.

Tuberculosis has affected man for thousands of years but was brought under control in the early part of this century by improved public health, and in the early 1950s with the discovery and widespread use of the anti-tuberculous drugs. TB used to be a major killer but today is rarely seen in Britain although it still occurs too frequently for us to be complacent about it.

Although TB can affect any part of the body, the most common and dangerous form in the UK affects the lungs and is spread by an infected person coughing up the bacteria which are then inhaled by someone else.

Until recently, almost every child was exposed to tuberculosis before he reached adulthood. The exposure was usually unnoticed because it caused no signs or symptoms of infection. A tiny scar might have been left on the lungs, only detectable by X-rays but remaining for the rest of life. Rarely, this trivial infection flared up to produce a full-blown attack of TB, meningitis or other symptoms but usually the child simply built up antibodies to tuberculosis.

TB used to be diagnosed only when it produced symptoms. Then mass X-rays were organized to pick up the first evidence of TB and so allow early treatment. The present rarity of the infection no longer justifies this costly arrangement. TB is now detected by a simple skin test and, as most younger people have not had the disease in the past, a positive test often indicates active TB.

The drugs available for treatment today are safe and effective and because of this most people with TB are treated as outpatients. The years spent in hospital and the expensive operations that were so common are nowadays rarely necessary.

Children are skin tested routinely at about the age of 12 to 13 years and if their skin test shows they have no immunity to TB, they are offered a vaccination (BCG) which gives life-long protection. In areas of the world where TB is still common, or if there is active TB in the family, newborn babies should be vaccinated. Special consideration is given to people coming into this country from any of these areas, and to those working with such immigrants.

Typhoid   *See* FOOD POISONING

U

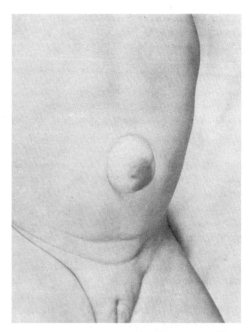

Umbilical hernia : hernias of this type usually disappear by themselves during the first few years.

Ulcerative colitis A chronic condition with inflammation and ulceration of the large bowel causing recurrent attacks of diarrhoea with the passage of blood and mucus in the loose stools. The disease continues into adult life though there may be long relapses.

The child with ulcerative colitis may have abdominal pain, a persistent but not always successful urge to open his bowels, loss of appetite with weight loss, and nausea and vomiting. The loss of blood and poor appetite can cause anaemia due to iron deficiency.

Once the diagnosis has been made, treatment is with diet and long-term drugs. If the child doesn't respond to drugs, an operation to bypass the large bowel can be performed by bringing the small intestine to the surface to empty its contents into a disposable bag (an ileostomy operation). Part of the large bowel may also have to be removed.

It has been suggested that ulcerative colitis may be due to infectious, psychological or immunological causes. Although the cause is as yet unknown, it is interesting that people with ulcerative colitis are twice as likely as people without it to have been bottle-fed. Another study showed that people with long-standing ulcerative colitis have high levels of antibodies to cows' milk protein in their blood. This suggests that complete breast feeding in the first four to six months of life may protect a child from getting ulcerative colitis.

Umbilical hernia A hernia is caused by a weakness or imperfect closure of the tissues around the UMBILICUS, which lets the underlying abdominal contents through. The soft lump usually contains part of the bowel which comes through the gap and into the space under the umbilical skin. An umbilical hernia is commonly seen in newborn babies (though it may not appear until some time after birth). The hernia becomes larger when the baby cries, coughs or strains but can easily be pushed back through the gap. There is no need to try to stop the baby doing any of these things.

One sort of umbilical hernia, seen most often in children of African origin, is just above the umbilicus. Children with such a 'supra-umbilical' hernia may have had abdominal skin extending half an inch or so up the umbilical cord.

Most umbilical hernias disappear spontaneously before the age of one year, and even some of the largest hernias have been known to go by the age of five or six years. An operation to close the gap is therefore only carried out if the hernia shows no signs of closing spontaneously by the age of five years, if it becomes larger after the age of one or two years, or if the child has any symptoms from it.

Strapping the hernia, with or without a coin under the strapping over the umbilicus, or with a special hernia belt, is frowned upon because it can damage the delicate bowel which lies so close to the skin surface. An umbilical hernia is best left alone unless it cannot be pushed back through the gap easily, in which case your child must quickly be seen by a doctor.

Umbilicus (navel, tummy button) The scar on the abdomen which marks the point where the umbilical cord was attached to the foetus. The umbilical cord carries the arteries and veins between the baby and the placenta while the baby is in the womb and so gives the baby all the nourishment and oxygen he needs to grow and develop. The umbilical cord occasionally becomes looped around the baby's neck during labour and, if the loop tightens, this may reduce the baby's blood supply so much that he becomes short of oxygen. If this happens early in labour, a caesarean section may be necessary, but if it happens towards the end, a forceps delivery can be done. If the loop is loose enough, the person delivering the baby may be able to slip it over the baby's head. Yet another mishap that can occur in labour is that the umbilical cord may enter the cervix before the baby. The pressure of the baby being pushed through the cervix against the umbilical cord during labour may then hazard his blood supply. Treatment for this condition is a caesarean section.

After birth, the cord is cut fairly close to the baby's abdomen, leaving the long end attached to the placenta which is still in the uterus. If the mother is rhesus negative, a sample of blood is taken from the umbilical cord to determine whether her baby is rhesus positive and whether or not the baby is already affected by rhesus haemolytic disease. (*See* BLOOD GROUPS.) The cut end of the umbilical cord attached to the newborn baby usually withers and drops off within six to eight days of birth. It doesn't matter if it takes longer. The raw surface scars and heals within a fortnight. Sometimes the umbilicus becomes mildly infected (usually with staphylococci) while the scar is healing, but the infection, with its pussy discharge, can usually be cleared up by cleaning with alcohol (surgical spirit) several times a day. Powder can be used, but may clog in the umbilicus and irritate the skin.

Occasionally some overactive scar tissue ('granulation tissue') is left but this can be treated at your doctor's surgery or at the baby clinic with silver nitrate, which soon clears it up. A more serious infection of the umbilicus is sometimes seen and as this can be potentially dangerous, antibiotics are necessary.

See UMBILICAL HERNIA

Urinary tract infection *See* CYSTITIS; NEPHRITIS

Urine The fluid produced by the kidneys and passed out of the body via the bladder and urethra. Urine is produced constantly 24 hours a day, stored in the bladder and passed at intervals.

Urine is usually a pale yellow, watery fluid but alters in various circumstances. After taking lots of fluid by mouth, a child will have

The kidneys are located one on each side of the backbone, and are connected with the bladder via the ureter.

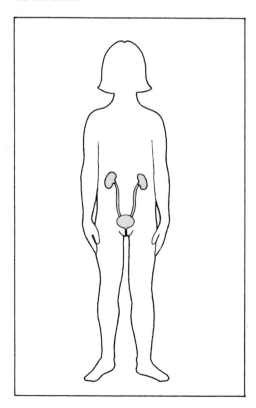

pale or even colourless urine, and after drinking very little will have dark yellow or even orange-brown urine. Children who have been sweating a lot also pass dark orange urine. Because it can be dangerous to pass dark, concentrated urine for long periods, it's wise to give your child plenty of fluid to drink if he has a temperature, has vomited a lot, or has diarrhoea, and to ask for your doctor's advice if you are worried.

Some mothers complain that their baby's urine has a strong smell. This is because the urine reacts with bacteria in the stools to produce ammonia. As well as smelling, ammonia can cause a NAPPY RASH. Infection of the urine may also cause it to smell unpleasant, and fishy.

Children sometimes pass red urine. If you are concerned that this might be due to blood in the urine, ask your doctor. The most usual cause of red urine is that the child has been eating red sweets, but beetroot and some laxatives can give rise to red urine too.

A child who is ill for no apparent reason may be suffering from a urinary infection. (*See* CYSTITIS; NEPHRITIS.)

Urticaria A skin condition of allergic origin characterized by well-defined, red, blotchy, raised, itching areas. The original area may disappear within 48 hours but new ones may continue to appear singly or in crops. As many as 20 per cent of the entire population suffer from urticaria at some time in their lives and it's seen more commonly in females.

Urticaria is caused by many different things. Commonly, it's something the child has eaten. Eggs, shellfish, nuts and several drugs can be responsible. Certain plants and drugs act on the skin directly to produce urticaria (hence the alternative name, nettlerash). Penicillin, insect stings, bites, certain infections, and cold and heat can also cause the condition. Urticaria is usually self-limiting, and only needs treatment if the itching is severe. Antihistamines usually relieve the condition quickly.

Sometimes urticaria can be very severe indeed and may involve the deeper tissues of the upper respiratory tract or even the intestine. In such cases steroid drugs may be needed.

Vaccination The inoculation with a vaccine to produce immunity against disease. The terms IMMUNIZATION and vaccination are now used almost synonymously, though originally vaccination applied to the inoculation of a person with a culture of the vaccinia (cowpox) virus to produce immunity against the disease smallpox. Today, a vaccine is a suspension of organisms (alive, modified, or dead), given by injection or by mouth to make the person immune to a particular disease.

Vaginal discharge A discharge of thick mucus is normal in the newborn baby and may even be accompanied by some bleeding. This is because of birth hormones still circulating in the baby's body after birth. It clears up within two weeks once the hormones have been naturally broken down in the body.

A year or so before a girl's periods begin, she may have a whitish vaginal discharge which again is quite normal. Reassurance and absorbent cotton pants are all that are necessary.

The VULVA and vagina of young girls may be infected with a variety of bacteria, causing a pussy discharge. A foreign body in the vagina or a threadworm infestation must always be thought of because both can cause a discharge. Mild symptoms in a baby can be cleared up simply by hygienic measures, including washing with soap and water at each nappy change, followed by the use of a zinc and castor oil barrier cream, or a cream containing oestrogens (available from your doctor if necessary). More severe infections need treatment with antibiotics and your doctor may choose the antibiotic on the basis of the results of the culture of a swab of the discharge. An infection with gonococci needs specific treatment with penicillin injections. This infection rarely

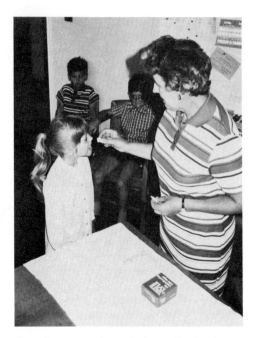

Carrying out routine polio immunization in school.

causes any permanent side effects in a young girl. (*See* GONORRHOEA.)

Newborn babies may suffer from vaginal MONILIASIS, as may older girls who are diabetic, on prolonged antibiotic treatment or on the Pill. Infection with trichomonas is rarely seen in children but can occur, as may any venereal infection, in teenagers having sexual intercourse.

Varicella   *See* CHICKENPOX

Verruca   *See* WART

Virus   A very small infective agent that grows and reproduces only in living cells. Viruses are very much smaller than bacteria and are usually much simpler structurally. They are antigenic and so produce antibodies in the host animal. Natural infection or IMMUNIZATION both increase the body's natural resistance to viruses (*see* IMMUNITY).

Diseases caused by viruses include colds, smallpox, chickenpox, shingles, polio, influenza, mumps, encephalitis, yellow fever, cold sores, rabies, measles and German measles

and typhus. They also cause some forms of hepatitis, respiratory illness and gastroenteritis. Some of the very biggest viruses are more like the bacteria and can be killed by antibiotics.

Most viruses, though, do not respond to antibiotic therapy. It is therefore a waste of time and money taking antibiotics for viral diseases. If there is a secondary bacterial infection *on top* of a viral one, then antibiotics are helpful (for example when bacterial pneumonia occurs in a person with 'flu). The search is on for effective anti-viral preparations but so far only one, idoxuridine, has proved useful on any kind of scale. The trouble with anti-viral agents as a group is that in order to have any effect on viruses they have, almost by definition, to be harmful to the body's normal cells, because viruses live within our cells. Because of this, there is still no cure for most of the infectious diseases listed above.

Vision testing   Under the National Health Service, the procedure for vision testing and for the treatment of visual defects is as follows: the child's eyes are examined either by the general practitioner or by the clinic doctor and if it is thought that further testing or treatment is necessary, the child is either referred to a doctor who is an eye specialist (an ophthalmic surgeon at a hospital, or an ophthalmologist at a hospital or special school clinic), or a special form is issued. This form enables the child to be seen by an optician or an ophthalmic medical practitioner (an ophthalmologist who may not be a hospital consultant and who works from his own premises or from a medical eye centre). Once the form has been issued, your child can return for further eye testing without getting another form.

Your doctor's choice of whether your child is referred to hospital or not depends not only on what he thinks is wrong with the eyes but also on the area in which you live: some hospital eye specialists routinely examine children with fairly minor visual defects while others deal only with more serious complaints.

Preliminary vision testing of the pre-school child requires expertise and many clinic doctors and some general practitioners and health visitors have been specially trained in the technique. Ideally, all children should be

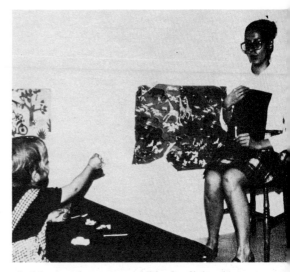

A vision test for a young child: the clinic doctor holds up a miniature toy, which the child is asked to match from the selection on the table.

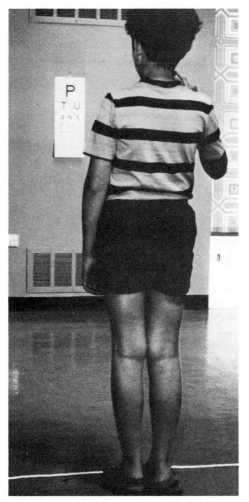

A school vision test for distant vision. The child holds a cover over one eye so that each eye can be tested separately.

screened for visual defects at intervals before school entry.

In some areas, only children 'at risk' are tested routinely and these include children from families in which one or more members squint or have defective eyesight, children with a difficult birth history and those that are mentally retarded.

All schoolchildren have routine eye tests, usually done by the health visitor or school nurse under the supervision of the school doctor, or by the school doctor himself.

Routine vision testing in pre-school and school children not only prevents children having undiagnosed refractive errors (long or short sight or astigmatism) causing difficulty in reading, seeing cars coming, and so on, but also prevents amblyopia – blindness in one eye. Amblyopia may develop in a remarkably short time and is due to the suppression by the brain of the image produced by an eye which is either squinting or not seeing clearly. The blindness is eventually permanent and so is very well worth preventing, especially as it is not a rare occurrence.

Children with poor eyesight in both eyes may be more clumsy than other children and may have obvious difficulty in seeing things at a distance (if shortsighted) or in seeing things close to (if longsighted). The child who has poor vision in one eye, however, is the one who is likely to become amblyopic. This is why both eyes should be tested separately.

It is possible to test the vision of each eye separately in a co-operative three-year-old in the baby clinic or GP's surgery, using simple tests which the child enjoys doing. Sometimes even younger children will do the tests. More sophisticated methods of testing, including refraction, are carried out by eye clinics and opticians.

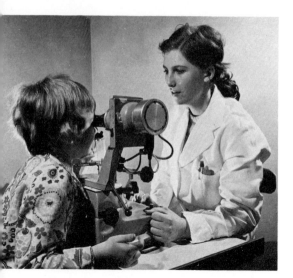

Testing for potential binocular vision.

The danger with testing the vision of young children is that a child with poor vision may be dismissed as being unco-operative, tired or bored, whereas in fact he simply cannot see.

The older child may cheat during a vision test at school for fear of his visual defect being shown up and having to wear glasses. It's important that the child should have his eye covered adequately during the test and also that he should not be able to learn by rote the letters on the test card as other children read them.

If your baby or young child squints, it's important to inform your doctor, even though the occasional squint of a new baby is likely to be of no significance. Many squints are not noticed by parents, so it is important for children to be tested for a squint at regular intervals from infancy onwards.

Routine vision testing is very worthwhile as children with poor eyesight are unlikely to tell their parents about it, parents will not necessarily notice it, and undiagnosed and untreated visual defects can cause permanent damage to the sight.

See BLINDNESS; EYES; SQUINT; VISUAL PROBLEMS

Visual problems *Shortsighted* (myopic) children have eyeballs that are longer than normal, so that the focused image of what the child is looking at falls in front of the retina instead of on it. The child cannot see properly in the distance, though he can accommodate (change the shape of) his lens to see things closer to him.

All children, and especially children whose parents have short sight, should be tested regularly for this condition, which can be treated with suitable glasses.

Longsighted (hypermetropic) children have eyeballs that are shorter than normal, so that the focused image falls behind the retina. Constant accommodation of the lens can lead to tiredness and even pain in the eye, and the child with severe long sight may be unable to see properly.

Regular testing identifies children with long sight as soon as possible, and suitable glasses correct the vision.

Astigmatism is a condition in which there is an irregularity in the normal spherical shape of the eyeball, usually due to a change in the curvature of the cornea and the lens. Light rays entering the eye are bent (refracted) by different amounts, and form a distorted image. Symptoms include difficulty in reading, headache, eye pain, tiredness, and redness of the eye. Glasses containing cylindrical lenses are helpful for children with moderate to severe astigmatism.

See BLINDNESS; EYES; VISION TESTING

Vitamin C   *See* BABY FEEDING; FOOD; SCURVY

Vitamin D   *See* BABY FEEDING; FOOD; RICKETS

Volvulus   *See* CYSTIC FIBROSIS

Vomiting   The forceful ejection of food from the stomach via the mouth.

Newborn babies sometimes vomit because they have swallowed amniotic fluid or mucus, though a doctor will rule out other more serious causes of vomiting before making this diagnosis. The normal and expected REGURGITATION of small amounts of milk down the chin is not true vomiting and needs no treatment.

Vomiting can be a sign that something serious is going on, even if it's only a minor infection such as a cold. Young children often swallow their nasal discharge as it trickles down the back of their throat and this may be vomited later. Similarly, the pus from an infection lower down the respiratory tract can be coughed up or swallowed, so making the child feel sick. The yellow, white or green pus in the vomit is easily distinguished.

Projectile vomiting is caused by PYLORIC STENOSIS. An infection of the baby's urine can cause vomiting when there may be no other symptoms. The baby with a blockage in his bowel may vomit and be constipated but may have few if any other symptoms and signs. Meningitis can also cause vomiting, as can almost any infection. Other causes of vomiting include APPENDICITIS, MOTION SICKNESS, emotional problems; drugs or poisons in overdose (see POISONING); MIGRAINE; GASTROENTERITIS; and FOOD POISONING.

Speak to your doctor if you are in doubt as to why your baby or young child is vomiting and especially if he also has diarrhoea, a fever, or any other symptoms; if his tummy is blown up; if he is dehydrated and so passing very little urine and not wetting his nappy as much as usual; if he is vomiting large volumes; if he vomits very forcibly; if you feel he is more unwell than the vomiting would account for; if he vomits repeatedly; or if you are worried.

The treatment of vomiting depends on the cause, but it's always important to make sure that a baby doesn't become dehydrated, so offer plenty of fluids. Don't worry if little or no food is taken for a day or two – children can survive for some time without food but not without fluids. If your baby or child won't drink or keeps little or no fluid down, get medical help.

See DEHYDRATION; RECURRENT ABDOMINAL PAIN

Vulva The external female genitals. The vulva consists of two outer lips and two inner lips, and covers the clitoris in front, the vaginal opening behind, and the urethra in between.

Just as a boy's penis can often look very small when he is first born, a girl's vulva can look unexpectedly large. Sometimes the clitoris looks large in proportion to the size of the child and very often the usually – in adults – smaller, inner lips are in fact bigger than the outer ones. In a few children the labia minora are fused to some degree but can be separated by a doctor if he thinks it necessary. The vaginal opening is very small or even completely closed over by the hymen and girls under about ten years old don't have much in the way of vaginal secretions. Your daughter's vulva may sometimes be inflamed. This can usually easily be cured by bathing, careful drying and the use of a barrier cream or one containing oestrogen. It's important to check that the child's bottom is wiped properly, from front to back, to avoid soreness. If there is any evidence of a VAGINAL DISCHARGE, see your doctor. MASTURBATION can make the vulva red in the absence of infection.

W

Walking *See* DEVELOPMENT; LIMP

Wart A small growth on the skin. Warts can occur anywhere on the body and are caused by viruses. They are acquired by direct infection from another person, from moist areas where someone with warts has been (such as a swimming pool or a bath mat), or by transfer by the sufferer to somewhere else on his body.

The commonest kind of wart is rough and yellowish and is found on the hand. Plane warts are flat, brown and smooth and are found on the face, neck and hands, while plantar warts (verrucae) occur on the soles of the feet and are often very painful. Verrucae frequently occur in epidemics in schoolchildren and can be difficult to control.

Eighty per cent of warts disappear on their own without treatment, which accounts for the success of many of the old wives' tales that surround warts and their treatment. However, simple remedies may be bought over the chemist's counter. Silver nitrate used carefully, according to the instructions, usually works in a short time. A verruca causing pain

A crop of warts on the hand.

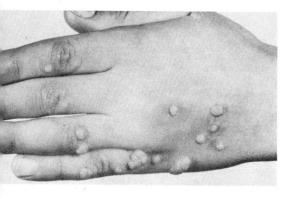

on weight-bearing that can't be treated satisfactorily with simple remedies may need to be excised. Cryotherapy in the form of dry ice (carbon dioxide snow), or liquid nitrogen, is used to treat warts in some hospitals.

There is no need to prevent children with verrucae from swimming if the verruca is adequately covered with a waterproof dressing that can't come off.

Wax A substance constantly produced by glands in the skin lining the external ear, which traps particles of dust and removes them from the ear. People make very different amounts of wax and in some it becomes so hard that it blocks the ear canal and may cause deafness. Only ever clean the easily visible wax from your child's ear. Never poke things down inside 'to get it really clean'. The dangers of doing this are great, especially in a young child who might move sharply and damage his ear on the instrument you are using. If your child's ears become really solid with wax, use special wax-softening oil, following the instructions provided. If absolutely necessary, and if there is no likelihood that the child has a perforated eardrum, your doctor may decide to syringe the wax-blocked ear following the use of wax-softening drops for a few days.

If you are ever in any doubt that the problem with your child's ear is wax, see your doctor, as a discharge caused by an inflammation of the outer ear, or a discharge from the middle ear via a perforated drum can both look like wax. Usually though, in either case, the child will have other symptoms of the underlying condition.

See EARACHE; OTITIS EXTERNA; OTITIS MEDIA

Weaning The accustoming of a baby to forms of nourishment other than MILK, either solid or liquid. The term is also used for giving up the breast or bottle.

There is no absolute 'law' concerning infant feeding, though a mother is sensible if she is guided by up-to-date recommendations which are based on research findings. The latest recommendations suggest that a baby should be breast-fed completely for the first four to six months. This avoids introducing foreign proteins in the way of cereals, cows' milk, egg, and so on, into the infant's bowel at a time when he is most susceptible to the development of food allergy. After this period, different foods can gradually be introduced in increasing amounts. It is said that you should wait a few days before giving each new food so that if the first sort is going to cause problems such as diarrhoea or eczema, it will have time to show. Many mothers believe they have insufficient milk to nourish their babies for this time, but a poor milk supply is nearly always due to insufficient stimulation of the breast by the baby. (*See* BREAST FEEDING.) The supply can be increased by feeding the baby more often and for as long as he wants to suck.

Bottle-fed babies should also be introduced to other foods at any time after the first four to six months. If milk alone doesn't satisfy your baby, you may decide to start him on other foods earlier than this. (*See* BOTTLE FEEDING.)

As the breast-fed baby takes more of his necessary calorie intake from solids and liquids other than breast milk, he will want less breast milk to drink and his mother's milk supply will automatically begin to decrease. Many mothers today do not want to stop breast feeding their babies as they are weaned on to other foods. The answer here is to provide most of your baby's drinks in the form of breast milk. As long as you are careful to avoid giving your baby sugar and refined flour products completely, he should not get fat and you will be able to maintain your milk supply for as long as you and your baby like. Babies allowed to wean themselves from the breast may do so at any time and some go on breast feeding for several years. The nourishment they get from breast milk is very important in the third world, where other food is in short supply, but in the West breast feeding into the second or third year or longer represents a source of comfort and pleasure to the baby rather than a necessary form of nourishment.

If you start weaning your baby before six months, give him spoonfuls of food that is moist and smooth in consistency. Small tastes may be all that he wants at first. After the age of six months, offer him food with more texture, gradually introducing lumps. As he soon develops the skill of chewing (with gums or

teeth), he will be able to cope with lumpy food. Babies also enjoy pieces of hard food (wholemeal bread rusks or pieces of carrot, for example) to bite on.

Your baby can be given any sort of food and giving him puréed or mashed teaspoonfuls of your own meal is the easiest way of weaning.

You can give your baby drinks from a cup as soon as you think he can manage. The breast milk supply can be maintained for as long as the mother and baby want if most drinks are from the breast. Both breast- and bottle-fed babies like to suck even though they may be capable of drinking from a cup.

For a long time it has been suggested that solids must be introduced at six months to avoid the development of ANAEMIA. However, it seems very likely from the results of recent research that breast milk in fact contains enough iron for the older baby and that babies can be breast-fed completely for longer than was thought, provided that the mother eats a well-balanced diet. Babies who were premature, however, should be tested from time to time to make sure they are not anaemic. Although the amount of iron in modified cows' milk is greater than that in breast milk, it is not nearly as well absorbed. The bottle-fed baby should therefore be given solids from six months on.

See BABY FEEDING; FOOD

Weight The weight of a newborn baby bears little relation to his eventual size as an adult, as it is affected so much by the conditions in the uterus during the last few weeks of pregnancy. There is much less emphasis on weight gain today and while the average baby may gain 5 to 7 ounces (140 to 200g) a week, many gain much less or more in any one week and are perfectly healthy. Any baby failing to thrive should be seen by a doctor. (*See* FAILURE TO THRIVE.) As a rough guide, a baby doubles its birth weight by five months and trebles it by a year. If you want a rule of thumb, the first month's gain is 4 to 7 ounces (115 to 200g) per week; the second to fourth month's gain is 6 to 8 ounces (170 to 225g) per week; from 6 to 9 months, 4 ounces (115g) per week and from 9 to 12 months, 2 to 3 ounces (50 to 85g) per week. Remember that a smaller weight gain in any one given week is no cause for alarm – the average over several weeks is more important.

Many babies, especially those breast-fed according to a strict schedule with short feeds in the first week, lose several ounces in weight and may not regain their birth weight for 10 to 14 days. Babies breast-fed on an unrestricted basis lose little, if any, weight, as the milk comes in sooner and there is more of it.

During the second year of life the average child puts on only half the weight it gained during the first year, which explains the apparent decrease in appetite in the second year that worries so many parents.

Weight, like height, is influenced by many variables, including family eating habits, the build of the child, the time of year, periods of illness and so on. Parents can do their children a great service by encouraging them to adopt sensible eating habits and a healthy attitude towards eating and food. OBESITY as a result of eating too many foods of the wrong kind is one of the greatest problems of the western world today. If children are offered a well balanced diet, there is rarely any need to worry if they refuse to eat, unless they are ill, in which case advice should be sought from your doctor. (See ANOREXIA.)

Weight measurements can be plotted on charts similar to the height charts mentioned under HEIGHT and again expert advice may be obtained from hospital paediatric clinics if the child is abnormally thin or fat.

See GROWTH; LOW BIRTH WEIGHT; SMALL CHILDREN

Wheezing A sound made during difficult breathing resulting from a narrowing of the respiratory passages.

Many children wheeze from time to time and the commonest cause of this is ASTHMA. However, many other conditions may be responsible, including a respiratory tract infection (especially BRONCHIOLITIS), some cases of whooping cough, an inhaled foreign body, the respiratory infection seen with cystic fibrosis, and even tuberculosis, though this is rare today. Your doctor's help will be needed to make the diagnosis, possibly with X-rays. It is usually impossible to differentiate between recurrent attacks of wheezy BRONCHITIS and asthma, and it is thought that these two conditions have a common asthmatic basis.

Any child wheezing badly enough to be short of oxygen will have a fast pulse rate, be restless, have obvious difficulty in drawing enough air in, and may be blue. He needs emergency treatment and you should lose no time getting him to a doctor or to hospital. (See ASPHYXIA.) He may be more comfortable sitting upright. You should try to keep as calm as possible while awaiting treatment, as any anxiety transmitted to him may make his wheezing worse.

CROUP is a certain type of wheezing caused by LARYNGITIS.

Whooping cough (pertussis) A serious infectious illness endemic in this country and causing deaths in up to 40 per cent of affected infants under the age of five months.

Whooping cough is caused by the bacillus Bordetella pertussis. Other closely related bacilli and certain viruses are responsible for milder and shorter illnesses causing an identical cough. Whooping cough is highly contagious and non-immune people in close contact with an infectious person are likely to become infected. It most commonly affects children under four years old, though older children and adults can also suffer from it. Immunity after immunization is not life-long, which explains why some adults who were immunized as children can get the disease again.

The bacilli are spread by the breathing out or coughing of infected droplets by one person and their inhalation by another. The incubation period is between 7 and 14 days, though the infected person is infectious for the last few days of this time. The illness itself lasts for six to eight weeks and there are three distinct stages.

In the first, catarrhal stage, the symptoms are those of the common cold: a runny nose, a cough and a slight temperature. In the second stage, the typical whooping cough is apparent: a series of short coughs followed by a 'whoop' as air is breathed in through a partially closed windpipe. Spasms of coughing may occur from two to dozens of times daily. The whoop is diagnostic but may not be present in young babies under six months and, in many cases, culture of swabs taken from the back of the mouth (during a spasm, preferably) is necessary to make a definite diagnosis. Children who have once had whooping cough may whoop again when they have an ordinary cough months later, if they get a cold, or simply out of habit. Vomiting after a coughing attack is common, especially in babies. In fact, a child may vomit so often that he loses a lot of weight during the illness. Giving some food and drink immediately after a coughing attack increases his chances of keeping it down. Babies may stop breathing and turn blue for short periods, and this can be followed by a convulsion. The third and last stage of whooping cough is the convalescent stage which lasts until the cough disappears. Sufferers should be isolated for 21 days from the onset of the characteristic cough to prevent spreading infection to others. Cough medicines are thought to be useless in whooping cough, but a medicine containing atropine may help relieve the muscle spasm. Putting a breast-fed baby to the breast at the beginning of a spasm of coughing may prevent the cough and subsequent vomiting. Sedatives may be given to allow the child to sleep at night.

Complications of whooping cough include acute and chronic lung disease: indeed, pneumonia is the main cause of death in affected babies. Otitis media and convulsions can also occur, while conjunctival haemorrhages – spots of blood in the eyes – may be brought on by a coughing attack. The outlook for complete recovery is, however, excellent in children over five months. Antibiotics are indicated if a treatable complication arises but there is no specific treatment for whooping cough. However, antibiotics are often prescribed even for uncomplicated whooping cough as they limit the period of infectivity, so making the child non-contagious sooner. They are also thought by some people to reduce the incidence of complications. Care must be taken that a baby does not become dehydrated through vomiting. Your doctor may consider that hospital is the safest place for your young child to be.

Discussions among experts over the advantages and disadvantages of IMMUNIZATION against whooping cough have been going on since it was suggested that some children suffered from brain damage as a result of the vaccine. The most recent (1977) Health Service recommendation is that babies should be immunized against whooping cough using a triple vaccine (whooping cough, diphtheria and tetanus vaccines in one suspension), given in three doses, as it is safer for most children to run the tiny risk of damage by the vaccine than to run the risk of getting the disease. It is recommended that the first dose of triple vaccine should be given at three months, not six months as was previously suggested, as young babies in particular are likely to be harmed by the disease. You may ask why it is that children over six months should be immunized at all. One answer is that older children with whooping cough may spread the illness to babies and although the illness is unlikely to be serious in older children, it can be deadly for younger infants. Another is that whooping cough can be an unpleasant illness even for an older child.

If you want your child to be immunized against whooping cough, bear in mind that there are five groups of children who should *not* be immunized. These are:
1) Those with a history of fits or convulsions, or irritation of the brain in the newborn period.
2) Those with a history (or family history) of epilepsy or other disease of the nervous system.
3) Those with a developmental neurological defect.
4) Those who have had a severe local or general reaction to a preceding dose of the vaccine.
5) Those with a feverish illness, particularly a respiratory one, who should not be immunized until they are fully recovered.

Some doctors advise against it if there is a history of allergy in the child or his family.

Wilms' tumour *See* KIDNEY

Wind All babies swallow some air as they suck and this accumulates in the stomach as an air bubble lying in whichever part of the stomach is uppermost, above the milk. Swallowing air is more likely if the teat of a bottle is not filled with milk properly because the bottle is not tilted enough.

The air either passes into the intestine along with the partially digested milk to be absorbed or passed out of the other end of the bowel later, or it may be brought up as 'wind' or a 'burp'.

There is no need to be overconcerned – or indeed concerned at all – about bringing the baby's wind up. If there is so much air in the stomach that the baby is uncomfortable, it is likely to come up anyway if the baby is held fairly upright so that the air bubble is somewhere near the opening of the gullet into the stomach. A baby put straight down to sleep after a feed may be restless simply because he can't get his wind up in that position. Some babies are obviously happier when they have brought up some wind, and a mother soon gets to know whether her baby usually has a bubble of air to get rid of. Many others virtually never burp, and their mothers never have to bother to hold them upright after a feed.

A large number of mothers hold their babies up to their shoulders or sit them on their laps after a feed and at the same time rub or pat their backs in an attempt to bring up the wind. There is no reason why this should have any effect – it is the position that does the trick.

A small amount of milk may be brought up as the baby burps (see REGURGITATION).

See COLIC

Word blindness *See* DYSLEXIA

Worms Several different sorts of worms can live in the human body and although many are commoner in tropical countries, they occur worldwide.

Threadworms (pinworms) are the commonest kind and are present in about 20 per cent of British children. They look like white, moving pieces of cotton in the stools or around the anus. They are said by some to cause abdominal pain and also itching around the anus, especially at night, when the worms come out of the bowel and lay their eggs. Threadworms can also inhabit the vagina, bladder and urethra and cause inflammation

with frequency of passing urine and pain on passing it. The affected child scratches a lot at night and by putting his hands with eggs on them to his mouth reinfects himself. He can also pass the infection on to another child.

The diagnosis can be confirmed (if worms are not obvious in the motions) by the microscopic examination of special swabs taken from the anal margin first thing in the morning.

Threadworms are harmless. A single dose of the right drug cures the condition and may need to be repeated after two or three weeks. The whole family has to be treated or the worms will come back again. Household infestation, including the adults, is the rule rather than the exception.

Make sure that your child understands about washing his hands after he has been to the lavatory, as worm eggs are often picked up by touching the lavatory seat or handle and transferred to the mouth and thence to the gut by the child licking his fingers. This is especially important in schools. Fingernails should be kept short. Threadworm eggs can survive in the air for two to three weeks at room temperature, and vacuum cleaning may help get rid of them. Bedding and clothing should be washed to stop reinfection.

Roundworms and whipworms are less common and are seen more often in tropical countries. As roundworms migrate round the body they can cause a variety of symptoms, some serious. A single dose of the right drug kills them all, but, again, the whole family should be treated.

Tapeworms are rare in Britain. They usually occur after eating undercooked pork and the first sign is the presence of moving pieces of the worm seen in the stool. Once again, drugs kill the worm and eventually it is passed in the stools.

Toxocariasis (*see* PETS), roundworms and whipworms can be spread by cats and dogs. Any worm infestation should be treated by a doctor.

Organizations providing further help and information

Great Britain

Advisory Centre for Education (ACE)
18 Victoria Park Square,
London E2 9PB
Tel: 01 980 4596

Association for All Speech Impaired Children
347 Central Markets,
Smithfield, London EC1A 9NH
Tel: 01 236 3632/6487

The Association of British Adoption and
Fostering Agencies
4 Southampton Row,
London WC1B 4AA
Tel: 01 242 8951

Association for Improvements in the
Maternity Services (AIMS)
Secretary: Ms Christine Beels,
19 Broomfield Crescent,
Leeds LS6 3DD
Tel: 0532 751911

Association of Parents and Friends of Mentally
Handicapped
Handicapped Children
St Michael's House,
Willowfield Park,
Goatstown, Dublin 14

Association for Spina Bifida and Hydrocephalus
Tavistock House North,
Tavistock Square,
London WC1H 9HJ
Tel: 01 388 1382

Asthma Research Council
12 Pembridge Square,
London W2 4EH
Tel: 01 229 1149

British Diabetic Association
10 Queen Anne Street,
London W1M 0BD
Tel: 01 323 1531

British Epilepsy Association
Crowthorne House,
New Wokingham Road,
Wokingham, Berkshire
Tel: Crowthorne 3122

British Institute for the Mentally Handicapped
Wolverhampton Road,
Kidderminister,
Worcester DY10 3PP
Tel: 0562 850251

British Migraine Association
Evergreen,
Ottermead Lane,
Ottershaw, Chertsey,
Surrey KT16 0BJ
Tel: 093 287 3242

British Polio Fellowship
Bell Close,
West End Road,
Ruislip,
Middlesex HA4 6LP
Tel: Ruislip 75515

British Pregnancy Advisory Service
Austy Manor,
Wootton, Wawen,
Solihull B15 6DA
Tel: 05642 3225

British Red Cross Society
National Headquarters,
9 Grosvenor Crescent,
London SW1X 7EJ
Tel: 01 235 5454
For County Branches throughout Britain, see local
directories.

British Rheumatism and Arthritis Association
6 Grosvenor Crescent,
London SW1X 7ER
Tel: 01 235 0902

Brittle Bones Association   c/o Mrs Grant,
63 Byron Crescent,
Dundee DD3 6SS
Tel: Dundee 87130

Cancer Information Association
Gloucester Green,
Oxford OX1 2EQ
Tel: Oxford 725223/46654

Children's Chest Circle
c/o Chest, Heart and Stroke Association,
Tavistock House North,
Tavistock Square,
London WC1H 9JE
Tel: 01 387 3012/3/4

Church of England Children's Society
Old Town Hall,
Kennington Road,
London SE11 4QD

The Coeliac Society
P.O. Box 181,
London NW2 2QY

The Compassionate Friends (support for bereaved parents)
c/o Mrs Charmion Mann,
25 Kingsdown Parade,
Bristol BS6 5UE
Tel: Bristol 47316

Cystic Fibrosis Research Trust
5 Blyth Road,
Bromley,
Kent BR1 3RS
Tel: 01 464 7211

Deaf/Blind Rubella Children
61 Senneleys Park Road,
Northfield, Birmingham
Tel: 021 475 1392

Disabled Living Foundation
346 Kensington High Street,
London W14 8NS
Tel: 01 602 2491

Dr Barnardo's
Tanner's Lane,
Barkingside,
Ilford, Essex
Tel: 01 550 8822

Family Planning Association
Margaret Pyke House,
27–35 Mortimer Street,
London W1N 7RJ
Tel: 01 636 7866

Foundation for the Study of Infant Deaths (Cot deaths)
23 St Peter's Square,
London W6 9NW
Tel: 01 748 7768

The Haemophilia Society
P.O. Box 9,
16 Trinity Street,
London SE1 1DE
Tel: 01 407 1010

Hyperactive Children's Support Group   c/o Sally Bunday,
59 Meadowside,
Angmering, West Sussex BN16 4BW
Tel: Rustington 6172

Invalid Children's Aid Association
126 Buckingham Palace Road,
London SW1W 9BR
Tel: 01 730 9891

Kith and Kids
c/o Maurice Collins
6 Grosvenor Road,
Muswell Hill,
London N10
Tel: 01 883 8762

Lady Hore Trust for Thalidomide & Other Physically
  Disabled Children
2 Milford House,
7 Queen Anne Street,
London W1M 9FD
Tel: 01 637 1545

La Leche League
P.O. Box 3424,
London WC1V 6XX

Leukaemia Society
45 Craigmore Avenue,
Queens Park,
Bournemouth, Hampshire
Tel: Bournemouth 37459

Migraine Trust
45 Great Ormond Street,
London WC1N 3HD
Tel: 01 278 2676

Muscular Dystrophy Group of Great Britain
Natrass House,
35 Macaulay Road,
London SW4 0QP
Tel: 01 720 8055

National Association for Deaf/Blind and Rubella
  Handicapped Children
164 Cromwell Lane,
Coventry CV4 8AP
Tel: Coventry 23308

National Association for Gifted Children
1 South Audley Street,
London W1Y 6JS
Tel: 01 499 1188

National Association for Maternal and Child Welfare
1 South Audley Street,
London W1Y 6JS
Tel: 491 1315

National Association for Mental Health (MIND)
22 Harley Street,
London W1N 2ED
Tel: 01 637 0741

National Association for Spina Bifida and Hydrocephalus
7 Spring Close View,
Gleadless Valley,
Sheffield 14

National Association for the Welfare of Children in
  Hospital
Exton House,
7 Exton Street,
London SE1 8VE
Tel: 01 261 1738

National Childbirth Trust
9 Queensborough Terrace,
London W2 3TB
Tel: W2 3TB
Tel: 01 229 9319

National Children's Bureau
8 Wakley Street,
London EC1
Tel: 01 278 9441

National Children's Home
85 Highbury Park,
London N5 1UD
Tel: 01 226 2033

National Council for One Parent Families
255 Kentish Town Road,
London NW5 2LX
Tel: 01 267 1361

National Council of Social Services
26 Bedford Square,
London WC1
Tel: 01 636 4066

National Deaf Children's Society
31 Gloucester Place,
London W1H 4EA
Tel: 01 486 3251

National Eczema Society
5 Tavistock Place,
London WC1H 9SR
Tel: 01 388 4097

National Marriage Guidance Council
Herbert Gray College,
Little Church Street,
Rugby, Warwickshire CV21 3AP
Tel: Rugby 73241

National Schizophrenia Fellowship
78–79 Victoria Road,
Surbiton,
Surrey KT6 4JT
Tel: 01 390 3651

National Society for Autistic Children
1a Golders Green Road,
London NW11 8EA
Tel: 01 458 4375/6

National Society for Epileptics
Chalfont Centre for Epilepsy,
Chalfont St Peter,
Gerrards Cross, Bucks SL9 0RJ
Tel: Chalfont St Giles 3991

National Society for Mentally Handicapped Children
Pembridge Hall,
17 Pembridge Square,
London W2
Tel: 229 8941

National Society for the Prevention of Cruelty to Children
1 Riding House Street,
London W1P 8AA
Tel: 01 580 8812

National Youth Bureau
17–23 Albion Street,
Leicester LE1 6GD
Tel: 0533 538811

Parents Anonymous: see local directories or local press,
  or telephone 01 668 4805 (24 hour service).

Patients Association
11 Dartmouth Street,
London SW1
Tel: 01 222 4992

Psoriasis Association
7 Milton Street,
Northampton NN2 7JG
Tel: Northampton 711129

Pregnancy Advisory Service
27 Fitzroy Square,
London W1P 5HH
Tel: 01 387 3057

Pre-School Playgroups Association
Alford House,
Aveline Street,
London SE11 5DH
Tel: 01 582 8871

Royal Society for the Prevention of Accidents (RoSPA)
Cannon House,
The Priory,
Queensway,
Birmingham B4 6BS
Tel: 021 233 2461

The Royal Association for Disability and Rehabilation
(incorporating The British Council for Rehabilitation
of the Disabled and The Central Council for the Disabled)
25 Mortimer Street,
London W1N 8AB
Tel: 01 637 5400

Royal National Institute for the Blind
224 Great Portland Street,
London W1N 6AA
Tel: 01 388 1266

Royal National Institute for the Deaf
105 Gower Street,
London WC1E 6AH
Tel: 01 387 8033

Safety in Playgrounds Action Group
85 Dalston Drive,
Didsbury,
Manchester M20 0LQ

The Samaritans
17 Uxbridge Road,
Slough SL1 1SN
Tel: Slough 32713

Schizophrenia Association of Great Britain
Hon Secretary: Mrs G. Hemmings BSc,
Tyr Twr,
Llanfair Hall,
Caenarvon LL55 1TT
Tel: Port Dinorwic 670 379

The Spastics Society
12 Park Crescent,
London W1N 4EQ
Tel: 01 636 5020

Spinal Injuries Association
General Secretary: Miss Bernice Wood,
126 Albert Street,
London NW1 7NF
Tel: 01 267 6111

Toy Libraries Association
Seabrook House,
Wyllyotts Manor,
Darkes Lane,
Potters Bar,
Herts EN6 5HL
Tel: 0707 44571

Twins Club
c/o Sue Wright,
Woodstock,
Heathdown Road,
Pyrford, Surrey
(Enclose s.a.e.)

Voluntary Council for Handicapped Children
National Children's Bureau,
8 Wakley Street,
London EC1
Tel: 01 278 9441

Australia

Asthma Foundation of New South Wales
249 Pitt Street,
Sydney,
NSW 2000

Autistic Children's Association
545 Pacific Highway,
Artarmon,
NSW 2064

Child Education Authority
Box N206,
Grosvenor Street Post Office,
Sydney
NSW 2000

Coeliac Society
4 Bull's Avenue,
Cronulla,
NSW 2230

Cystic Fibrosis Association
21–3 Belmore Street,
Burwood,
NSW 2134

Deaf and Blind Children's Association
361 North Rocks Road,
North Rocks,
NSW 2151

Deaf and Dumb Society of New South Wales
5 Elizabeth Street,
Sydney,
NSW 2000

Diabetic Association of New South Wales
P.O. Box A6,
Sydney South,
NSW 2001

Disabilities Unlimited Association
c/o Lidcombe Hospital,
Joseph Street,
Lidcombe,
NSW 2141

Epileptic Welfare Association
158 Pacific Highway,
North Sydney,
NSW 2060

Haemophilia Association of New South Wales
54B Grove Avenue,
Narraweena,
NSW 2099

Muscular Dystrophy Association of New South Wales
c/o New South Wales Society for Crippled Children,
Cnr Chalmers and Bedford Streets,
Sydney,
NSW 2000

Spastic Centre of New South Wales
189 Allambie Road,
Allambie Heights,
NSW 2100

Spina Bifida Association
P.O. Box 15,
Carlingford,
NSW 2118

Subnormal Children's Welfare Association
8 Junction Street,
Ryde,
NSW 2112

Sudden Infant Death Association
P.O. Box 172,
St Ives,
NSW 2075

Tuberculosis: contact the Tuberculosis Service Division of
the Health Commission in each State.

New Zealand

Association for Deaf Children Inc.
21 Roseneath Terrace,
Wellington 3

Cystic Fibrosis Association of New Zealand
P.O. Box 241,
Auckland

Deaf-Blind Rubella Society Ltd
11 Tirimoana Road,
Te Atau

New Zealand Asthma Society Inc.
P.O. Box 40 333,
Upper Hutt,
Wellington

New Zealand Crippled Children's Society Inc.
P.O. Box 15021,
Mirimar,
Wellington

New Zealand Society to the Intellectually Handicapped
Inc.
P.O. Box 4155,
Wellington

Royal New Zealand Society for the Health of Women
and Children Inc. (Plunket Society)
P.O. Box 6042,
Dunedin

Society for Aid to Mentally Affected Children
P.O. Box 9220,
Newmarket,
Auckland

Spastic Fellowship of New Zealand Inc.
57A Moa Road,
Pt Chevalier,
Auckland

Spina Bifida Association
P.O. Box 68454,
Newton,
Auckland

South Africa

Child Welfare Society
168 Fox Street,
Johannesburg
2001

Institute for Public Health
P.O. Box 4623,
Johannesburg
2000

The National Council for the Care of Cripples in
South Africa
P.O. Box 10173,
Johannesburg
2000

South African National Council for the Blind
P.O. Box 1343,
Pretoria
0001

South African National Council for the Deaf
P.O. Box 31663,
Braamfontein,
Johannesburg
2017

South African Nursing Association
707 Union Centre,
Pritchard Street,
Johannesburg
2001

South African Orthopaedic Association
Secretary,
12 Jameson Road,
Cape Town
8001

South African Red Cross Society
11 Inez Street,
Sunnyside,
Pretoria
0002

South African Speech and Hearing Association
1 Jan Smuts Avenue,
Johannesburg
2001

South African Tuberculosis Association (SANTA)
P.O. Box 10501,
Johannesburg
2000

Illustrations Acknowledgements

The producers of this book gratefully acknowledge the help
of all the organizations who supplied illustrations. Special
thanks are due to Croydon Area Health Authority for the
loan of material. The diagrams were drawn by Peter Sarson
and Tony Bryan.

JACKET *Top and bottom left* Picturepoint Ltd
        Top right John Watney
        Bottom right Andrew Stanway
3 *Left* Institute of Dermatology
  Right Camera Talks Limited
12 Richard and Sally Greenhill
19 Royal Society for the Prevention of Accidents
22 John Watney
24 Medical Recording Service Foundation
25 Alan Hutchinson/Camera Press
27 Richard and Sally Greenhill
31 James Webb/Bruce Coleman Ltd
34 *Left* Treat Davidson/Frank W. Lane
  Top right Jane Burton/Bruce Coleman Ltd
  Centre right Stephen Dalton/Bruce Coleman Ltd
  Bottom right Dr Frieder Sauer/Bruce Coleman Ltd
37 Parents Magazine
39 *Both pictures* Henry Grant
44 Parents Magazine
50 David Kilpatrick/Camera Press
51 Richard and Sally Greenhill
60 G. M. Villermet
61 Henry Grant
63 Camera Press
70 John Watney
81 *Both pictures* Peter Gordon
82 Institute of Dermatology
86 *Top* Hounslow, Ealing and Hammersmith Health
  Authority
  Bottom Richard and Sally Greenhill
89 *Left* Camera Press
  Right Colin Davey/Camera Press
90 Richard and Sally Greenhill
91 British Diabetic Association
95 Paul Almasy/Camera Press
97 Parents Magazine
99 N. Shah
100 Institute of Dermatology
107 John Watney
108 *Left* James Webb/Bruce Coleman Ltd
   Right Gene Cox/Bruce Coleman Ltd
121 N. Shah
123 Institute of Dermatology
124 *Top* Peter Gordon
   Bottom Hounslow, Ealing and Hammersmith Health
   Authority
130 B. Edsall & Co Ltd, Publishers, London
132 Picturepoint Ltd
143 Hamlyn Group
145 Institute of Dermatology
160 Jonathan and Sally Harris
170 *Top* Institute of Dermatology
173 *Left* Medical Recording Service Foundation
   Right Hounslow, Ealing and Hammersmith Health
   Authority
177 Medical Recording Service Foundation
180 *All pictures* David Barnett
185 *Both pictures* Institute of Dermatology
187 *Top* Richard and Sally Greenhill
   Bottom Institute of Dermatology
188 *Both pictures* Institute of Dermatology
192 *Both pictures* John Drysdale/Camera Press
197 Hamlyn Group
205 Picturepoint Ltd
207 Institute of Dermatology
208 Institute of Dermatology
214 N. Shah
221 *Top and centre right* Institute of Ophthalmology
223 Institute of Ophthalmology
228 John Watney
231 Peter Miles/Camera Press
238 Picturepoint Ltd
239 *Both pictures* Medical Recording Service Foundation
240 Department of Health and Social Security